Student Workbook

Health Insurance Today:
A Practical Approach

Sixth Edition

Student Workbook

Health Insurance Today: A Practical Approach

Sixth Edition

Janet I. Beik, AA, BA, MEd
Southeastern Community College
Administrative Instructor (retired)
Medical Assistant Program
West Burlington, Iowa

ELSEVIER

3251 Riverport Lane
St. Louis, Missouri 63043

WORKBOOK FOR HEALTH INSURANCE TODAY: ISBN: 978-0-323-40073-2
A PRACTICAL APPROACH, SIXTH EDITION

Notices

Knowledge and best practice in this field are constantly changing. As new research and experience broaden our understanding, changes in research methods, professional practices, or medical treatment may become necessary.

Practitioners and researchers must always rely on their own experience and knowledge in evaluating and using any information, methods, compounds, or experiments described herein. In using such information or methods they should be mindful of their own safety and the safety of others, including parties for whom they have a professional responsibility.

With respect to any drug or pharmaceutical products identified, readers are advised to check the most current information provided (i) on procedures featured or (ii) by the manufacturer of each product to be ad-ministered, to verify the recommended dose or formula, the method and duration of administration, and con-traindications. It is the responsibility of practitioners, relying on their own experience and knowledge of their patients, to make diagnoses, to determine dosages and the best treatment for each individual patient, and to take all appropriate safety precautions.

To the fullest extent of the law, neither the Publisher nor the authors, contributors, or editors, assume any liability for any injury and/or damage to persons or property as a matter of products liability, negligence or otherwise, or from any use or operation of any methods, products, instructions, or ideas contained in the ma-terial herein.

Content Strategist: Linda Woodard
Content Development Manager: Luke Held
Content Development Specialist: Jennifer Bertucci
Publishing Services Manager: Deepthi Unni
Project Manager: Janish Ashwin Paul
Designer: Patrick Ferguson

Printed in United States of America

Last digit is the print number: 9   8   7   6   5   4   3

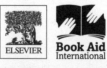

Working together
to grow libraries in
developing countries

www.elsevier.com • www.bookaid.org

Acknowledgments

I would like to express my appreciation and gratitude to those who assisted me in editing and updating this student workbook, especially Jennifer Bertucci and Janish Ashwin Paul, as well as the distinguished members of the Advisory Board, who were integral in making sure the entire product suite stayed as up to date as possible with this new edition. Also, I would like to thank several of my former students and peers, now working in healthcare facilities, who so kindly let me run some of these exercises by them to see if the exercises were appropriate for preparing students for their health insurance careers.

Janet I. Beik, AA, BA, MEd

Introduction to the Workbook

OBJECTIVES

After completing the workbook exercises and activities, the student should be able to:

- Define the **terms** used in the chapters.
- Answer the **review questions** within the evaluation criteria set by the instructor.
- Demonstrate the ability to use analytical logic to draw rational conclusions from facts and information in **critical thinking** exercises.
- Use individual and group thinking techniques to reach valid conclusions on **problem-solving** issues and collaborative (group) activities.
- Complete assigned **projects** as directed by the instructor.
- Assume an active and productive role in **group discussions.**
- Analyze hypothetical situations, applying logical concepts for rational decision-making to **case studies** and health insurance scenarios.
- Perform **Internet searches and exploration** to access information needed to complete assigned activities.
- Achieve the required proficiency on all **performance objectives.**
- Complete the **application exercises** as assigned.
- Generate information and guidelines of major payers for inclusion in the Health Insurance Professional's Notebook.
- Access the Evolve website for updates.
- Conduct a **self-evaluation** on achievement of successful content mastery and classroom performance.
- Perform basic mathematical computations.
- Generate both paper and electronic CMS-1500 claims in an accurate and timely manner.
- Apply reasoning and problem-solving skills (individually or in a group) to arrive at practical solutions to common health insurance issues.
- Interpret a variety of computer-generated accounting reports.
- Create appropriate correspondence for fees and collection.
- Abstract relevant information (from health record documents) necessary for completing various forms used in healthcare billing and claims.
- Integrate knowledge necessary for interpreting payer documents (e.g., EOBs and RAs).
- Apply exact processes for accurate coding (ICD-10, CPT, and HCPCS).

TO THE STUDENT

This workbook accompanies the textbook titled *Health Insurance Today: A Practical Approach,* sixth edition, and is intended to supplement the material presented in the book. Each chapter follows a precise structure that begins with a short introduction and builds to application activities that allow the student to apply what he or she has learned to today's healthcare environment. The workbook chapters are organized as follows:

- *Introduction to the Workbook Chapter*. The introduction gives a brief statement regarding what the student can expect in the specific workbook chapter.
- *Workbook Chapter Objectives*. These objectives are different from those listed in the textbook. They are designed to encourage the student to meet the challenges presented in each chapter of the workbook.
- *Defining Chapter Terms*. In this section, the chapter terms are listed, and the student is expected to generate clear and precise definitions (in his or her own words), after which a comparison should be made to the correct definitions in the textbook glossary.
- *Assessment*. Each workbook chapter has a review test. These tests may be in the form of multiple choice, true/false, matching, fill-in-the-blanks, or short answer or essay. In general, tests promote deeper thinking instead of "surface" learning, and the benefits are twofold: (1) Tests benefit students because they provide feedback on discrimination of important material and course relevance, and (2) tests benefit instructors because they provide feedback on what students have accomplished in the chapter, at course intervals, or at course end. This level of learning is mainly recall; the student, if he or she has read and studied the material in the textbook, should be able to answer the questions correctly.

- *Critical Thinking Activities*. These activities require that the student use his or her abilities to analyze and evaluate information and reach a conclusion or answer by using logic and reasoning skills. Each chapter presents anywhere from one to four critical thinking exercises.
- *Problem-Solving and Collaborative (Group) Activities*. In this step, students use thought processes in which previously learned principles are applied to case-specific situations. Problem solving can be accomplished either individually or collaboratively in groups, as directed by the instructor.
- *Projects and Discussion Topics*. Several topics are listed as suggestions for in-class discussions or oral presentations. As with problem solving, projects and discussion topics will be assigned according to the discretion of the instructor.
- *Case Studies*. Real-world "scenarios" are presented to further stimulate critical thinking and problem-solving skills. As with problem solving, case studies allow the student to apply information he or she has learned to resolve a similar situation that may present itself after the student becomes employed in a healthcare facility.
- *Internet Exploration*. Many of today's learners rely heavily on the Internet for research and up-to-date information on a particular subject. In the constantly changing world of healthcare, textbooks are often somewhat outdated by the time they are published. Students must use caution, however, to make sure that the information found on the Internet is not biased or political in nature; this is an area in which critical thinking skills can be used.
- *Performance Objectives*. Most workbook chapters present at least one "Performance Objective." A performance (or learning) objective is a statement of what the learners will be expected to do when they have completed a specified course of instruction. It prescribes the conditions, behavior (action), and standard of task performance for the training setting. Performance objectives must be mastered to the predetermined criteria set by the instructor, institution, or organization. If the course is competency based, performance objectives may be repeated up to three times or until the student successfully meets the predetermined grading criteria.
- *Application Exercises*. Application, a higher level of learning, asks the learner to take the knowledge and skills he or she has acquired and apply them to "real-world" situations. In this workbook, there is at least one application exercise per chapter.
- *Creating a Health Insurance Professional's Notebook*. The purpose of this notebook is to allow the student to access information quickly and accurately when preparing insurance claims for some of the major third-party payers.
- *Self-Evaluation*. At the end of each workbook chapter, there are two documents that the student must complete to allow him or her to conduct a self-evaluation. These are the following:
  - A *Chapter Checklist* to make sure the student has completed all activities and assignments associated with the chapter.
  - A *Performance Evaluation*, which the student will use to evaluate his or her performance in the classroom. This is then compared with the instructor's evaluation. The performance evaluation can also be used by the student to track his or her grade.

TIPS FOR SUCCESSFUL STUDYING

When they enroll in a college course, many students don't know how to study effectively. Some tend to do too much, and others do too little. The ideal is to find a happy medium. The following are some practical tips on how to get the most out of study time.

Listening in Class

Engage in *active* listening. Involve yourself in the lecture. Research shows that the average college student listens at approximately 35 percent efficiency. Here are some tips to maximize active listening:

- Choose a seat where you can see and hear well, away from distractions.
- Have a pen ready to take notes—it helps you focus.
- Watch the instructor as he or she talks. Watch for signals that will help you recognize the difference between important key points and supporting information.
- Think about what the speaker is saying. Think: "What would be a good test question on this material?" or "How could I use this information?" or "What can I ask to clarify what is being said?"
- Try not to let your mind wander. Pull your concentration back when you have a lapse.
- Be open to learning something new—it can be exciting.
- Try to guess what the instructor might say next.

  Some experts say it's helpful to use the mnemonic LISAN:

- **L**ead: Think ahead; don't just follow.
- **I**deas: Watch and listen for the main ideas.
- **S**ignals: Be aware of the instructor's nonverbal cues.
- **A**ctive: Stay focused.
- **N**otes: They are your summary of the lecture.

Reading, Highlighting, and Taking Notes

Read the assigned material before class. As you read, use a highlighter to mark important points. If you have read the material before class and focused on the key points, you will understand the lecture much better. More important, you will know what questions to ask to clarify any confusing concepts in the reading. Then, as the instructor progresses through the lecture, note any points missed in the reading, paraphrasing (translating to your own words) what the lecturer is saying.

Briefly review your notes from the last class so that you will be able to connect the new material to what you already know. This helps you sort and categorize information mentally and makes information easier to remember.

Some students ask, "Why should I take notes in class?" Here are some good reasons:

- Memory can be unreliable.
- Notes provide a summary from which to study.
- Note taking encourages you to put the main ideas down on paper, in your own words, making them easier to remember.
- Notes expand on the information in the textbook.
- Instructor lectures and class discussions add current real-life ideas, examples, and explanations.

Many students, especially those new to college, are tempted to write down every word the instructor says. Anyone who has taken a college course knows that this is not practical. What you need to do is distinguish between what is and is not important. This is not an easy task.

Example:

The instructor says: "The goal of the health insurance professional is to submit clean claims—those that can be processed for payment quickly and with the maximum reimbursement allowed without being returned for clarification or omissions or rejected for incorrect information."

The student might note: Goal—clean claims; complete, no errors, omissions, or wrong information; prompt, maximum reimbursement.

The student has reduced a nearly 40-word paragraph to 13 words.

Develop your own note-taking style so that your notes make sense to you when you review them later. Think of your notes as an outline.

- Use headings and subheadings.
- List items 1, 2, 3, and so on.
- Use a phrase or word rather than a sentence.
- Note examples with a one-word reminder.
- Develop your own abbreviations (e.g., INS for insurance; PIF for patient information form).
- Don't spend time rewriting your notes to make them look better. As long as you can read them and they make sense to you, that's what is important.

Watch for signals. Good note taking depends on your ability to listen actively in class. Listen and watch for signals that will help you select the main ideas. For example, the instructor may:

- Repeat a point several times.
- Speak loudly to emphasize.
- Write on the board or put on an overhead.
- Distribute a handout.
- Say things such as, "There are three reasons for this . . ." or "The most important thing to remember is. . . ."

Review your notes that same day, when the class is still fresh in your mind. Add important points you might have missed, if necessary. Recalling material that day signals to the brain that this material must be stored for future use.

A good test of effective note taking is: Could you summarize the lecture to someone who wasn't there, using your own words? If you can, you've done a good job of taking notes.

WRITING ESSAYS

When instructors assign an essay writing exercise, many students panic. Writing is often not a student's strong point. The best tip about writing an essay is not to leave it to the last minute! As soon as the instructor assigns the essay topic, think about it, start forming ideas in your mind, and begin your research.

Most essay writing assignments in this course are relatively short—typically 250 to 500 words. This should not be too daunting for most students. This section looks at an example essay topic and some ideas on how to "flesh it out."

Let's say the instructor assigned a 350- to 400-word essay on health insurance reform or the importance of HIPAA compliance. Think about the topic, remembering what you've read and what the instructor has said in his or her lectures.

ix

Then begin your research. Log on to the Internet and get some ideas. *Do not* copy any information you find; just use it as a source and then form your own ideas and opinions around it. The following steps can help guide you through the essay writing process:

- Decide on your topic (or use the topic assigned by the instructor).
- Prepare an outline or diagram of your ideas.
- Form a thesis statement.

  NOTE: A **thesis statement** tells the reader what the essay is about and what point you, the author, will be making. A thesis statement has two parts:

- The first part states the topic; for example:
  - Insurance reform . . .
  - HIPAA compliance . . .
- The second part states the point of the essay; for example:
  - . . . is taking a toll on the American middle class.
  - . . . is crucial in today's medical practices.

  Once a thesis statement is formed, begin writing your essay:

- Write the introduction.
- Write the body:
  - Write the main points.
  - Write the subpoints.
  - Elaborate on the subpoints.
- Write the conclusion.
- Proofread, edit, and add the finishing touches (e.g., name, date).

The essay illustrated in Box 1 demonstrates the principles of writing a basic essay. The different parts of the essay have been labeled. The thesis statement is in bold, the topic sentences are in italics, and each main point is underlined. When you write your own essay, you will probably not need to identify the different parts of the essay unless your instructor asks you to do so. They are marked in this example so that you can more easily identify them.

BOX 1: SAMPLE ESSAY

The New Revolution in Healthcare: Electronic Medical Records

Electronic medical records (EMRs) have been around in one form or another for a long time, but **recent advances in technology and continued efforts to streamline and improve the healthcare system have brought EMRs to center stage of the current healthcare debate**. Many "experts" have suggested ways that computerized databases can improve the care of patients and reduce costs at all levels of the healthcare system.

<u>There are many benefits of EMRs.</u> For instance, a recent EMR system installed at Icon Medical Center allows patient records to be viewed anytime from anywhere in the complex. Records can be accessed concurrently by hospital staff and physicians in adjacent office buildings. *Greater coordinated care has been achieved by interfacing the EMR system with hospital clinical applications.* This has resulted in a more complete care assessment and reduced critical errors. Compliance with HIPAA and other government regulations has also been improved.

<u>There is a downside to EMRs.</u> *The risk of breaching patient confidentiality and medico legal concerns head the top of the list of disadvantages.* Another disadvantage is the cost and time expended to convert existing paper records to an electronic system.

<u>There will be a need for more uniform national standards for data entry and security if EMRs are to become the norm.</u> *If an EMR system is to provide a comprehensive solution for today's practice environment, it must accomplish multiple functions.* These functions include streamlining workflow efficiency, improving adherence to treatment standards, providing detailed financial practice analysis, enhancing patient education and interaction, and optimizing compliance with regulatory and managed care guidelines.

NOTE: When you use Times New Roman Font, 12-point size type, 1-inch margins, double-spaced text, and a title, a one-page essay is approximately 325 to 350 words, depending on paragraphing. When you type in a document, Microsoft Word automatically counts the number of pages and words in your document and displays them on the status bar at the bottom of the workspace. If you don't see the word count in the status bar, right-click the status bar, then and click "Word Count."

PREPARING FOR TESTS

There are three stages of test preparation:

- *Long-term*—from the beginning of school to the test
- *Short-term*—the time leading up to the test when study and review become crucial (often the week or so before)
- *Immediate*—the day or night before

Long-Term Preparation

From day one, keep the final exam or test in mind by asking yourself, "What do I need to know?" Some useful strategies include the following:

- Looking at the objectives stated in the course outlines
- Reviewing regularly
- Looking at old tests or exams, if available
- Trying to understand the material rather than just memorizing it

Short-Term Preparation

Use these strategies as you begin your test-studying in earnest:

- Organize your information.
- Combine related information to help you understand it.
- Practice "active study" techniques (e.g., paraphrasing your notes [saying them in your own words]).
- Pace and schedule your study.
- Use memory aids such as mnemonics and acronyms (e.g., PIF for patient information form) to aid recall of hard-to-remember lists and terms. An example of a typical mnemonic that allows someone to remember the musical bass clef is **G**ood **B**oys **D**o **F**ine **A**lways (g-b-d-f-a).

Immediate Preparation

By the time you get to the day or night immediately before your test, your study technique should be review (as opposed to relearning). Keep these guidelines in mind as you refresh your knowledge:

- Get enough sleep.
- Eat properly.
- Take breaks, relax, and exercise.
- Focus your attention.
- Keep a positive attitude.

Cramming

Cramming is not learning; rather, it is short-term remembering. However, when time is short, you may occasionally have to cram. If that is the case, do the following:

- Make choices—don't attempt to remember everything.
- Turn what you're studying into questions.
- Recite.
- Relax; take some long, deep breaths (being nervous and upset will not help).

Before You Begin

- **Preview the test before you answer anything.** This gets you thinking about the material. Make sure to note the point value of each question. This will give you some ideas on how to budget your time.
- **Do a "mind dump."** Using what you remember from your study sessions, make notes of anything you think you might forget. Write down things that you used in learning the material that might help you remember. Outline your answers to discussion questions.
- **Quickly calculate how much time you should allow for each section** according to the point value. (You don't want to spend 30 minutes on an essay question that counts only 5 points.)

Taking the Test

- **Read the directions.** Can more than one answer be correct? Are you penalized for guessing? Never assume that you know what the directions say.

- **Answer the easy questions first.** This will give you the confidence and momentum to get through the rest of the test because you are sure these answers are correct.
- **Go back to the difficult questions.** When looking over the test and doing the easy questions, your subconscious mind will have been working on the answers to the harder ones. Also, later items on the test might give you useful or needed information for earlier items.
- **Answer all questions** (unless you are penalized for wrong answers).
- **Ask the instructor to explain any items that are not clear.** Do not ask for the answer, but phrase your question in a way that shows the instructor that you have the information but are not sure what the question is asking.
- **Try to answer the questions from the instructor's point of view.** Try to remember what the instructor emphasized and believed was important.
- **Use the margin to explain why you chose the answer** if the question does not seem clear or if the answer seems ambiguous.
- **Circle key words in difficult questions.** This will force you to focus on the central point.
- **Express difficult questions in your own words.** Rephrasing can make it clear to you, but be sure you don't change the meaning of the question.
- **Use all of the time allotted for the test.** If you have extra time, cover up your answers and actually rework the question.

Student Software

HOW TO USE THE STUDENT SOFTWARE

The following section introduces and briefly walks you through the software element located on the Evolve site. After going to the site (http://evolve.elsevier.com/Beik/Today), open the CMS-1500 Software (available in Chapters 6, 8, 9, and 10) and the loading screen will pop up. Please note that your information (name and email address) will automatically feed from your Evolve log-in, so there is no need to sign into the software.

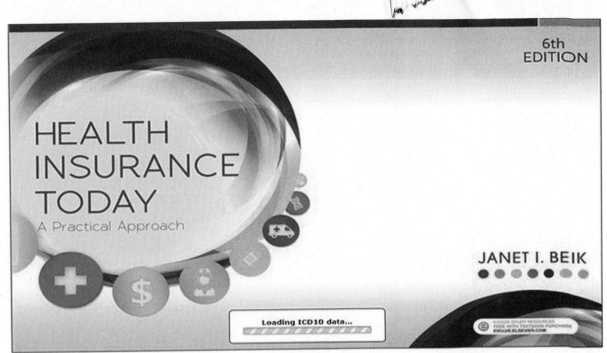

Loading Screen.

CASES

When the software opens, you will be taken to a screen that shows all the available cases (six guided patient cases that are included in the Workbook) that allow you to fill out the CMS-1500 (02/12) form for each case, one block at a time. Accompanying case documents are available for each case, which contain vital information for filling out the claim form. You are able to fill out the form in study mode (with "hints") or exam mode (in which you can test yourself on your progress). In study mode, you will have unlimited attempts to input the correct information. You may also click on the "show hints" button at any time to reveal customized instructions for your case. In exam mode, your work will be graded, and a score will print out on the completed form for your instructor. Once you have completed the form and graded your work, you can print out a copy to turn into your instructor.

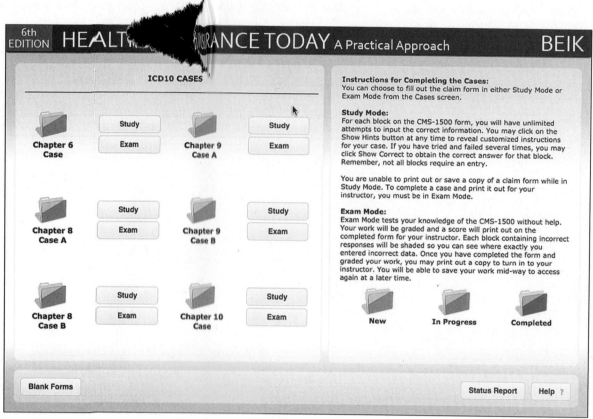

Cases.

Contents

1 The Origins of Health Insurance

Chapter 1 of the textbook *Health Insurance Today: A Practical Approach* provides a brief history and background of medical insurance, how it got started, and its transformation into what we know today as modern health insurance. It is important to know this information to have a complete understanding of the topic.

These accompanying workbook activities are intended to enhance the student's knowledge and understanding of the material included in Chapter 1. Students should follow the instructor's directions for completing each section. A checklist and a student evaluation are included with the end of the chapter exercises to help both the instructor and the student assess the student's comprehension of the material covered in the corresponding chapter.

WORKBOOK CHAPTER OBJECTIVES

After completing the workbook activities for Chapter 1, the student should be able to:
1. Define the terms used in the chapter.
2. Answer the review questions according to the evaluation criteria set by the instructor.
3. Evaluate and provide rational opinions regarding the critical thinking issues.
4. Use individual or group thinking techniques to reach valid conclusions on problem-solving issues and scenarios.
5. Complete assigned projects or participate in class discussions as directed by the instructor.
6. Achieve the required proficiency on all performance objectives.
7. Perform Internet exploration and searches as assigned.
8. Do the enrichment activities as assigned.

DEFINING CHAPTER TERMS

Using the computer, students should write an accurate definition for each of the chapter terms listed. These definitions should be in the students' own words. When finished, students should compare their definitions with those listed in the glossary at the back of the textbook and correct any inaccuracies.

Accountable Care Organization (ACO)
Affordable Care Act
Consolidated Omnibus Budget Reconciliation Act (COBRA)
cost sharing
deductible
entity/entities
fee-for-service
health (medical) insurance
health insurance exchanges
Health Insurance Portability and Accountability Act (HIPAA)
Health Maintenance Organization (HMO) Act
indemnify
indemnity insurance
indigent
insurance
insured
insurer
maintenance of effort (MOE)
managed healthcare
medical insurance
Patient Protection and Affordable Care Act
Patient-Centered Medical Home (PCMH)
policy
preexisting conditions
premium
preventive medicine
subsidies
tiering

ASSESSMENT

The activities and exercises in this section are intended to present a variety of learning opportunities for mastering the information presented in the text and to prepare the student for on-the-job performance. The instructor will tailor these activities and exercises to meet the specific needs and time requirements of the course.

1

Review tests help the instructor measure the extent to which the student has learned the chapter material. Before attempting to complete the test, the student should review the chapter.

Multiple Choice

Directions: In the questions and statements presented, choose the response that **best** answers or completes the stem by circling the letter that precedes it.

1. Financial protection against loss or harm basically is referred to as:
   a. An event
   b. Insurance
   c. A premium
   d. Preventive medicine

2. Medical insurance narrows down "undesired events" to:
   a. Illnesses
   b. Injuries
   c. Preventive medicine
   d. a and b

3. Keeping a person well or catching and treating an emerging illness in its early stages is referred to as:
   a. Outpatient care
   b. Preventive medicine
   c. Emergency medicine
   d. Individualized treatment

4. The beginning of modern health insurance began in 1850 in:
   a. Italy
   b. Russia
   c. England
   d. Germany

5. Health insurance was "born" in the United States in 1929 with a plan that later became known as:
   a. Medicare
   b. Blue Cross
   c. Managed care
   d. National healthcare

6. Blue Cross and Blue Shield plans traditionally established premiums wherein everybody in the community paid the same premium, called:
   a. A premium set
   b. Standard rating
   c. Community rating
   d. Equalizing premium rating

7. A profound change in form from one stage to the next in the life history of an organism is referred to scientifically as:
   a. Change
   b. Mutation
   c. Adulteration
   d. Metamorphosis

8. Congress passed the Health Maintenance Organization (HMO) Act in:
   a. 1850
   b. 1925
   c. 1973
   d. 1991

9. A type of insurance that provides comprehensive major medical benefits and allows insured individual(s) to choose any provider when seeking medical care is called:
   a. A fee-for-service plan
   b. Managed care
   c. Indemnity insurance
   d. a and c

10. The government provides health insurance programs to specific groups, such as the elderly, the disabled, and people who qualify because their income is lower than:
    a. The federal poverty level
    b. The federal minimum wage
    c. Allowable COBRA levels
    d. HIPAA recommendations

11. The Affordable Care Act became fully implemented in:
    a. 2010
    b. 2012
    c. 2013
    d. 2014

12. Under the Affordable Care Act, individuals who have not had health insurance for 6 months receive a subsidy allowing them to enroll in:
    a. High-risk insurance pools
    b. Uninsurable groups
    c. "Watch dog" categories
    d. Risk assessment clusters

13. _____ contains protections for health coverage offered in connection with employment (group health plans) and for individual insurance policies sold by insurance companies (individual policies).
    a. Blue Cross and Blue Shield
    b. Medicare
    c. Medicaid
    d. HIPAA

14. Experts believe that increasing healthcare costs are due to:
    a. The "graying of America"
    b. Advances in medical technology
    c. More demand for healthcare
    d. All of the above

15. Any system of healthcare that attempts to control or coordinate the use of healthcare to contain expenditures, improve quality, or both falls under the category of:
    a. Managed healthcare
    b. A fee-for-service plan
    c. An indemnity plan
    d. All of the above

16. Two new healthcare laws enacted in 2010 that represent significant changes in America's healthcare industry are (choose two):
    a. Consolidated Omnibus Budget Reconciliation Act (COBRA)
    b. Health Care and Education Reconciliation Act
    c. Health Maintenance Organization (HMO) Act
    d. Patient Protection and Affordable Care Act

17. The three major changes that the laws listed in question 16 brought about include all *except:*
    a. Insurance companies cannot deny coverage to children with preexisting illnesses.
    b. Children can remain on their parents' insurance policies until age 26.
    c. Qualifying Medicare recipients will get a $250 rebate.
    d. HMOs and managed care plans will be eliminated.

3

18. Before the Affordable Care Act took effect, the estimated number of Americans who were without healthcare coverage numbered in the:
    a. Hundreds
    b. Thousands
    c. Millions
    d. Billions

19. The program that provides insurance for qualifying children who are ineligible for Medicaid but cannot afford private insurance is called:
    a. CHIP
    b. COBRA
    c. ARRA
    d. HIPAA

20. The two relatively new types of healthcare plans that the text mentions that provide additional options for coverage are:
    a. Medicare and Medicaid
    b. Health Insurance Exchanges and Accountable Care Organizations
    c. CHIP and COBRA
    d. HMOs and HIPAA

True/False

Directions: Place a "T" in the blank preceding the statement if it is true; place an "F" if it is false.

_T_ 1. *Medical insurance* and *health insurance* are interchangeable terms.

_T_ 2. Medical insurance narrows down the "undesirable events" to illnesses and injuries.

_F_ 3. Health insurance in the United States began shortly after the turn of the 19th century, when physicians agreed to provide certain services to all Texans for a nominal fee.

_F_ 4. Politics has never played a role in the growth and change of health insurance.

_F_ 5. The Affordable Care Act significantly limits an individual's choice of healthcare options.

_T_ 6. Effective as of 2014, all Americans with incomes up to 133% of federal poverty guidelines are covered under the Affordable Care Act's new, expanded Medicaid program.

_F_ 7. Advances in medical technology have tended to keep healthcare costs down.

_T_ 8. People buy health insurance to protect them from financial loss or ruin.

_F_ 9. COBRA and HIPAA were enacted by Congress in the same year—1996.

_T_ 10. The two main categories of private health insurance plans are indemnity (fee-for-service) and managed care.

_T_ 11. One way the Affordable Care Act aims to cut healthcare costs is to cut down on Medicare waste and fraud.

_F_ 12. The new healthcare reform laws make it more difficult for Americans to qualify for state Medicaid programs.

Fill-in-the-Blank

Directions: Insert the word(s) in these sentences that best completes the statement.

1. The word "insurance" comes from the Latin word _securitas_.

2. The beginnings of modern health insurance occurred in _England_ (country) in _1880_ (year).

3. The name of the Massachusetts company that first offered medical expense coverage similar to today's health insurance is _FHAC_.

4. In 1929, Justin Kimball, a Baylor University professor in Dallas, introduced a plan that evolved into _Blue Cross_.

5. The Blue Shield plan got its start in the _Pacific Northwest_ (geographical area of United States).

6. _Medicare_ and _Medicaid_ are the federal healthcare programs that began during President Johnson's term in 1965.

7. A(n) _HMO_ is a plan that provides healthcare from specific physicians and hospitals who contract with that plan.

8. The "traditional" or "standard" type of healthcare plan is called a(n) _indeminity_ plan or _fee_ - _for_ - _service_ plan.

9. The model in which a patient's treatment is coordinated through his or her primary care physician to ensure that care is received when and where they need and want it and delivered in a culturally and linguistically appropriate manner is known as the _patient_ _centered_ _medical_ _home_.

10. Name the two new healthcare laws that were enacted in 2010.

Affordable care act

Health care and Education Reconciliation Act

CRITICAL THINKING ACTIVITIES

A. Think about the term *cost sharing*. Give some examples and explain how cost sharing can help curb the rising cost of healthcare.

B. Explain how the Affordable Care Act changed how Americans can get access to affordable healthcare.

C. Why and how does "media intervention" affect healthcare costs?

PROBLEM-SOLVING/GROUP ACTIVITY

Your instructor will separate the class into groups. Each group will be assigned a particular decade or time period from the PBS website chart. Research the particular decades your group has been assigned and prepare a short presentation on the important developments and acts of that period.

PROJECTS/DISCUSSION TOPICS

A. Research and be prepared to discuss the theory of cost containment in healthcare. Focus on specific methods of keeping healthcare costs under control on the federal level and on the level of the individual states.

B. Prepare for (or lead) a class discussion on one of these key medical insurance issues:
   1. How people get affordable health insurance
   2. How the new healthcare "reform" legislation affects Americans
   3. Why healthcare costs so much
   4. How cost sharing helps keep healthcare expenditures down

CASE STUDY

Margaret and Jeremy Tinsman were, so they thought, in the prime of their lives. Margaret was a homemaker, and Jeremy was a successful used car salesman. Both were covered under a group healthcare plan through Jeremy's employer. At 53, Jeremy had a debilitating stroke, which left him completely paralyzed on his left side and unable to speak. Subsequently, Jeremy had to quit his job. What options are open to Margaret and Jeremy as far as health insurance is concerned? What role, if any, do HIPAA and the Affordable Care Act play in this scenario?

INTERNET EXPLORATION

A. Browse the Internet to learn more about the major factors that are contributing to the increased costs of healthcare insurance.

B. Using the Internet, find out how "group insurance plans" differ from "individual/private" plans.

C. Research "Healthcare Reform" on the Internet at http://www.hhs.gov/healthcare/rights/law/index.html or at http://www.healthcare.gov type the key words "Healthcare Reform" in the search engine block.

APPLICATION EXERCISES

Create a Health Insurance Professional's Notebook.

1. Supplies needed:
   a. Black, three-ring, 1-inch binder
   b. Prepunched, color-coded, tabbed dividers
   c. Self-adhesive labels for dividers

2. Create a title page for the notebook (Fig. 1.1).

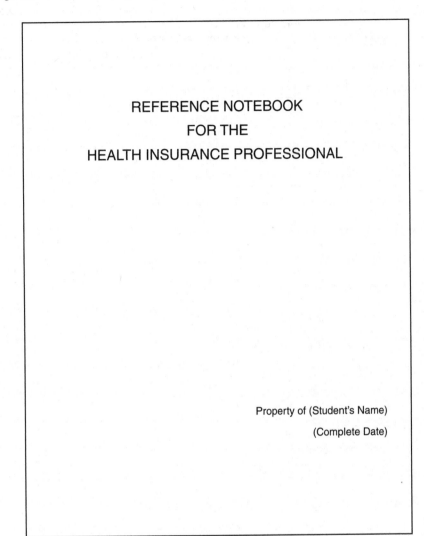

REFERENCE NOTEBOOK

FOR THE

HEALTH INSURANCE PROFESSIONAL

Property of (Student's Name)

(Complete Date)

Fig. 1.1 Sample cover sheet.

3. Prepare six individual labels as follows:
   a. COMMERCIAL/BCBS
   b. MEDICAID
   c. MEDICARE
   d. TRICARE/CHAMPVA
   e. WORKERS' COMPENSATION
   f. MISCELLANEOUS CARRIERS

4. Place labels on tabbed dividers and insert into notebook.

SELF-EVALUATION

Chapter Checklist

Student Name: _____

Chapter Completion Date: _____

Evaluate your classroom performance. Complete the self-evaluation and submit it to your instructor. When your instructor returns this form to you, compare your self-evaluation with the evaluation completed by your instructor.

1.	Record	Your start time and date: _____
2.	Read	The assigned chapter in the text
3.	View	PowerPoint slides (if available)
4.	Complete	Exercises in the workbook as assigned
5.	Compare	Your answers with the answers posted on the bulletin board, website, or handout
6.	Correct	Your answers
7.	Complete	All tests and required activities
8.	Read	Assigned readings (if any)
9.	Complete	Chapter performance objectives (competencies), if any
10.	Evaluate	Chapter performance and submit to your instructor
11.	Record	Your ending time and date: _____
12.	Move on	Begin next chapter as assigned

PERFORMANCE EVALUATION

Student Name: _____

Chapter Completion Date: _____

Evaluate your classroom performance. Compare this evaluation with the one provided by your instructor.

Skill	Student Self-Evaluation			Instructor Evaluation		
	Good	Average	Poor	Good	Average	Poor
Attendance/punctuality						
Personal appearance						
Applies effort						
Is self-motivated						
Is courteous						
Has positive attitude						
Completes assignments in timely manner						
Works well with others						

Student's Initials: _____

Date: _____

Points Possible: _____

Points Awarded: _____

Chapter Grade: _____

Instructor's Initials: _____

Date: _____

2 Tools of the Trade: A Career as a Health (Medical) Insurance Professional

Chapter 2 addresses what "tools" the student needs to succeed in his or her career as a health insurance professional. These tools include skills and interests applicable to the world of health insurance. Although job duties and responsibilities differ from one facility to another, certain core skills are the same across the field. Additionally, students should realize that the term *health insurance professional* encompasses diverse specialties in which credentialing is possible, further heightening their career success and potential. Students are encouraged to explore the Internet to focus on the particular specialty of interest.

WORKBOOK CHAPTER OBJECTIVES

After completing the workbook activities for Chapter 2, the student should be able to:
1. Define the terms used in the chapter.
2. Answer the review questions according to the evaluation criteria set by the instructor.
3. Use critical thinking skills to evaluate, make decisions, and communicate his or her viewpoint clearly and accurately for the scenarios presented.
4. Demonstrate college entry-level core skills in five of the six areas listed in the textbook.
5. Identify and discuss job duties and responsibilities of various specialties under the umbrella of "health insurance professional."
6. Explore career prospects.
7. Investigate certification possibilities.

DEFINING CHAPTER TERMS

Using the computer, students should write an accurate definition for each of the chapter terms listed. These definitions should be in the students' own words. When finished, students should compare their definitions with those listed in the glossary at the back of the textbook and correct any inaccuracies.

application
autonomy
certification
CMS-1500 claim form
communication
comprehension
covered entity
diagnosis
diligence

electronic data interchange (EDI)
enthusiasm
initiative
integrity
objectivity
paraphrase
prioritize
professional ethics
trading partners

ASSESSMENT

Multiple Choice
Directions: In the questions and statements presented, choose the response that **best** answers or completes the stem by circling the letter that precedes it.

1. The nationally recognized title for a health insurance professional is:
   a. Nationally Certified Health Insurance Professional (NCHIP)
   b. Health Insurance Professional of America (HIPA)
   c. Academy of Health Insurance Professionals (AHIP)
   d. Nonexistent for this broad specialty

2. To increase the potential for success, candidates entering the health insurance field should possess which of these college entry-level skills?
   a. Reading and comprehension
   b. Basic business math
   c. English and grammar
   d. All of the above

3. Typical program length for a career as a health insurance professional in community colleges and technical schools can range from:
   a. 2–4 months
   b. 6–8 months
   c. 1–2 years
   d. 2–4 years

4. The concept that learning will not stop when individuals graduate from a college or career program but that they will continue to learn for the rest of their lives is called:
   a. Career identity
   b. Job dedication
   c. Lifelong learning
   d. Permanent commitment

5. The process of arranging daily tasks and activities by the order of their importance is called:
   a. Organizing
   b. Prioritizing
   c. Multitasking
   d. Categorizing

6. Self-discipline, possessing a positive attitude, and diligence best describe examples of:
   a. Desirable personality traits
   b. Qualities of character
   c. Behavioral characteristics
   d. All of the above

7. Writing down important facts from lectures and readings *in your own words* is called:
   a. Paraphrasing
   b. Active listening
   c. Paying attention to detail
   d. Two-way communication

8. Possessing the ability to work without direct supervision is called:
   a. Freedom from restraint
   b. A workplace "right"
   c. Endorsement
   d. Autonomy

9. The growth of certain types of medical facilities has greatly increased the demand for employees with a solid background in coding and excellent computer skills. These are:
   a. Outpatient clinics
   b. Inpatient hospitals
   c. Ambulatory care facilities
   d. Both a and c

10. As an alternative to working in a medical office, health insurance professionals have the option of working *independently* from:
    a. Computer "cafes"
    b. Home-based offices
    c. Contract associations
    d. Health information networks

11. Graduates of a health insurance professional program can enhance their careers through:
    a. Autonomy
    b. Certification
    c. Preauthorization
    d. Computerization

12. The standard insurance form used by all government and most commercial insurance payers is:
    a. CMS-1400
    b. CMS-1500
    c. HIPAA Standard Form
    d. Nonexistent

13. The focus of the health insurance professional's career is:
    a. Submitting clean insurance claims
    b. Becoming certified
    c. Patient account collections
    d. Medical records documentation

14. The new version of HIPAA's standard for filing electronic claims is:
    a. 1500
    b. ASCX12
    c. 5010
    d. 4010A1

15. All covered entities were to be in full compliance with the new HIPAA standards version by:
    a. June 30, 2012
    b. January 6, 2013
    c. December 15, 2014
    d. March 1, 2020

True/False

Directions: Place a "T" in the blank preceding the statement if it is true; place an "F" if it is false.

___T___ 1. To succeed as a health insurance professional, an individual should possess specific college entry-level skills in several areas.

___F___ 2. All learning institutions offer programs in which students can receive extensive hands-on training and practice in medical insurance billing and coding.

___T___ 3. The length for a typical health insurance professional program varies from several months to several years.

___F___ 4. A 4-year degree is not offered in any medical field except nursing.

___T___ 5. Preparation is a crucial key for success in any career.

___T___ 6. "Lifelong learning" means that learning does not stop when an individual completes college or a career program.

___F___ 7. Autonomy—doing things on your own without supervision—is frowned on in medical facilities.

___T___ 8. A career as a health insurance professional offers the individual a variety of tasks and responsibilities.

___F___ 9. The career prospects of a health insurance professional are limited to physicians' offices.

___F___ 10. HIPAA has limited the amount of jobs available in healthcare because of its encouragement of computer-to-computer claim filing.

___T___ 11. One of the biggest rewards of a career in the healthcare field is the knowledge that you are helping people.

___F___ 12. There is no nationally recognized certification specifically referred to as a *health insurance professional*.

___F___ 13. Health insurance professionals never have direct contact with patients.

_____T_____ 14. The law requires that only certified coders make changes to a patient's medical codes after it is determined an error has occurred.

_____F_____ 15. There are no exceptions to Medicare's "mandatory" electronic claim file requirements.

Short Answer

Note: If space provided is not adequate, use a separate piece of blank paper.

1. List the six college entry-level skills that candidates should possess to maximize success as health insurance professionals.

_____

_____

_____

_____

_____

_____

2. Explain why each of these "core" courses is typically included in a health insurance professional program.

Anatomy and Physiology: _____

Medical Terminology: _____

Keyboarding: _____

Microsoft Word: _____

Business English: _____

Medical Office Administrative Skills: _____

3. List at least five types of facilities that offer a graduate of a health insurance professional or billing and coding program opportunities for entry-level employment.

_____

_____

_____

_____

_____

4. In addition to the essential classroom skills, individuals experienced in working as health insurance professionals suggest that candidates for this field should also possess certain job skills. Choose three of these "on-the-job" skills listed in the textbook and write them on the lines below. Then use a blank sheet of paper to write a short paragraph explaining why these skills are important to a health insurance professional.

a. _____

b. _____

c. _____

CRITICAL THINKING ACTIVITIES

Fig. 2.1 shows an article that appeared in a recent newspaper, which contains a mixture of facts and opinions. Read the article and then label the bracketed areas as "fact" or "opinion." When you have finished, make up a title representing the main idea of the article.

Exercise

The following are excerpts from an article that appeared recently in *The Hawkeye* that contains a mixture of facts and opinions. Read the article and then label the bracketed areas as fact or opinion. When you have finished, make up a heading to show the main idea of the article.

_____ Healthcare in America is fast becoming a matter of stock prices, CEOs' salaries, cost savings, and cutbacks–not new cancer therapies, breakthrough drugs, or new help for intractable diseases. Its heroes and role models aren't the white-coated scientists who discover new cures but the suits who put together the big deals; not the physicians who save lives but the corporate honchos who cut healthcare jobs and find innovative ways to deny treatment.

_____ Millions of Americans will be pushed into managed-care organizations of various types in the next few years. Many of them will be vulnerable to a pattern of abuses that is emerging as healthcare becomes just another business opportunity for investors and executives, and doctors are being told, in essence, to put up and shut up.

_____ To get away with curtailing high-tech and expensive care, some HMOs force physicians to sign agreements that contain "gag" orders forbidding them to tell patients about treatments or referrals to specialists the HMO will not provide, even though they might be successful. The American Medical Association calls gag orders "unethical" and "harmful to patients."

_____ Some emerging remedies are worrisome. For example, state legislatures are hurrying to pass laws to give more protection to HMO patients. Two states have made gag rules illegal, and several others are considering such laws. Many states now require HMOs to pay for two days of hospital care for mothers after childbirth, instead of pushing them out in half that time.

But this process is a slow and difficult way to assure patients will get the necessary care they used to take for granted. And it's troubling that there seems to be a need for legislators to intervene in what should be private, professional relationships between patient and doctor.

Fig. 2.1 Critical thinking exercise.

PROBLEM-SOLVING/COLLABORATIVE (GROUP) ACTIVITIES

Your instructor will assign groups and give instructions for oral presentations or discussions on one or more of these topics:

- Employment prospects for the healthcare professional are increasing.
- Alternative career prospects exist for the healthcare professional other than working in physicians' offices or clinics.
- The recent HIPAA laws have created new job opportunities for health insurance professionals.
- Personal and professional rewards can be gained from a career as a health insurance professional.

PROJECTS/DISCUSSION TOPICS

A. Select someone you know who is working in a health career. Prepare a list of 10 questions to ask this person regarding his or her job. Interview this individual, using the question list as a guide. Develop a short, 3- to 5-minute oral presentation explaining this individual's role in healthcare and any other information you were able to gather from the interview.

B. In anticipation of completing your education as a health insurance professional, generate a list of career opportunities available in your area for which you would be qualified. Outline the skills and traits you will need for each and the approximate beginning wages.

CASE STUDY

You are having lunch with Carrie Phillips, a long-time friend, and you inform her that you have en-rolled in a college program to pursue a career in healthcare. She is excited for you and informs you that she herself is interested in this field, but because of obligations that keep her house-bound, she feels she cannot spend time away from home attending classes. As a favor to your friend and for your own information, investigate what *distance learning* opportunities are available in the medical billing and insurance field. Prepare a short report of your findings to tell Carrie the next time you have lunch.

INTERNET EXPLORATION

A. Use the Internet to find out what career certifications are available in the various specialties associated with a health insurance professional.

B. Using search words such as "health career opportunities in (your state)," search the Internet for information on what is currently available for a health insurance professional. Note any specific requirements for the positions available.

C. As an alternate to "B," focus on your specific area of interest in healthcare and search the Internet for job opportunities either in your area or elsewhere in the United States if you are considering or are willing to relocate. Also note the various wage scales that different areas of the United States offer.

PERFORMANCE OBJECTIVES

The **Secretary's Commission on Achieving Necessary Skills (SCANS)** states that a "high-performance" workplace requires workers who have a solid foundation in the *basic literacy and computational skills,* in the *thinking skills* neces-sary to put knowledge to work, and in the *personal qualities* that make workers dedicated and trustworthy. Next, your instructor will administer the performance objective you will be taking to determine competency in the "thinking skills" category, which include:

- Creative thinking—generates new ideas
- Decision-making—specifies goals and constraints, generates alternatives, considers risks, and evaluates and chooses the best alternative
- Problem solving—recognizes problems and devises and implements plan of action
- Seeing things in the mind's eye—organizes and processes symbols, pictures, graphs, objects, and other information
- Knowing how to learn—uses efficient learning techniques to acquire and apply new knowledge and skills
- Reasoning—discovers a rule or principle underlying the relationship between two or more objects and applies it when solving a problem

PERFORMANCE OBJECTIVE 2.1: THINKING SKILLS

Conditions: Student will develop a 250-word written composition using this topic as the subject: "Modern Healthcare Is a Team Effort."

Instructions: In your essay, discuss what you think this means and how you believe you will fit into a "high-performance" workplace. After doing a self-evaluation and some serious introspection, discuss some of your personal attributes that might have to be modified to perform effectively in a team setting, indicate what you would change about yourself, and describe how you would go about making these changes. Use the six thinking skills outlined previously in developing your essay. Compositions must be typed and double spaced, using 1-inch margins all around and 12-point Times New Roman font. Proofread your document before submission. Remember, using spell check does not catch all errors. Pay close attention to grammar and punctuation rules using reference manuals available.

Supplies/Equipment: Internet-ready computer, printer, textbook, and reference material

Time Allowed: To be determined by instructor

Accuracy Needed to Pass: 70%

Procedural Steps	Points Earned	Comments
Evaluator: Note time began: _____		
Carefully read and study the applicable documents.		
1. Student adequately defined the topic and gave reasons why he or she would or would not fit into a "high-performance" workplace. (10)		
2. Student listed and discussed necessary modifications/changes in personal attributes. (20)		
3. Student discussed how these modifications would be accomplished. (20)		
4. Essay shows evidence that the student used all or most of the six "thinking skills." (20)		
5. Student used proper sentence structure, English grammar, and punctuation and spacing in essay using rules from reference materials. (15)		
6. Proofread and edited essay. (10)		
7. Essay is properly identified according to instructions. Print a hard copy. (5)		
Optional: May deduct points for taking more time than allowed.		

Total Points = 100

Student's Score: _____

Evaluator: _____

Comments: _____

_____

_____

_____

Reference Notebook Assignment

Using the Table of Contents in the textbook as a reference along with Fig. 2.2 as a guide, create a table of contents for your reference notebook. Save this table of contents as an electronic file to add information as the course progresses. For now, page numbers will be blank.

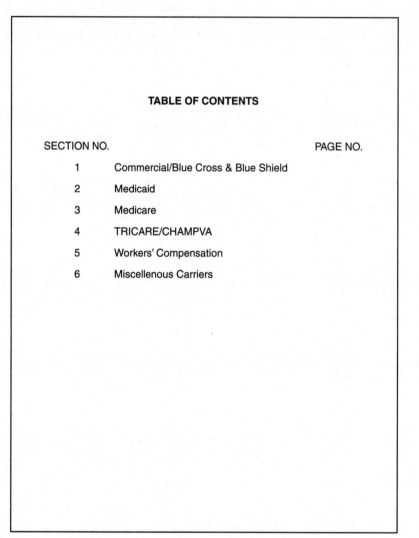

Fig. 2.2 Example of reference notebook table of contents.

Chapter Checklist

Student Name: _____

Chapter Completion Date: _____

Evaluate your classroom performance. Complete the self-evaluation and submit it to your instructor. When your instructor returns this form to you, compare your self-evaluation with the evaluation completed by your instructor.

1.	Record	Your start time and date: _____
2.	Read	The assigned chapter in the textbook
3.	View	PowerPoint slides (if available)
4.	Complete	Exercises in the workbook as assigned
5.	Compare	Your answers to the answers posted on the bulletin board, website, or handout
6.	Correct	Your answers
7.	Complete	All tests and required activities
8.	Read	Assigned readings (if any)
9.	Complete	Chapter performance objectives (competencies), if any
10.	Evaluate	Chapter performance and submit to your instructor
11.	Record	Your ending time and date: _____
12.	Move on	Begin next chapter as assigned

PERFORMANCE EVALUATION

Student Name: _____

Chapter Completion Date: _____

Evaluate your classroom performance. Compare this evaluation with the one provided by your instructor.

Skill	Student Self-Evaluation			Instructor Evaluation		
	Good	Average	Poor	Good	Average	Poor
Attendance/punctuality						
Personal appearance						
Applies effort						
Is self-motivated						
Is courteous						
Has positive attitude						
Completes assignments in timely manner						
Works well with others						

Student's Initials: _____

Date: _____

Points Possible: _____

Points Awarded: _____

Chapter Grade: _____

Instructor's Initials: _____

Date: _____

3 The Legal and Ethical Side of Medical Insurance

Chapter 3 addresses the legal and ethical issues regarding the protection of the rights of patients, the healthcare provider, and the entire healthcare team. When patients visit a medical facility, healthcare professionals (and patients, too) are governed by basic guidelines. Some of these guidelines are of a legal nature, such as those set by governmental licensing agencies and state and federal laws, and others are ethical, such as those imposed by professional organizations that define appropriate conduct.

Legal and ethical issues that health insurance professionals are exposed to daily have taken on new meaning with the advent of the federal Health Insurance Portability and Accountability Act (HIPAA) privacy rule, especially the important aspect of patient confidentiality. Students should be able to understand lawful and ethical medical conduct and apply this conduct to the workplace to promote practice policies and goals. In addition, students need to understand the relationship between law and ethics and foster a deeper consideration of legal and ethical issues and issues of quality of care, patient safety, and prevention of medical errors. These workbook activities are intended to enhance the material presented in the textbook and help the student attain the previously mentioned workplace goals.

WORKBOOK CHAPTER OBJECTIVES

After completing the workbook activities for Chapter 3, the student should be able to:
1. Define the terms used in the chapter.
2. Answer the review questions according to the evaluation criteria set by the instructor.
3. Evaluate and provide rational opinions regarding critical thinking issues.
4. Analyze data, make decisions, and communicate his or her beliefs (either individually or collaboratively) clearly and accurately regarding certain legal or ethical issues.
5. Complete assigned exercises and actively participate in group discussions.
6. Achieve the stated competency level in all performance objectives.
7. Perform all application exercises to required accuracy.
8. Conduct a self-evaluation on classroom performance.

DEFINING CHAPTER TERMS

Using the computer, students should write an accurate definition for each of the chapter terms listed. These definitions should be in the students' own words. When finished, students should compare their definitions with those listed in the glossary in the back of the textbook and correct any inaccuracies.

abandonment
abuse
acceptance
accountability
ancillary
binds
breach of confidentiality
confidentiality
consideration
durable power of attorney
emancipated minor
ethics
etiquette
fraud
implied contract
implied promises
incidental disclosure

The Joint Commission
litigious
medical ethics
medical etiquette
medical (health) record
mentally competent
negligence
offer
party of the first part (first party)
party of the second part (second party)
party of the third part (third party)
portability
privacy
privacy statement
respondeat superior
subpoena *duces tecum*

21

Multiple Choice

Directions: In the questions and statements presented, choose the response that **best** answers or completes the stem by circling the letter that precedes it.

1. The practice of medicine is:
   a. A business
   b. Always profitable
   c. Supported by tax dollars
   d. Often considered a charity

2. The primary goal(s) of the health insurance professional is (are):
   a. To complete and submit insurance claims
   b. To conduct billing and collection procedures
   c. To generate as much money for the practice as legally and ethically possible
   d. All of the above

3. A breach of medical care can result in:
   a. A denied claim
   b. A malpractice lawsuit
   c. Cancellation of an insurance policy
   d. The health insurance professional losing his or her license

4. Loosely translated, the Latin term *respondeat superior* means:
   a. The physician is always the boss
   b. Failure to exercise a reasonable degree of care
   c. The physician must respond to all legal accusations
   d. The employer is ultimately responsible for employee actions

5. Failure to exercise a reasonable degree of care is referred to as:
   a. Negligence
   b. *Respondeat superior*
   c. Omission by default
   d. Employer liability

6. A health insurance policy and the relationship between a healthcare provider and a patient are considered:
   a. Dual agreements
   b. Legal contracts
   c. Faultless covenants
   d. All of the above

7. In terms of contract law, when an individual completes an application for health insurance, he or she is:
   a. Making an offer
   b. Completing an acceptance
   c. Submitting a consideration
   d. Proving competency

8. When the insurance company agrees to grant health insurance coverage to an individual, this is called:
   a. Making an offer
   b. Completing an acceptance
   c. Submitting a consideration
   d. Proving competency

9. The binding force in any contract that gives it legal status—the *thing of value* that each party gives to the other—is the:
   a. Offer
   b. Acceptance
   c. Consideration
   d. Legal object

10. For a contract to be enforceable, it must be:
    a. Legal
    b. In writing
    c. At least 48 hours old
    d. All of the above

11. The parties to a legal contractual agreement must be:
    a. Emancipated
    b. At least 21 years old
    c. Mentally competent
    d. A citizen of the United States

12. Individuals younger than 18 years of age who are independent and living away from home are:
    a. Uninsurable
    b. Illegal minors
    c. Emancipated minors
    d. Unable to enter into a contract

13. The contract between a healthcare provider and a patient is referred to as a(n):
    a. Overt contract
    b. Implied contract
    c. Contract by default
    d. Representative contract

14. Ceasing to provide care to a patient without taking prudent steps is a breach of the physician–patient contract referred to as:
    a. Disclosure
    b. Negligence
    c. Abandonment
    d. Infringement

15. The act that regulates disclosure of Social Security numbers or other confidential information is the:
    a. Fraud and Abuse Act
    b. Federal Privacy Act of 1974
    c. Federal False Claim Amendments Act of 1986
    d. Federal Omnibus Budget Reconciliation Act (OBRA) of 1980

16. The act allowing current or former employees or dependents younger than age 65 to become eligible for Medicare because of end-stage renal disease is the:
    a. Federal Privacy Act of 1974
    b. Federal False Claim Amendments Act of 1986
    c. Consolidated Omnibus Budget Reconciliation Act (COBRA) of 1986
    d. Federal Omnibus Budget Reconciliation Act (OBRA) of 1987

17. The Patient Protection and Affordable Care Act (PPACA) along with the Health Care and Education Reconciliation Act make up the:
    a. Healthcare Reform Act
    b. Federal Omnibus Budget Reconciliation Act
    c. Consolidated Omnibus Budget Reconciliation Act
    d. Health Insurance Privacy and Portability Act

Chapter **3** **The Legal and Ethical Side of Medical Insurance**

18. Standards of human conduct—sometimes called *morals*—of a particular group or culture are also known as:
    a. Mores
    b. Ethics
    c. Etiquette
    d. Conventions

19. Adhering to the rules and conventions governing correct or polite behavior in society is called:
    a. Mores
    b. Ethics
    c. Etiquette
    d. Conventions

20. Timeliness, according to The Joint Commission, is within _____ hours of the encounter.
    a. 6
    b. 12
    c. 24
    d. 48

21. An chronological account of a patient's medical assessment, investigation, and course of treatment is called a:
    a. Contract
    b. Medical record
    c. Consultation report
    d. History and physical

22. A medical record is considered privileged communication; information in it should not be divulged to anyone without a patient's:
    a. Approval
    b. Knowledge
    c. Implied consent
    d. Written consent

23. If additional information needs to be added to a patient's record, it should be in the form of a(n):
    a. Appropriate addendum
    b. Separate typewritten page
    c. Computer-generated document
    d. Penciled note in the margin of the history and physical

24. Adequate and complete documentation helps to:
    a. Determine the level of service
    b. Establish medical necessity
    c. Justify the fees charged
    d. All of the above

25. Lack of proper documentation often results in:
    a. Denied claims
    b. Reduced claim payments
    c. Patients losing their healthcare benefits
    d. Both a and b

26. HIPAA's objective stating that employees cannot be denied health insurance coverage when moving from one group health plan to another is called:
    a. Portability
    b. Preexisting conditions
    c. Unfair competition
    d. Covered expenses

27. If medical personnel in a reception room call a patient by name, HIPAA refers to this exposure as:
    a. Defendable circumstances
    b. Incidental disclosure
    c. Unavoidable contact
    d. Accidental events

28. Situations that do not come under the umbrella of patient confidentiality include:
    a. Communicable diseases
    b. Abuse of a child (or an adult)
    c. Wounds inflicted by firearms
    d. All of the above

29. A signed release of information may not be required when:
    a. The patient is a Medicaid recipient
    b. The patient is a Medicare recipient
    c. The patient is being treated as a result of an on-the-job injury
    d. Both a and c

30. A legal document that requires an individual to appear in court with a piece of evidence that can be used or inspected by the court is called a(n):
    a. Judgment
    b. Arrest warrant
    c. Small claims suit
    d. Subpoena *duces tecum*

True/False

Directions: Place a "T" in the blank preceding the sentence if it is true; place an "F" if it is false.

__T__ 1. Health insurance professionals should be knowledgeable in the area of medical law and liability.

__F__ 2. Medical laws regulating insurance are the same from state to state.

__T__ 3. Direct and indirect patient contact involves ethical and legal responsibility.

__T__ 4. A health insurance professional can be a party to legal action in the event of error or omission.

__T__ 5. In contract law, the promise to pay the premium is the consideration of the individual seeking health insurance coverage.

__F__ 6. All states require that all types of insurance policies be filed with, and approved by, the state regulatory authorities before the policy may be sold.

__F__ 7. A contract between an insurance company and the insured party cannot be terminated.

__T__ 8. A patient can terminate the contract with the physician simply by paying all incurred charges and not returning to the practice.

__F__ 9. The healthcare provider can terminate the physician–patient contract simply by dismissing the patient without reason.

__T__ 10. If the physician wants to withdraw from a particular case, he or she must notify the patient by a letter sent by certified mail with a return receipt.

__T__ 11. An insurance company is often referred to as the *third party* to a contract.

__T__ 12. Laws are universal rules to be observed by everyone, but different cultures follow different moral and ethical codes.

__F__ 13. It is now commonly accepted that patients are the legal owners of their medical records.

__T__ 14. How long medical records are kept and how they are stored and disposed of varies from practice to practice and state to state.

__T__ 15. A medical (health) record is considered a legal document.

Chapter **3** **The Legal and Ethical Side of Medical Insurance**

_F_ 16. Records are the property of the healthcare provider and must be preserved as long as the patient is alive.

_T_ 17. Timely, accurate, and complete documentation in patient records is a crucial element to good patient care.

_F_ 18. All patient record documentation must be performed by the physician.

_T_ 19. Appropriate documentation serves as the basis for the defense of malpractice claims and lawsuits.

_F_ 20. HIPAA's influence is felt only in medical facilities.

_T_ 21. One significant change HIPAA has made for businesses is that health records must be kept separate from routine personnel records.

_T_ 22. Each member of a healthcare team has a responsibility to uphold confidentiality for patients.

_F_ 23. HIPAA does not allow billing insurance companies without a written release of information.

_F_ 24. There are never any exceptions to patient confidentiality.

_F_ 25. A written release form is usually not required for an on-the-job illness or injury.

Short Answer/Fill-in-the-Blank

Note: If space provided is not adequate, use a separate piece of blank paper.

1. Explain in your own words what is meant by a "litigious" society.

_____

_____

2. List and explain each of the five elements necessary to establish a legal contract.

_____

_____

_____

_____

_____

3. Explain the contractual relationship between a healthcare provider and a patient.

_____

_____

_____

4. Under what circumstances and how might a healthcare provider terminate a contract between the provider and a patient?

_____

_____

_____

5. How do medical ethics differ from medical etiquette?

_____

_____

_____

6. List HIPAA's four primary objectives.

_____

_____

_____

_____

7. List six physical safeguards required by HIPAA for guarding data confidentiality, integrity, and availability.

_____

_____

_____

_____

_____

_____

8. A breach of confidentiality occurs when patient information is released to relatives without the patient's consent, except when the relative has a(n) _____, meaning he or she has been named as an agent to handle the individual's affairs if the patient becomes incapacitated.

CRITICAL THINKING ACTIVITIES

A. You receive a telephone call from an attorney asking for information on Eric Downs, a patient who was recently treated in your office for injuries resulting from an automobile accident. How would you handle this phone call?

B. Write a paragraph detailing how an implied contract is created between a healthcare provider and a patient. Explain why this type of contract is binding and what must transpire for it to be "set aside."

PROBLEM-SOLVING/COLLABORATIVE (GROUP) ACTIVITIES

A. Medical ethics is a current area of concern for practitioners and consumers alike. The textbook lists several debatable topics on ethical issues, such as:

- Abortion
- Experimentation
- Prolongation of life
- Quality of life
- Euthanasia

Your instructor will assign teams to discuss or debate one or more of these issues. Choose a topic of interest and be prepared to discuss the pro or con side of the issue.

B. At Broadmoor Medical Clinic, the staff takes turns manning the telephone during the noon lunch break. Today, it is your turn. Patient Sally Albright phones and requests a refill on her prescription for captopril (high blood pressure medicine). List all the information you should get from Sally.

C. Now, assume that Sally's healthcare provider has authorized a prescription refill: captopril, 25 mg, 1 by mouth in the morning, #100 × 2 refills. Additionally, the physician has told you that Sally needs to come in for a weekly blood pressure check. Should Sally's telephone call, the resulting prescription refill, and the physician's request of weekly blood pressure checks be documented in her health record? If so, illustrate an appropriate method of documentation.

PROJECTS/DISCUSSION TOPICS

A. **Individual or Group:** The textbook lists several exceptions to confidentiality. List these and explain in your own words why you think they should, or should not, be exceptions.

B. **Individual:** Research a current article regarding healthcare fraud and abuse. Prepare a one-page (200-word) essay or a 2- to 3-minute oral presentation summarizing the information.

CASE STUDIES

Read each of the case studies presented and explain, on a separate sheet of paper, what your opinion is and how you arrived at it.

A. Brent Underwood, a health insurance professional in the Beach Front Medical Clinic, is convinced by Bertha Parker, a 60-year-old patient of the clinic, that she is a "financial hardship" case. Brent tells Ms. Parker that he will send in a claim to her insurance company and "write off" any balance that they do not pay. Determine whether Brent is within his legal rights as a health insurance professional to do this for Bertha. If not, decide if his actions constitute fraud or abuse.

B. Mary Larson visits Dr. Jacob Astor, her obstetrician, for a suspected pregnancy. Dr. Astor performs an examination; determines Mary is pregnant; and asks you, one of his versatile healthcare professionals, to arrange for an ultrasound. The office is busy, so you inform Mary that you will schedule the procedure later and call her with the appointment date and time. Later that day, you telephone Mary's residence, and her husband answers the telephone. You inform him of the appointment time that has been set up for Mary's ultrasound. Is this a breach of confidentiality? Why or why not?

C. You are employed as a health insurance professional for Dr. Gail Lorber, a family practice physician. Dr. Ian Sutton telephones from the state university epidemiology laboratory. He informs you that he is doing a clinical study on infectious diseases and is requesting a list of all patients who have been treated for hepatitis A, B, and C in the past 5 years. Do you need to procure a written release from each patient to give this information to Dr. Sutton? Why or why not?

INTERNET EXPLORATION

A. **Preventing Fraud and Abuse:** Using search words such as "preventing healthcare fraud and abuse," search the Internet and find some good websites that discuss this topic. Generate a list of at least five ways a health insurance professional can help to curb this growing problem.

B. **Criminal versus Civil Law:** Conduct research on the Internet to determine the difference between criminal law and civil (tort) law. Make your findings detailed and specific.

C. **"The 4 Ds of Negligence":** Search the Internet, determine what the 4 Ds of negligence are, and briefly explain each. To enhance your definitions, give an example for further explanation.

D. The textbook mentions the Affordable Care Act's "Patient's Bill of Rights." Research the Internet using http://www.healthreform.gov/newsroom/new_patients_bill_of_rights.html or type these key words into your search engine to learn more about this topic.

Performance Objective 3.1: Documenting Information Accurately

Conditions: The student will read the following case study, after which he or she will generate an entry in the patient's health record that illustrates the fundamentals of accurate documentation.

Instructions: In this case study, determine the important information that requires documentation in the patient's health record. Using your computer, write a "chart note" illustrating proper and adequate documentation.

Case Study: Helen Arbuckle telephones the office at 9:45 AM on 04/06/XX and informs you that she was in the office a week ago. At that time, Dr. Herschell prescribed Xanax for her anxiety episodes. She was instructed by the doctor to take the medication as he prescribed and let him know in 1 week how she was doing. If she felt her condition had not improved significantly, she was to schedule another appointment as soon as there was an opening. She has not noticed any improvement and wants to schedule another appointment as soon as possible, which you do.

Supplies/Equipment: Computer, printer, notes, textbook, reference materials

Time Allowed: _____

Accuracy Needed to Pass: 90%

Procedural Steps	Points Earned	Comments
Evaluator: Note time began: _____		
Student read the case study in the instructions given.		
1. Student correctly generated the proper heading for the "chart note" (wrote patient's name and date at the top of the document). (10)		
2. Student accurately recorded the required information from Mrs. Arbuckle's telephone call. (50)		
3. Student affixed the proper signature/identification to the chart note. (5)		
4. Student proofread, edited, and printed hard copy. (10)		
Optional: May deduct points for taking more time than allowed.		

Total Points = 75

Student's Score: _____

Evaluator: _____

Comments: _____

_____

_____

_____

_____

Performance Objective 3.2: Identifying, Documenting, and Reporting Abuse and Fraud

Conditions: The student will research and generate an **outline** to present at a "staff meeting" for creating a policy for identifying, documenting, and reporting abuse and fraud in the medical office.

Instructions: The policy outline should include but not be limited to:

- A general definition of fraud and abuse
- Purpose of the policy
- Reasons for the policy
- Examples of fraud and abuse that frequently occur in medical facilities
- Methods used to discourage fraud and abuse
- How to gather evidence
- Responsibilities of team members
- Mandatory reporters
- Identify individuals and firms to report incidents to

Write and print a hard copy of your outline using your computer and printer. Use 1-inch margins all around and 12-point Times New Roman font. Double-space outline entries. Identify your document according to instructions. *Cite your references.*

Supplies/Equipment: Internet-ready computer, printer, notes, textbook, reference materials

Time Allowed: 50 minutes

Accuracy Needed to Pass: 70%

Procedural Steps	Points Earned	Comments
Evaluator: Note time began: _____		
1. Student generated document in acceptable outline form for presentation at "staff meeting." (10)		
2. Document included the required number of "relevant" topics listed in "logical" order. (25)		
3. Student followed specific formatting guidelines as noted in the instructions. (10)		
4. Student properly cited references. (10)		
5. Student proofread, edited, and printed hard copy. (10)		
6. Student affixed proper identification to document. (5)		
Optional: May deduct points for taking more time than allowed.		

Total Points = 70

Student's Score: _____

Evaluator: _____

Comments: _____

_____

_____

_____

APPLICATION EXERCISES

Reference Notebook Assignment

Prepare a section in your notebook for filing information on specific laws and regulations in your state that govern insurance. Include pertinent telephone and fax numbers, websites, and addresses for contacting agencies that can help you with insurance questions.

SELF-EVALUATION

Chapter Checklist

Student Name: _____

Chapter Completion Date: _____

Evaluate your classroom performance. Complete the self-evaluation and submit it to your instructor. When your instructor returns this form to you, compare your self-evaluation with the evaluation completed by your instructor.

1.	Record	Your start time and date: _____
2.	Read	The assigned chapter in the textbook
3.	View	PowerPoint slides (if available)
4.	Complete	Exercises in workbook as assigned
5.	Compare	Your answers to the answers posted on the bulletin board, website, or handout
5.	Correct	Your answers
7.	Complete	All tests and required activities
8.	Read	Assigned readings (if any)
9.	Complete	Chapter performance objectives (competencies), if any
10.	Evaluate	Your personal performance and submit it to your instructor
11.	Record	Your ending time and date: _____
12.	Move on	Begin next chapter as assigned

PERFORMANCE EVALUATION

Student Name: _____

Chapter Completion Date: _____

Evaluate your classroom performance. Compare this evaluation with the one provided by your instructor.

Skill	Student Self-Evaluation			Instructor Evaluation		
	Good	Average	Poor	Good	Average	Poor
Attendance/punctuality						
Personal appearance						
Applies effort						
Is self-motivated						
Is courteous						
Has positive attitude						
Completes assignments in timely manner						
Works well with others						

Student's Initials: _____

Date: _____

Points Possible: _____

Points Awarded: _____

Chapter Grade: _____

Instructor's Initials: _____

Date: _____

4 Healthcare Reform: Coverage Types and Sources

Chapter 4 introduces the student to healthcare reform, types and sources of health insurance, and terms common to third-party carriers. The changing face of healthcare is presented in this chapter with emphasis on the health insurance marketplace and its role in today's healthcare system. The major carriers are briefly addressed along with miscellaneous healthcare coverage options. (Major carriers are discussed in more depth in later chapters of the textbook.) Additionally, the various types of healthcare models are presented. Students are introduced to the universal healthcare insurance paper claim form—the CMS-1500. These workbook exercises have been developed to reinforce the concepts and materials in Chapter 4.

WORKBOOK CHAPTER OBJECTIVES

After completing the workbook activities for Chapter 4, the student should be able to:
1. Define the terms used in the chapter.
2. Answer the review questions to within the evaluation criteria set by the instructor.
3. Use critical thinking skills to evaluate, make decisions, and communicate his or her viewpoint clearly and accurately.
4. Redefine and use collaborative learning skills.
5. Research the Internet successfully for up-to-date information on relevant topics.
6. Perform basic mathematical computations.
7. Apply learning experiences to applicable circumstances.

DEFINING CHAPTER TERMS

Using the computer, students should write an accurate definition for each of the chapter terms listed. These definitions should be in the students' own words. When finished, students should compare their definitions with those listed in the glossary at the back of the textbook and correct any inaccuracies.

Accountable Care Organization (ACO)
Affordable Care Act (ACA)
annual dollar limit
balance billing
birthday rule
cafeteria plan
capitation
Civilian Health and Medical Program of the Department of Veterans Affairs (CHAMPVA)
CMS-1500 claim form
coinsurance
comprehensive plan
Consolidated Omnibus Budget Reconciliation Act (COBRA)
coordination of benefits (COB)
copayment
cost-sharing
deductible
disability insurance
enrollees
episode-of-care
essential health benefits

exclusions
fee-for-service (FFS)
flexible spending account (FSA)
grandfathered plans
group plan
hardship exemption
health insurance exchanges
Health Insurance Marketplace
Health Reimbursement Arrangements (HRAs)
health savings account (HSA)
indemnity (fee-for-service)
insured
lifetime limits
long-term care
managed care
Medicaid
medical savings account (MSA)
medically necessary
Medicare
Medicare Supplement plans
Medigap
metal plans (metal levels)

nonparticipating (nonPAR) provider
out-of-pocket maximum
participating (PAR) provider
policyholder
preexisting condition
premium
premium reimbursement arrangement (PRA)

preventive services
resource-based relative value scale (RBRVS)
Social Security Disability Insurance (SSDI)
TRICARE
usual, customary, and reasonable (UCR)
value-based care
workers' compensation

ASSESSMENT

Multiple Choice

Directions: In the questions and statements presented, choose the response that **best** answers or completes the stem by circling the letter that precedes it.

1. The traditional healthcare delivery system relies heavily on what type of reimbursement model?
   a. Capitation
   b. Fee-for-service (indemnity)
   c. Managed care
   d. Commercial

2. If an insurer negotiates to pay a healthcare provider $300 per year for 1000 people enrolled in a plan, the healthcare reimbursement model would be:
   a. Indemnity
   b. Capitation
   c. Indemnity
   d. UCR

3. With an indemnity policy, patients:
   a. Can choose any provider they want
   b. Can change physicians at any time
   c. Pay a monthly "premium"
   d. Pay no yearly deductible
   e. a, b, and c

4. Under an FFS plan, the value of a provider's service is based on specific historical data, referred to as:
   a. The usual, customary, and reasonable (UCR) fee
   b. Medically necessary charge
   c. Average provider fee
   d. Geographical data fee

5. The universal form used to submit claims to third-party payers is:
   a. CMS-1100
   b. HCFA-1000
   c. CMS-1500
   d. Nonexistent

6. Under the _____ system, a formula established by CMS assigns a value to every medical procedure to calculate Medicare's fee schedule allowance.
   a. Capitation
   b. Fee-for-service
   c. RBRVS
   d. Episode-of-care

7. The percentage amount (typically 20%) a patient is required to pay out of pocket toward the cost of healthcare when a health insurance claim is filed is called:
   a. Indemnity
   b. Copayment
   c. Deductible
   d. Coinsurance

8. Minimum coverage requirements for all plans in the Health Insurance Marketplace are referred to as:
   a. Preventive health benefits
   b. Essential health benefits
   c. Mutual health benefits
   d. Common health benefits

9. Which of the following is NOT a "metal plan" under the ACA?
   a. Gold
   b. Bronze
   c. Lead
   d. Silver

10. Under a(n) _____ plan, patients are told which healthcare providers they can see and their medications and treatments are monitored, thus ensuring enrollees that their costs will remain as low as possible.
   a. Managed care
   b. Grandfathered
   c. Indemnity
   d. UCR

11. The federal health insurance program that provides healthcare benefits to individuals age 65 or older and individuals younger than 65 with certain disabilities is called:
   a. Medicare
   b. Medicaid
   c. Disability insurance
   d. TRICARE/CHAMPVA

12. The name of the federal entitlement program that covers certain categories of low-income individuals and certain disabled individuals is called:
   a. Medicare
   b. Medicaid
   c. Disability insurance
   d. TRICARE/CHAMPVA

13. Insurance that pays workers who are injured or disabled on the job or experience job-related illnesses is called:
   a. Workers' compensation
   b. Medicare
   c. Medicaid
   d. TRICARE/CHAMPVA

14. The type of plan available to self-employed individuals that works in conjunction with special low-cost, high-deductible health insurance is called a(n):
   a. Self-employed savings account (SESA)
   b. Flexible spending account (FSA)
   c. Health savings account (HSA)
   d. Investment retirement account (IRA)

15. A network of doctors and hospitals that shares responsibility for managing the healthcare needs of a minimum of 5000 Medicare beneficiaries for at least 3 years is a(n):
   a. Accountable Care Organization
   b. Health Insurance Exchange
   c. Health Savings Plan
   d. Health Maintenance Organization

16. Which of these organizations are instrumental in recognizing and assessing healthcare plans and certifying the quality of the care they provide? (Choose all that apply.)
   a. The Joint Commission
   b. National Committee for Quality Assurance
   c. American Medical Association
   d. Consumer Coalition for Quality Health Care

True/False

Directions: Place a "T" in the blank preceding the statement if it is true; place an "F" if it is false.

_____ 1. Fee-for-service and indemnity insurance are the same.

_____ 2. The portion of the medical fee that the patient is responsible for is called *coinsurance*.

_____ 3. All third-party insurers have the same UCR rates.

_____ 4. The traditional healthcare delivery system relies heavily on the FFS payment method in which a provider is paid a fee for rendering a specific service.

_____ 5. All managed care plans allow patients to choose any healthcare provider they want.

_____ 6. Under RBRVS, the cost of providing each service is divided into three components: (1) physician work, (2) practice expense, and (3) professional liability insurance.

_____ 7. Managed care is medical care that is provided by a corporation established under state and federal laws.

_____ 8. Catastrophic plans are available only to people who are under 65 years old or have a hardship exemption.

_____ 9. Medicaid is a joint federal-state health program run by the individual states.

_____ 10. Medicare is the military's comprehensive healthcare program.

_____ 11. SSDI is an insurance program administered by HIPAA for individuals who are unable to work.

_____ 12. Workers' compensation laws are designed to ensure injured or disabled employees are provided with monetary awards, eliminating the need for litigation.

_____ 13. Health insurance plans typically cover dental restoration work caused by disease or accident.

_____ 14. Most healthcare plans cover routine vision care, such as refractions.

_____ 15. If a medical service is not listed as "covered" in the policy, the insurance company normally will not pay any portion of the charge.

Matching

Directions: Insert the letter of the definition that correctly corresponds to the terms listed.

_____ 1. COBRA

_____ 2. Indemnity insurance

_____ 3. FSA

_____ 4. Preexisting condition

_____ 5. Coinsurance

_____ 6. HSA

_____ 7. Nonparticipating (nonPAR) provider

_____ 8. Premium

_____ 9. Deductible

_____ 10. UCR

a. The amount the insured must pay before insurance coverage begins

b. The part of a provider's charge that the insurance carrier will allow as covered expenses

c. The portion of the fee (usually a percentage) that the insured must pay

d. A provider who is under no contractual agreement with the insurance carrier to accept reimbursement as payment in full

e. A special tax shelter set up for the purpose of paying medical bills

f. An IRS Section 125 cafeteria plan

g. Traditional healthcare in which patients can choose any provider they want (including specialists) and change physicians at any time

h. Illnesses or injuries that occurred before the start of a health insurance contract

i. A law that provides continuation of group health coverage when an individual leaves his or her place of employment

j. A periodic fee that is paid to an insurer for healthcare coverage

CRITICAL THINKING ACTIVITIES

A. Compare and contrast an HSA with an FSA.

B. Write a "news event" on a current health insurance topic. This should be a paragraph of at least 150 words, and it should explain the "event" thoroughly enough for your peers to understand.

C. Express your opinion (pro or con) of "managed care" in one to two paragraphs.

D. The textbook talks about health insurance "watchdogs" and lists several organizations that are instrumental in recognizing and assessing healthcare plans and certifying the quality of the care they provide. Discuss why you think organizations such as these are important to healthcare in general.

PROBLEM-SOLVING/COLLABORATIVE THINKING ACTIVITIES

A. Imagine you are married with two minor children. Your spouse comes home from work and announces that his or her employer has offered a choice of health insurance policies. One is an indemnity plan with a $250 yearly deductible and an 80/20 copayment. The other is a managed care plan (HMO) requiring only a $25-per-encounter payment.
   1. Do you have enough information for making an educated choice?
   2. If so, which plan would you choose and why?
   3. If not, what further information do you need before you can make a decision?

PROJECTS/DISCUSSION TOPICS

Choose one of these topics and, according to your instructor's guidelines, prepare an outline for an oral discussion:
   1. What does it mean to not have health insurance?
   2. The costs versus the benefits of health insurance
   3. Which of the four "metal plans" works best for you?
   4. Consolidated Omnibus Budget Reconciliation Act (COBRA)
   5. Health insurance in other countries (e.g., Canada, Great Britain)
   6. Compare and contrast participating (PAR) and nonPAR providers.

CASE STUDIES

A. Sally and Joe Barnes have three children, ages 12, 8, and 5. Sally has a 60% teaching contract with the Oak Crest County School System, and Joe works full time for Amex Auto Sales. Both have a group policy through their respective employers. Sally's date of birth is 08/17/64, and Joe's is 03/10/65. Which policy is primary for their children?

B. Dr. Maxwell Stark is a PAR provider with Blue Cross and Blue Shield; Dr. Forrest Wilson is nonPAR with the same insurer. Both providers are specialists in gastroenterology. Both physicians charge $1000 for a colonoscopy. Blue Cross and Blue Shield allows $700 as its UCR fee for this procedure. Assuming each provider has a patient who undergoes a colonoscopy, each patient has satisfied his or her yearly deductible, and each has paid the same amount of coinsurance (20% of the "allowable" charge—$140), how much can Dr. Stark bill his colonoscopy patient? How much can Dr. Wilson bill his patient?

Chapter **4** **Healthcare Reform: Coverage Types and Sources**

INTERNET EXPLORATION

A. Research and analyze long-term care insurance. Compose a list of advantages and disadvantages of this type of health insurance. Imagine you are having a discussion with your 62-year-old aunt. What would you tell her about long-term care insurance?

B. Investigate the healthcare coverage options available in your state (including the new healthcare exchanges) by entering applicable key words into your Internet search engine. You may even refine your search to healthcare options available in your state if a resident is unemployed or is employed in a business that does not offer healthcare.

PERFORMANCE OBJECTIVE

A basic foundation skill for any career is mathematics. Individuals seeking entry-level positions should be able to "perform basic computations and approach practical problems by choosing appropriately from a variety of mathematical techniques."

Performance Objective 4.1: Math Skills

Conditions: Read the following math problem and choose an appropriate method to arrive at the correct answer (you must show your work).

Supplies/Equipment: Calculator, pencil, sheet of plain paper, and (allowed) reference materials

Time Allowed: 15 minutes

Accuracy Needed to Pass: 100%

Problem: You are employed as a health insurance professional by Bright Horizons Medical Center. You note that your supply of CMS-1500 forms is getting low, and it is time to reorder. According to the catalog, these forms can be ordered two ways: a case containing 250 forms priced at $0.20 each or a case of 1500 (quantity) forms priced at $195 per 1000. Which is the more economical method for purchasing these forms?

Procedural Steps	Points Earned	Comments
Evaluator: Note time began: _____		
1. Carefully read the problem.		
2. Using an appropriate mathematical technique, calculate the correct answer.		
3. Insert your answer in the blank provided. (10)		
4. Show your calculations and make sure the method you used to arrive at the solution is accurate. (10)		
Optional: May deduct points for taking more time than allowed.		

Total Points = 20

Student's Score: _____

Evaluator: _____

Comments: _____

_____

_____

_____

Health Insurance Professional's Notebook

If your instructor has chosen this project for you to complete, you now should have these items generated for your notebook:

- A cover page
- Six tabbed and labeled dividers
- A Table of Contents (not final)

Now, create a cover sheet for each of the six main sections (Fig. 4.1). After these documents have been created, insert them in your notebook behind the tabbed dividers.

MEDICAID

TABLE OF CONTENTS

    I.   Federal regulations

    II.   State regulations for _____ (insert your state here)

   III. Eligibility chart/table

   IV. Sample forms

    V. Sample identification card(s)

   VI. Current fiscal intermediary name/address/phone

  VII. Guidelines for completing the CMS-1500

 VIII. CMS-1500 template

(List other pertinent topics.)

Fig. 4.1 Sample section cover sheet.

Chapter Checklist

Student Name: _____

Chapter Completion Date: _____

Evaluate your classroom performance. Complete the self-evaluation and submit it to your instructor. When your instructor returns this form to you, compare your self-evaluation with the evaluation completed by your instructor.

1.	Record	Your start time and date: _____
2.	Read	The assigned chapter in the textbook
3.	View	PowerPoint slides (if available)
4.	Complete	Exercises in the workbook as assigned
5.	Compare	Your answers to the answers posted on the bulletin board, website, or handout
6.	Correct	Your answers
7.	Complete	All tests and required activities
8.	Read	Assigned readings (if any)
9.	Complete	Chapter performance objectives (competencies), if any
10.	Evaluate	Chapter performance and submit to your instructor
11.	Record	Your ending time and date: _____
12.	Move on	Begin next chapter as assigned

PERFORMANCE EVALUATION

Student Name: _____

Chapter Completion Date: _____

Evaluate your classroom performance. Compare this evaluation with the one provided by your instructor.

Skill	Student Self-Evaluation			Instructor Evaluation		
	Good	Average	Poor	Good	Average	Poor
Attendance/punctuality						
Personal appearance						
Applies effort						
Is self-motivated						
Is courteous						
Has positive attitude						
Completes assignments in timely manner						
Works well with others						

Student's Initials: _____

Date: _____

Points Possible: _____

Points Awarded: _____

Chapter Grade: _____

Instructor's Initials: _____

Date: _____

5 Claim Submission Methods

Chapter 5 introduces the student to the two basic methods for submitting health insurance claims: electronically (using electronic data interchange [EDI] transactions standards) or the CMS-1500 "universal" paper claim form—formerly used by all government and most third-party payers—for those providers who meet the specific guidelines for a "waiver" of the electronic claim submission directive. These workbook exercises familiarize students further with these two methods of submitting claims and guide them through the multistage process of collecting and "abstracting" the necessary information from various documents to complete and submit a "clean" claim. Some exercises can be completed using practice management software (available in an optional package upgrade) that will provide students with real-time experience of entering the necessary patient information into a series of screens that ultimately generates electronic claims.

WORKBOOK CHAPTER OBJECTIVES

After completing the workbook activities for Chapter 5, the student should be able to:
1. Define the terms used in the chapter.
2. Answer the review questions according to the evaluation criteria set by the instructor.
3. Analyze hypothetical situations, applying logical concepts for rational decision-making to health insurance scenarios.
4. Apply reasoning and problem-solving skills (individually or in a group) to arrive at practical solutions to common health insurance issues.
5. Conduct Internet research to learn more about selected topics.
6. Abstract information from healthcare documents for the purpose of accurate claims completion.
7. Collect information and documents for inclusion in the Health Insurance Professional's Notebook.
8. Perform self-evaluation on successful content mastery for Chapter 5.

DEFINING CHAPTER TERMS

Using the computer, students should write an accurate definition for each of the chapter terms listed. These definitions should be in the students' own words. When finished, students should compare their definitions with those listed in the glossary at the back of the textbook and correct any inaccuracies.

American Standard Code for Information Interchange (ASCII)
assign(s) benefits
beneficiary
claim attachments
claims clearinghouse
clean claims
CMS-1500 form
demographic information
dial-up(s)
direct claim submission
electronic protected health information (e-PHI)
employer identification number (EIN)
encounter form

guarantor
HIPAA-covered entity
insurance billing cycle
medical necessity
monospaced fonts
national provider identifier (NPI)
optical character recognition (OCR)
patient ledger card
practice management software
protected health information (PHI)
release of information
small (entity) provider
third-party payer
waiver

ASSESSMENT

Multiple Choice

Directions: In the questions and statements presented, choose the response that **best** answers or completes the stem and circle the letter that precedes it.

1. The two basic methods of submitting health insurance claims are (choose two):
   a. Electronic
   b. Fax modem
   c. Paper form
   d. Wireless router

2. The health insurance claims process is an interaction between the healthcare provider and a(n):
   a. Patient
   b. Insurance company
   c. Guarantor
   d. Beneficiary

3. Services or supplies that are appropriate and necessary for the symptoms, diagnosis, and treatment of the medical condition and meet the standards of good medical practice is the definition for:
   a. Medical necessity
   b. Demographic information
   c. Principles of morality
   d. Value-based medicine

4. A modern innovation that has made claims submission faster and more accurate at a cost savings to a medical practice is:
   a. ASCII bit converter
   b. Optical character recognition
   c. Computer technology
   d. Universal paper claim form

5. A "small provider" of services is one with fewer than:
   a. 5 full-time equivalent employees
   b. 15 full-time equivalent employees
   c. 20 full-time equivalent employees
   d. 25 full-time equivalent employees

6. The patient information form is considered a legal document and should be updated no less often than:
   a. Once a month
   b. Once a year
   c. Every 2 years
   d. Every 5 years

7. A patient's name, address, Social Security number, and employment data are commonly referred to as:
   a. Viable data
   b. Pertinent facts
   c. Transient statistics
   d. Demographic information

8. An individual covered under Medicare is referred to as a(n):
   a. Enrollee
   b. Beneficiary
   c. Recipient
   d. Covered entity

9. An insurance policy that covers an individual, his or her spouse, and eligible dependents is referred to as a(n):
   a. Dual plan
   b. Family plan
   c. Multiple plan
   d. Individual plan

10. A multipurpose form used by most medical practices for billing is called a(n):
    a. Superbill
    b. Encounter form
    c. Routing form
    d. All of the above

11. In noncomputerized practices, patient charges and payments can be tracked manually on a(n):
    a. Encounter form
    b. CMS-1500 form
    c. Patient ledger card
    d. Patient information form

12. Identify which of these is considered a HIPAA-covered entity:
    a. Healthcare plans
    b. Healthcare providers
    c. Healthcare clearinghouses
    d. All of the above

13. The standard unique identifier that was adopted to identify all healthcare providers and health plans is the:
    a. PHI
    b. EIN
    c. OCR
    d. NPI

14. An example of a method for manual claims follow-up is using an:
    a. Insurance log
    b. Encounter form
    c. Insurance register
    d. Both a and c

15. A company that receives claims, consolidates them, and transmits them in batches to third-party payers is called a:
    a. Third-party payer
    b. Clearinghouse
    c. Claims consolidator
    d. Covered entity

16. After January 2010, a new version of the HIPAA standards was implemented called:
    a. 4010A1
    b. Version 5010
    c. Standard X12
    d. Version 4010/4010A1

17. This new HIPAA standards version addresses many of the deficiencies in the former version and accommodates the reporting of (choose two):
    a. National Provider Identifiers (NPIs)
    b. The new CPT codes
    c. Employer identification numbers (EINs)
    d. The new ICD-10 codes

18. According to the text, the two methods of submitting electronic claims are (choose two):
    a. The IVR system
    b. Through a claims clearinghouse
    c. Directly to the insurance carrier
    d. An Internet-based eligibility check system

19. The CMS-1500 form is an 8½- × 11-inch, two-sided document, the front side of which is printed in:
    a. OCR scannable red ink
    b. Both English and Spanish
    c. Italicized 12-point font
    d. ASCII control characters

20. Medicare claims must be submitted electronically unless the secretary of HHS grants a(n):
    a. Penalty exclusion
    b. Forfeiture
    c. Waiver
    d. Exclusion pledge

True/False

Directions: Read these sentences. If the statement is true, place a "T" in the blank preceding the number. If it is false, place an "F" in the blank and then rewrite the sentence in the space provided beneath so that it is true. The first one is done for you as an example.

___F___ 1. The American Medical Association is responsible for creating the universal claim form known as the CMS-1500.

The Health Care Financing Administration is responsible for creating the universal claim form known as the CMS-1500.

_____ 2. The CMS-1500 form (originally known as the *HCFA-1500*) was developed for the purpose of submitting Medicare claims.

_____ 3. Practice management software allows users to enter patient demographic information, schedule appointments, maintain lists of insurance payers, perform billing tasks, and generate reports.

_____ 4. The Centers for Medicare and Medicaid Services (CMS) initiated changes to promote uniformity in healthcare claim submission by adopting standards for electronic health information transactions.

_____ 5. Roster billing of Medicare-covered vaccinations for multiple beneficiaries must be submitted electronically.

_____ 6. Small entity providers are those with 25 or fewer full-time employees (FTEs) and physicians, practitioners, and suppliers with 10 or fewer FTEs.

_____ 7. The intent of HIPAA's Administrative Simplification legislation was to provide consumers with lower healthcare costs.

_____ 8. HIPAA allows providers who conduct business electronically to use their own established healthcare transactions, code sets, and identifiers.

_____ 9. The health insurance professional's most important responsibility is to obtain the maximum amount of reimbursement in the minimal amount of time that the patient's health record will support.

_____ 10. The HIPAA Administrative Simplification Compliance Act (ASCA) prohibits the Department of Health and Human Services (HHS) from paying all claims that are not submitted electronically, without exception.

_____ 11. The patient information form typically lists both demographic and insurance information.

_____ 12. The health insurance professional must obtain written permission from the patient to release healthcare information to any person or business entity except the patient's insurance carrier.

_____ 13. If a claim requires an attachment to provide additional medical information to the claims processor, neither the claim nor the attachment can be submitted electronically; both must be mailed.

_____ 14. The insurance claim process begins when the health insurance professional submits the claim to the insurance processor.

_____ 15. A clearinghouse is an independent, centralized service available to healthcare providers for the purpose of simplifying medical insurance claims submission for multiple carriers.

Short Answer/Fill-in-the-Blank

Note: If space provided is not adequate, use a separate piece of blank paper.

1. List four exceptions identified by the Administrative Simplification Compliance Act (ASCA) of 2001 for submitting Medicare claims electronically.

_____

_____

_____

_____

2. Name the four parts to HIPAA's Administrative Simplification Act.

_____

_____

_____

_____

3. HIPAA has identified 10 standard transactions for electronic data interchange (EDI) for the transmission of healthcare data. Name three.

_____

_____

_____

4. What is the health insurance professional's most important task?

_____

5. Who uses the paper CMS-1500 form?

_____

6. ASCA prohibits HHS from paying Medicare claims that are not submitted electronically unless the Secretary grants

a(n) _____ for this requirement.

7. Define a "small provider."

_____

8. List three reasons why healthcare facilities use a patient information form.

_____

_____

_____

9. Explain the rationale for making a photocopy of both sides of a patient's insurance ID card.

_____

10. What is the significance of a patient "assigning benefits"?

_____

11. Define a *medical record*.

_____

12. List six things a complete medical record should provide.

_____

_____

_____

_____

_____

_____

13. List at least six types of information typically found on an encounter form.

_____

_____

_____

_____

_____

_____

14. List at least five reasons why a claim might be rejected.

_____

_____

_____

_____

_____

15. What are three advantages of electronic claims filing?

_____

_____

_____

16. Identify three technological methods for verifying a patient's insurance coverage.

_____

_____

_____

17. Explain the process used by a claims clearinghouse.

_____

_____

_____

18. How does the direct claims submission method work?

_____

_____

_____

CRITICAL THINKING ACTIVITIES

A. You are employed as a health insurance professional in a family practice facility. Eloise Grafton, the office supervisor, asks you to generate a document for the office procedures manual explaining the steps involved in the insurance claims and billing process. Begin with the patient's arrival at the office through the checkout process at the reception area when the encounter is concluded. Include a diagram or a flow chart to enhance understanding.

B. Write a paragraph explaining the purpose and function of the **encounter form.** Be specific and thorough. Use examples as needed.

PROBLEM-SOLVING/COLLABORATIVE (GROUP) ACTIVITIES

A. Your instructor will give you two blank patient information forms. Along with a partner, role-play a health insurance professional and patient. When you play the part of the "patient," complete the patient information form using your own personal information or create a fictitious character. Then ask your partner, the "health insurance professional," to check the form for omissions or errors. Reverse roles and repeat the procedure.

B. Carefully examine the completed claim form (Adam Rogers) in Fig. 5.1. Highlight or circle any shaded blocks that contain errors. Then, in Table 5.1, insert a "C" in Column 2 if the information in the block is correct; insert an "I" if it is incorrect. Last, illustrate how the information should be entered correctly in Column 3.

HEALTH INSURANCE CLAIM FORM

APPROVED BY NATIONAL UNIFORM CLAIM COMMITTEE (NUCC) 02/12

PICA — PICA — CARRIER

1. MEDICARE (Medicare#) ☐ MEDICAID (Medicaid#) ☐ TRICARE (ID#DoD#) ☐ CHAMPVA (Member ID#) ☐ GROUP HEALTH PLAN (ID#) ☒ FECA BLK LUNG (ID#) ☐ OTHER (ID#) ☐

1a. INSURED'S I.D. NUMBER (For Program in Item 1): XQS123456789

2. PATIENT'S NAME (Last Name, First Name, Middle Initial): ROGERS ADAM L

3. PATIENT'S BIRTH DATE MM DD YY: 10 21 54 — SEX M ☒ F ☐

4. INSURED'S NAME (Last Name, First Name, Middle Initial): SAME

5. PATIENT'S ADDRESS (No., Street): 1500 WEST 50TH ST

6. PATIENT RELATIONSHIP TO INSURED: Self ☒ Spouse ☐ Child ☐ Other ☐

7. INSURED'S ADDRESS (No., Street)

CITY: MILTON — STATE: XY

8. RESERVED FOR NUCC USE

CITY — STATE

ZIP CODE — TELEPHONE (Include Area Code) ( )

ZIP CODE — TELEPHONE (Include Area Code) ( )

9. OTHER INSURED'S NAME (Last Name, First Name, Middle Initial)

10. IS PATIENT'S CONDITION RELATED TO:

11. INSURED'S POLICY GROUP OR FECA NUMBER

a. OTHER INSURED'S POLICY OR GROUP NUMBER

a. EMPLOYMENT? (Current or Previous) ☐ YES ☐ NO

a. INSURED'S DATE OF BIRTH MM DD YY — SEX M ☐ F ☐

b. RESERVED FOR NUCC USE

b. AUTO ACCIDENT? ☐ YES ☐ NO — PLACE (State)

b. OTHER CLAIM ID (Designated by NUCC)

c. RESERVED FOR NUCC USE

c. OTHER ACCIDENT? ☐ YES ☐ NO

c. INSURANCE PLAN NAME OR PROGRAM NAME

d. INSURANCE PLAN NAME OR PROGRAM NAME

10d. CLAIM CODES (Designated by NUCC)

d. IS THERE ANOTHER HEALTH BENEFIT PLAN? ☐ YES ☐ NO *If yes*, complete items 9, 9a, and 9d.

READ BACK OF FORM BEFORE COMPLETING & SIGNING THIS FORM.

12. PATIENT'S OR AUTHORIZED PERSON'S SIGNATURE I authorize the release of any medical or other information necessary to process this claim. I also request payment of government benefits either to myself or to the party who accepts assignment below.

SIGNED *Adam L Rogers* DATE 9/10/XX

13. INSURED'S OR AUTHORIZED PERSON'S SIGNATURE I authorize payment of medical benefits to the undersigned physician or supplier for services described below.

SIGNED

PATIENT AND INSURED INFORMATION

14. DATE OF CURRENT ILLNESS, INJURY, or PREGNANCY(LMP) MM DD YY: 09 10 20XX QUAL.

15. OTHER DATE QUAL. MM DD YY

16. DATES PATIENT UNABLE TO WORK IN CURRENT OCCUPATION FROM MM DD YY TO MM DD YY

17. NAME OF REFERRING PROVIDER OR OTHER SOURCE: HORNER WILLIAMS MD

17a. G2 655432112

17b. NPI 231314800

18. HOSPITALIZATION DATES RELATED TO CURRENT SERVICES FROM MM DD YY TO MM DD YY

19. ADDITIONAL CLAIM INFORMATION (Designated by NUCC)

20. OUTSIDE LAB? ☐ YES ☐ NO — $ CHARGES

21. DIAGNOSIS OR NATURE OF ILLNESS OR INJURY Relate A-L to service line below (24E) ICD Ind.

A. S91.301A B. C. D.
E. F. G. H.
I. J. K. L.

22. RESUBMISSION CODE — ORIGINAL REF. NO.

23. PRIOR AUTHORIZATION NUMBER

24. A. DATE(S) OF SERVICE From MM DD YY	To MM DD YY	B. PLACE OF SERVICE	C. EMG	D. PROCEDURES, SERVICES, OR SUPPLIES (Explain Unusual Circumstances) CPT/HCPCS	MODIFIER	E. DIAGNOSIS POINTER	F. $ CHARGES	G. DAYS OR UNITS	H. EPSDT Family Plan	I. ID. QUAL.	J. RENDERING PROVIDER ID. #
1 09 10 XX	09 10 XX	11		99202	1	A	60 00	1		NPI	0020202 / 231314800
2 09 10 XX	09 10 XX	11		90703	1	A	20 00	1		NPI	0020202 / 231314800
3										NPI	
4										NPI	
5										NPI	
6										NPI	

PHYSICIAN OR SUPPLIER INFORMATION

25. FEDERAL TAX I.D. NUMBER: 421898989 — SSN ☐ EIN ☒

26. PATIENT'S ACCOUNT NO.

27. ACCEPT ASSIGNMENT? (For govt. claims, see back) ☒ YES ☐ NO

28. TOTAL CHARGE $ 80 00

29. AMOUNT PAID $

30. Rsvd for NUCC Use $

31. SIGNATURE OF PHYSICIAN OR SUPPLIER INCLUDING DEGREES OR CREDENTIALS (I certify that the statements on the reverse apply to this bill and are made a part thereof.)
HORNER WILLIAMS MD
Horner Williams MD 09/14/20XX
SIGNED DATE

32. SERVICE FACILITY LOCATION INFORMATION
BROADMOOR MEDICAL CLINIC
4353 PINE RIDGE DRIVE
MILTON XY 12345-0001
a. X100XX1000 b.

33. BILLING PROVIDER INFO & PH # ( )
BROADMOOR MEDICAL CLINIC
4353 PINE RIDGE DRIVE
MILTON XY 12345-0001
a. X100XX1000 b.

NUCC Instruction Manual available at: www.nucc.org — PLEASE PRINT OR TYPE — APPROVED OMB-0938-1197 FORM 1500 (02-12)

Fig. 5.1 CMS-1500 form for Adam Rogers.

Table 5.1 Table of Corrections

Block No.	C/I	Corrected Information
2		
3		
5		
10		
11d		
17		
17a		
24b		
24g		
25		
32b		
33		
33a		
33b*		

Block 33b is not to be reported.

C. Study the insurance ID card in Fig. 5.2. Answer these questions with regard to the information on the card.
   1. In whose name is this insurance policy written?
   2. What identification code should be entered in Block 1a of the CMS-1500 form?
   3. What is the name of the insured's primary care physician?
   4. When was this primary care physician assigned to the insured?
   5. Explain what the numbers mean in the last line of the card: **Copay $10 Office/$50 ER/$100 Hosp**

BlueCross BlueShield of Iowa   Preferred Blue

Mary K Smith
XQB 918 89 2910   Group #2014
Bill D Jones MD (PCP)
PCP Eff Date: 01/01/94
Copay $10 Office/$50 ER/$100 Hosp

BS Plan Code - 640   BC Plan Code - 140

Fig. 5.2 Insurance ID card for Mary K. Smith.

Your instructor will assign one or more of these topics:

A. Discuss the pros and cons of filing claims electronically.

B. Create a table comparing and contrasting direct claims filing versus using a claims clearinghouse. Include advantages and disadvantages of both methods.

C. Following is a list of tips for filing electronic claims successfully. Study this list and see if you can add additional items to it. (You may want to use the Internet for this exercise or interview a health insurance professional from a local office.) When you are finished, print and file the document in your Health Insurance Professional Notebook.
- Verify, file, and keep all transmission reports.
- Track clearinghouse claims to ensure successful transmission.
- Ensure that your computer software is consistent with the clean claims rules.
- Call your software vendor, if needed, to address the previous item.

In the event you are eventually employed in a medical office that still uses the CMS-1500 claim form, create an additional list of tips for filing paper claims using the "universal" paper form.

D. Fig. 5.3 illustrates the back of an insurance ID card. Discuss the function and importance of each line of information on this ID card.

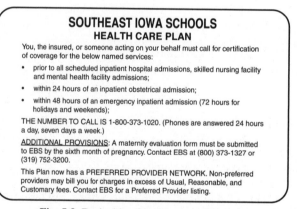

Fig. 5.3 Back side of an insurance ID card.

A. Using the information on Mary K. Smith's patient information form (Fig. 5.4) and her insurance ID card (see Fig. 5.2), complete Blocks 1 through 13 in the top half of the CMS-1500 claim form (Fig. 5.5). *Note: This patient has a group policy.*

PATIENT INFORMATION SHEET

Today's date: ___6/12/XX___

HEAD OF HOUSEHOLD

Head of household: __Mary K. Smith__

Social Security #: __918-89-2910__

Sex: __F__   Date of birth: __7/24/68__

Address: __409 Oak St.__

City, St: __Milton, XY__   Zip __12345__

Home phone #: __SSS-765-1234__

Occupation: __waitress__

Employer's name: __Grover's Pizza__

Employer's address: __1516 Main St.__

Employer's City, St: __Milton, XY__   Zip __12345__

Employer's phone #: __SSS-766-4321__

PATIENT INFORMATION

Patient's legal name: __Mary K. Smith__   Nickname: ___   Relationship to head of household: __same__

Date of birth ___   Age ___   Sex ___   Marital Status __S__

Employer name / Employer address: __SAME AS ABOVE__

Social Security / Employer phone #: __SAME AS ABOVE__

City, St: ___   Zip ___   Workers' Compensation Carrier (If applicable): __-N/A__

Referring Physician: __none__   Allergies: ___

EMERGENCY INFORMATION

Other contact not living with you: __Betty Keyes__   Home phone# ___   Work phone# ___

Address: __Rt 63 Box 112__   City __Milton__   St __XY__   Zip __12345__

Patient relationship to other contact: __daughter__   If patient is a child, parent name: __N/A__

INSURANCE INFORMATION

Primary insurance: __BlueCross/BlueShield__   Subscriber: __Mary K. Smith__

ID #: __XQB 918-89-2910/Group # 2014__   Relationship to subscriber: __self__

Secondary insurance: __none__   Subscriber: ___

ID #: ___   Relationship to subscriber: ___

OTHER FAMILY MEMBERS:

Name __Darrell P. Beckett__   Date of birth: __2/21/90__

Name __Cathy M. Beckett__   Date of birth: __4/6/95__

Name ___   Date of birth: ___

Name ___   Date of birth: ___

I understand that it is my responsibility that any incurred charges are paid.

To the extent necessary to determine liability for payment to obtain reimbursement, process claim forms, I authorize the release of any medical information necessary to process claims.

I hereby assign all medical and/or surgical benefits, to include major medical benefits to whichI am entitled, including Medicare, private insurance, and other health plans to Family Medicine of Mt. Pleasant, P.C.

This assignment will remain in effect until revoked by me in writing, a photocopy of this assignment is to be considered as valid as an original. I hereby authorize said assignee to release all information necessary to secure the payment.

Signed __Mary K. Smith__   Date __6/12/XX__

If patient is a minor, parent or guardian signature.

Fig. 5.4 Patient information sheet for Mary K. Smith.

HEALTH INSURANCE CLAIM FORM

APPROVED BY NATIONAL UNIFORM CLAIM COMMITTEE (NUCC) 02/12

| | PICA | | | | | | | | | PICA | |

1. MEDICARE ☐ (Medicare#) MEDICAID ☐ (Medicaid#) TRICARE ☐ (ID#DoD#) CHAMPVA ☐ (Member ID#) GROUP HEALTH PLAN ☐ (ID#) FECA BLK LUNG ☐ (ID#) OTHER ☐ (ID#)
1a. INSURED'S I.D. NUMBER (For Program in Item 1)

2. PATIENT'S NAME (Last Name, First Name, Middle Initial)

3. PATIENT'S BIRTH DATE MM DD YY SEX M ☐ F ☐

4. INSURED'S NAME (Last Name, First Name, Middle Initial)

5. PATIENT'S ADDRESS (No., Street)

6. PATIENT RELATIONSHIP TO INSURED Self ☐ Spouse ☐ Child ☐ Other ☐

7. INSURED'S ADDRESS (No., Street)

CITY STATE

8. RESERVED FOR NUCC USE

CITY STATE

ZIP CODE TELEPHONE (Include Area Code) ( )

ZIP CODE TELEPHONE (Include Area Code) ( )

9. OTHER INSURED'S NAME (Last Name, First Name, Middle Initial)

10. IS PATIENT'S CONDITION RELATED TO:

11. INSURED'S POLICY GROUP OR FECA NUMBER

a. OTHER INSURED'S POLICY OR GROUP NUMBER

a. EMPLOYMENT? (Current or Previous) YES ☐ NO ☐

a. INSURED'S DATE OF BIRTH MM DD YY SEX M ☐ F ☐

b. RESERVED FOR NUCC USE

b. AUTO ACCIDENT? YES ☐ NO ☐ PLACE (State)

b. OTHER CLAIM ID (Designated by NUCC)

c. RESERVED FOR NUCC USE

c. OTHER ACCIDENT? YES ☐ NO ☐

c. INSURANCE PLAN NAME OR PROGRAM NAME

d. INSURANCE PLAN NAME OR PROGRAM NAME

10d. CLAIM CODES (Designated by NUCC)

d. IS THERE ANOTHER HEALTH BENEFIT PLAN? YES ☐ NO ☐ If yes, complete items 9, 9a, and 9d.

READ BACK OF FORM BEFORE COMPLETING & SIGNING THIS FORM.
12. PATIENT'S OR AUTHORIZED PERSON'S SIGNATURE I authorize the release of any medical or other information necessary to process this claim. I also request payment of government benefits either to myself or to the party who accepts assignment below.

SIGNED _____ DATE _____

13. INSURED'S OR AUTHORIZED PERSON'S SIGNATURE I authorize payment of medical benefits to the undersigned physician or supplier for services described below.

SIGNED _____

CARRIER / PATIENT AND INSURED INFORMATION

Fig. 5.5 Top half of CMS-1500 form for Mary K. Smith.

B. Using the information in the encounter form (Mary K. Smith) shown in Fig. 5.6, complete the bottom half of the CMS-1500 claim form (Fig. 5.7). Use this information:

Provider Block	
Broadmoor Medical Clinic 4353 Pine Ridge Drive Milton, XY 12345-0001 Clinic NPI # X100XX1000 Telephone: 555-656-7890	Clinic EIN # 42 1898989 Dr. Robert L. Jones NPI 1234567890 Dr. Marilou Lucerno NPI 2907511822 Date claims 1 day after examination Referring provider = DN Ordering provider = DK Supervising provider = DQ

Note: For this exercise, use Qualifier 454 (initial treatment) between the vertical dotted lines in Block 14, qualifier DK (ordering provider) between the vertical dotted lines in Block 17, qualifier 0B between the vertical dotted lines in Block 17a, and the provider's NPI in Block 17b.

56

Chapter 5 **Claim Submission Methods**

Broadmoor Medical Clinic

Date of service: 6/12/XX	Waiver? ☐
Patient name: Mary K. Smith	Insurance: Blue Cross/Blue Shield
	Subscriber name: Mary K. Smith
Address: 409 Oak St., Milton, XY 12345	Group #: 2014 | Previous balance: 0
	Copay: | Today's charges: 185.00
Phone: 555-765-1234	Account #: XOB 918-89-2910 | Today's payment: 35.00
DOB: 7/24/68 Age: Sex: F	Physician name: R. L. Jones | Balance due: 150.00

RANK	Office visit	New	Est	RANK	Office procedures			RANK	Laboratory		
	Minimal		99211		Anoscopy		46600		Venipuncture		36415
	Problem focused	99201	99212		Audiometry		92551		Blood glucose, monitoring device		82962
	Expanded problem focused	99202	99213		Cerumen removal		69210		Blood glucose, visual dipstick		82948
	Detailed	99203	99214		Colposcopy		57452	✓	CBC, w/ auto differential	5.00	85025
	Comprehensive	99204	99215		Colposcopy w/biopsy		57455		CBC, w/o auto differential		85027
	Comprehensive (new patient)	99205			ECG, w/interpretation		93000		Cholesterol		82465
	Significant, separate service	-25	-25		ECG, rhythm strip		93040		Hemoccult, guaiac		82270
	Well visit	New	Est		Endometrial biopsy		58100		Hemoccult, immunoassay		82274
	< 1 y	99381	99391		Flexible sigmoidoscopy		45330		Hemoglobin A1C		85018
	1-4 y	99382	99392		Flexible sigmoidoscopy w/biopsy		45331		Lipid panel		80061
	5-11 y	99383	99393		Fracture care, cast/splint	29___			Liver panel		80076
	12-17 y	99384	99394		Site: ___				KOH prep (skin, hair, nails)		87220
	18-39 y	99385	99395		Nebulizer		94640		Metabolic panel, basic		80048
✓	40-64 y	130.00 99386	99396		Nebulizer demo		94664		Metabolic panel, comprehensive		80053
	65 y +	99387	99397		Spirometry		94010		Mononucleosis		86308
	Medicare preventive services				Spirometry, pre and post		94060		Pregnancy, blood		84703
✓	Pap	25.00	Q0091		Tympanometry		92567		Pregnancy, urine		81025
	Pelvic & breast		G0101		Vasectomy		55250		Renal panel		80069
	Prostate/PSA		G0103		Skin procedures		Units		Sedimentation rate		85651
	Tobacco counseling/3-10 min		99406		Burn care, initial	16000			Strep, rapid		86403
	Tobacco counseling/>10 min		99407		Foreign body, skin, simple	10120			Strep culture		87081
	Welcome to Medicare exam		G0344		Foreign body, skin, complex	10121			Strep A		87880
	ECG w/Welcome to Medicare exam		G0366		I&D, abscess	10060			TB		86580
	Flexible sigmoidoscopy		G0104		I&D, hematoma/seroma	10140			UA, complete, non-automated		81000
	Hemoccult, guaiac		G0107		Laceration repair, simple	120___			UA, w/o micro, non-automated		81002
	Flu shot		G0008		Site: ___ Size: ___			✓	UA, w/ micro, non-automated	5.00	81003
	Pneumonia shot		G0009		Laceration repair, layered	120___			Urine colony count		87086
	Consultation/preop clearance				Site: ___ Size: ___				Urine culture, presumptive		87088
	Expanded problem focused		99242		Lesion, biopsy, one	11100			Wet mount/KOH		87210
	Detailed		99243		Lesion, biopsy, each add'l	11101			Vaccines		
	Comprehensive/mod complexity		99244		Lesion,destruct.,benign,1-14	17110			DT, <7 y		90702
	Comprehensive/high complexity		99245		Lesion,destruct.,premal.,single	17000			DTP		90701
	Other services				Lesion,destruct,premal.,ea.add'l	17003			DtaP, <7 y		90700
	After posted hours		99050		Lesion, excision, benign	114___			Flu, 6-35 months		90657
	Evening/weekend appointment		99051		Site: ___ Size: ___				Flu, 3 y +		90658
	Home health certification		G0180		Lesion, excision, malignant	116___			Hep A, adult		90632
	Home health recertification		G0179		Site: ___ Size: ___				Hep A, ped/adol, 2 dose		90633
	Post-op follow-up		99024		Lesion, paring/cutting, one	11055			Hep B, adult		90746
	Prolonged/30-74 min		99354		Lesion, paring/cutting, 2-4	11056			Hep B, ped/adol 3 dose		90744
	Special reports/forms		99080		Lesion, shave	113___			Hep B-Hib		90748
	Disability/Workers comp		99455		Site: ___ Size: ___				Hib, 4 dose		90645
	Radiology				Nail removal, partial	11730			HPV		90649
					Nail removal, w/matrix	11750			IPV		90713
					Skin tag, 1-15	11200			MMR		90707
	Diagnoses				Medications		Units		Pneumonia, >2 y		90732
1	200.00				Ampicillin, up to 500mg	J0290			Pneumonia conjugate, <5 y		90669
2					B-12, up to 1,000 mcg	J3420			Td, >7 y		90718
3					Epinephrine, up to 1ml	J0170			Varicella		90716
4					Kenalog, 10mg	J3301			Immunizations & Injections		Units
Next office visit					Lidocaine, 10mg	J2001			Allergen, one	95115	
Recheck | Prev | PRN |___| D W M (Y)					Normal saline, 1000cc	J7030			Allergen, multiple	95117	
Instructions:					Phenergan, up to 50mg	J2550			Imm admin, one	90471	
					Progesterone, 150mg	J1055			Imm admin, each add'l	90472	
					Rocephin, 250mg	J0696			Imm admin, intranasal, one	90473	
					Testosterone, 200mg	J1080			Imm admin,intranasal,each add'l	90474	
					Tigan, up to 200 mg	J3250			Injection, joint, small	20600	
Referral					Toradol, 15mg	J1885			Injection, joint, intermediate	20605	
To:					Miscellaneous services				Injection, joint, major	20610	
Instructions:									Injection, ther/proph/diag	90772	
									Injection, trigger point	20552	
Physician signature									Supplies		
X R.L. Jones, MD											

Fig. 5.6 Encounter form for Mary K. Smith.

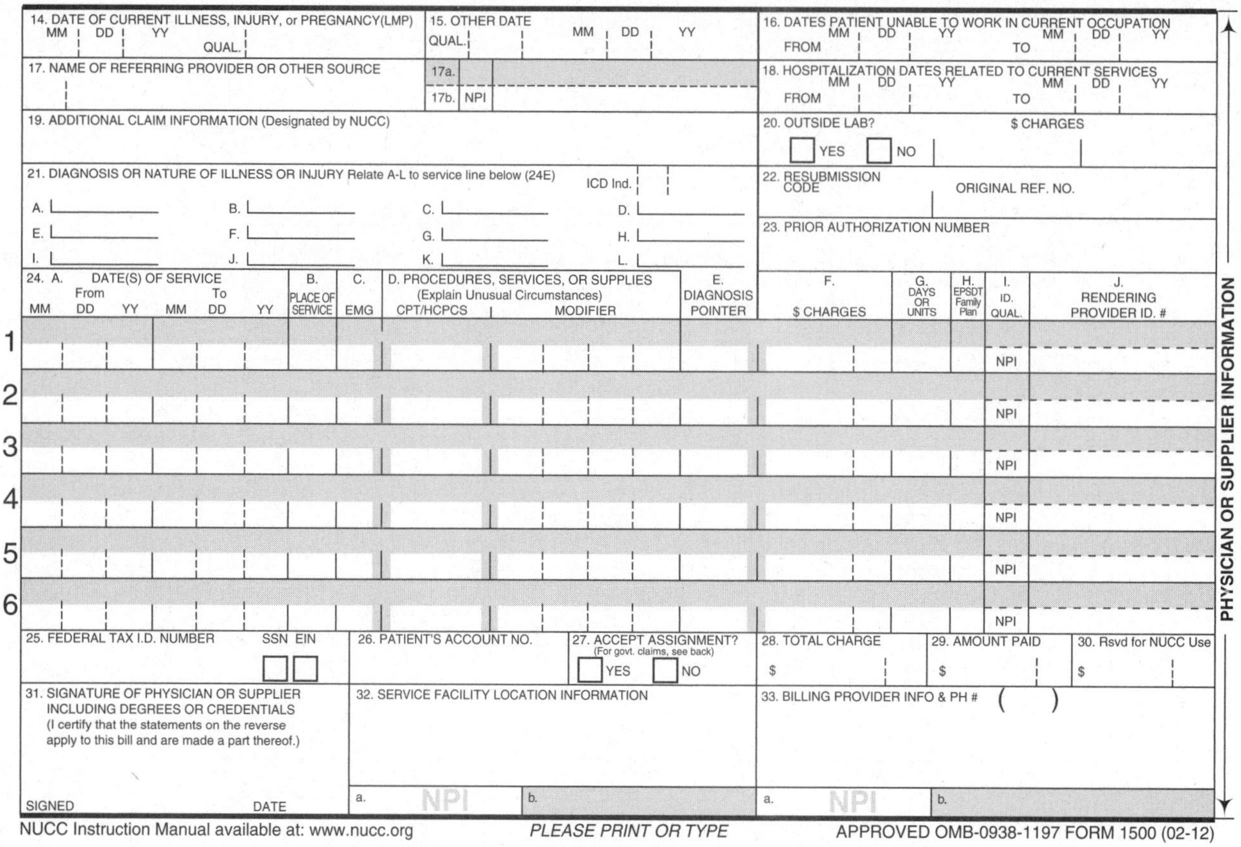
14. DATE OF CURRENT ILLNESS, INJURY, or PREGNANCY(LMP) MM DD YY QUAL.
15. OTHER DATE QUAL. MM DD YY
16. DATES PATIENT UNABLE TO WORK IN CURRENT OCCUPATION MM DD YY FROM TO
17. NAME OF REFERRING PROVIDER OR OTHER SOURCE
17a.
17b. NPI
18. HOSPITALIZATION DATES RELATED TO CURRENT SERVICES MM DD YY FROM TO
19. ADDITIONAL CLAIM INFORMATION (Designated by NUCC)
20. OUTSIDE LAB? YES NO $ CHARGES
21. DIAGNOSIS OR NATURE OF ILLNESS OR INJURY Relate A-L to service line below (24E) ICD Ind.
A. B. C. D.
E. F. G. H.
I. J. K. L.
22. RESUBMISSION CODE ORIGINAL REF. NO.
23. PRIOR AUTHORIZATION NUMBER
24. A. DATE(S) OF SERVICE From MM DD YY To MM DD YY
B. PLACE OF SERVICE
C. EMG
D. PROCEDURES, SERVICES, OR SUPPLIES (Explain Unusual Circumstances) CPT/HCPCS MODIFIER
E. DIAGNOSIS POINTER
F. $ CHARGES
G. DAYS OR UNITS
H. EPSDT Family Plan
I. ID. QUAL.
J. RENDERING PROVIDER ID. #
1 NPI
2 NPI
3 NPI
4 NPI
5 NPI
6 NPI
PHYSICIAN OR SUPPLIER INFORMATION
25. FEDERAL TAX I.D. NUMBER SSN EIN
26. PATIENT'S ACCOUNT NO.
27. ACCEPT ASSIGNMENT? (For govt. claims, see back) YES NO
28. TOTAL CHARGE $
29. AMOUNT PAID $
30. Rsvd for NUCC Use $
31. SIGNATURE OF PHYSICIAN OR SUPPLIER INCLUDING DEGREES OR CREDENTIALS (I certify that the statements on the reverse apply to this bill and are made a part thereof.)
SIGNED DATE
32. SERVICE FACILITY LOCATION INFORMATION
a. NPI b.
33. BILLING PROVIDER INFO & PH # ( )
a. NPI b.
NUCC Instruction Manual available at: www.nucc.org PLEASE PRINT OR TYPE APPROVED OMB-0938-1197 FORM 1500 (02-12)

Fig. 5.7 Bottom half of CMS-1500 form for Mary K. Smith.

INTERNET EXPLORATION

A. Research the Internet and locate a specific example of an HIPAA-compliant authorization form for use or disclosure of protected health information (PHI).

B. Your office manager has informed you that the practice is considering electronic claims submission. She has asked you to do some research to find the names of two or three clearinghouses and compare what they have to offer, specifically considering services offered, software and equipment needed, and corresponding costs. Research the Internet using "claims clearinghouse" as your search phrase and create a memo to your office manager providing him or her with at least two clearinghouse companies to show a comparison of services provided by the companies, their costs, and required equipment and software.

Performance Objective 5.1: Patient Ledger Card

Conditions: Student will create a ledger card for a new patient using the information abstracted from the patient information form and the insurance ID card for Adam Rogers.

Supplies/Equipment: Pen or computer, patient information form (Fig. 5.8), insurance ID card (Fig. 5.9), blank ledger card (Fig. 5.10)

Time Allowed: 20 minutes

Accuracy Needed to Pass: 90%

Procedural Steps	Points Earned	Comments
Evaluator: Note time began: _____		
1. Carefully read and study the applicable documents.		
2. Type the patient's correct name and address in the appropriate position. (10)		
3. Type the insurance information in the upper, left-hand corner of the ledger card (ensure none of the information falls within the address block). (20)		
4. Type the amount of coinsurance the patient must pay for each office visit in the upper right-hand corner. (5)		
5. Type the number to call for preadmission certification beneath the coinsurance amount. (5)		
Optional: May deduct points for taking more time than allowed.		

Total Points = 40

Student's Score: _____

Evaluator: _____

Comments: _____

_____

_____

_____

PATIENT INFORMATION SHEET

Today's date: 9/10/XX

HEAD OF HOUSEHOLD

Head of household: patient

Occupation: night watchman

Social Security #: 123-45-6789

Employer's name: Raritan Hydraulics

Sex: M Date of birth: 12/21/54

Employer's address: 1500 W. 60th St.

Address: 400 Maple Av

Employer's City, St: Milton, XY Zip: 12345

City, St: Milton, XY Zip: 12345

Employer's phone #: 555-800-3210

Home phone #: 555-800-2222

PATIENT INFORMATION

Patient's legal name: Adam L. Rogers

Nickname: _____

Relationship to head of household: self

Date of birth: 12/21/54 Age: _____ Sex: M Marital Status: S

Employer name: Raritan Hydraulics

Social Security #: 123-45-6789

Employer address: 1500 W. 60th St.

Employer phone #: 555-800-6611

City, St: Milton, XY Zip: 12345

Workers' Compensation Carrier (If applicable): NA

Referring Physician: _____

Allergies: NONE

EMERGENCY INFORMATION

Other contact not living with you: Phillip Rogers

Home phone#: SSS-800-2104 Work phone#: SSS-800-3210

Address: 2925 Sunnylawn City: Milton St: XY Zip: 12345

Patient relationship to other contact: son

If patient is a child, parent name: _____

INSURANCE INFORMATION

Primary insurance: BlueCross & BlueShield

Subscriber: Adam L. Rogers patient

ID #: XQS 123456789

Relationship to subscriber: self

Secondary insurance: _____

Subscriber: _____

ID #: _____

Relationship to subscriber: _____

OTHER FAMILY MEMBERS:

Name _____ Date of birth: _____

Name _____ Date of birth: _____

Name _____ Date of birth: _____

Name _____ Date of birth: _____

I understand that it is my responsibility that any incurred charges are paid.

To the extent necessary to determine liability for payment to obtain reimbursement, process claim forms, I authorize the release of any medical information necessary to process claims.

I hereby assign all medical and/or surgical benefits, to include major medical benefits to which I am entitled, including Medicare, private insurance, and other health plans to Family Medicine of Mt. Pleasant, P.C.

This assignment will remain in effect until revoked by me in writing, a photocopy of this assignment is to be considered as valid as an original. I hereby authorize said assignee to release all information necessary to secure the payment.

Signed: Adam L. Rogers Date: 9/10/XX

If patient is a minor, parent or guardian signature.

Fig. 5.8 Patient information sheet for Adam Rogers.

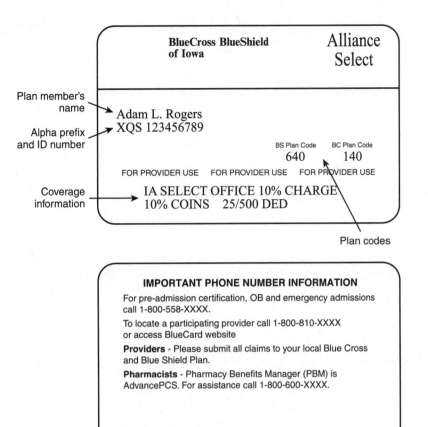

Plan member's name

Alpha prefix and ID number

Coverage information

Plan codes

BlueCross BlueShield of Iowa

Alliance Select

Adam L. Rogers
XQS 123456789

BS Plan Code   BC Plan Code
640   140

FOR PROVIDER USE   FOR PROVIDER USE   FOR PROVIDER USE

IA SELECT OFFICE 10% CHARGE
10% COINS   25/500 DED

IMPORTANT PHONE NUMBER INFORMATION

For pre-admission certification, OB and emergency admissions call 1-800-558-XXXX.

To locate a participating provider call 1-800-810-XXXX or access BlueCard website

Providers - Please submit all claims to your local Blue Cross and Blue Shield Plan.

Pharmacists - Pharmacy Benefits Manager (PBM) is AdvancePCS. For assistance call 1-800-600-XXXX.

Fig. 5.9 front and back of id card for adam rogers.

STATEMENT

BROADMOOR MEDICAL CLINIC
4353 Pine Ridge Drive
Milton, XY 12345-0001
Telephone: 555-656-7890

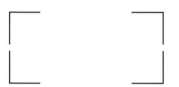

DATE	PROFESSIONAL SERVICE DESCRIPTION	CHARGE		CREDITS			CURRENT BALANCE	
				PAYMENTS	ADJUSTMENTS			

Due and payable within 10 days.   **Pay last amount in balance column** ⇧

Fig. 5.10 Blank ledger card.

Performance Objective 5.2: Patient Ledger Card

Conditions: Using the ledger card created in Performance Objective 5.1, student will enter the procedures and charges abstracted from the encounter form for Adam Rogers.

Supplies/Equipment: Pen, patient encounter form (Fig. 5.11)

Time Allowed: 20 minutes

Accuracy Needed to Pass: 100%

Procedural Steps	Points Earned	Comments
Evaluator: Note time began: _____		
1. Carefully read and study the applicable documents.		
2. Enter the correct date. (5)		
3. Enter the descriptions for the professional services rendered along with the applicable codes. (20)		
4. Post the corresponding charges for each service rendered. (10)		
5. Post the amount of coinsurance collected on this date from the patient. (5)		
6. Enter the current balance in the proper column. (10)		
Optional: May deduct points for taking more time than allowed.		

Total Points = 50

Student's Score: _____

Evaluator: _____

Comments: _____

_____

_____

_____

_____

Broadmoor Medical Clinic

Date of service: 9/10/20XX		Waiver? ☐		
Patient name: Adam L. Rogers		Insurance: Blue Cross/Blue Shield		
		Subscriber name: Adam L. Rogers		
Address: 400 Maple Avenue, Milton, XY 12345		Group #:		Previous balance: 0
		Copay:		Today's charges: 80.00
Phone: 555-800-2222		Account #: XQS 123456789		Today's payment: 6.00
DOB: 10/21/54 Age: Sex: M		Physician name: Horner Williams		Balance due: 74.00

RANK	Office visit	New	Est	RANK	Office procedures			RANK	Laboratory		
	Minimal		99211		Anoscopy		46600		Venipuncture		36415
	Problem focused	99201	99212		Audiometry		92551		Blood glucose, monitoring device		82962
✓	Expanded problem focused 60.00	99202	99213		Cerumen removal		69210		Blood glucose, visual dipstick		82948
	Detailed	99203	99214		Colposcopy		57452		CBC, w/ auto differential		85025
	Comprehensive	99204	99215		Colposcopy w/biopsy		57455		CBC, w/o auto differential		85027
	Comprehensive (new patient)	99205			ECG, w/interpretation		93000		Cholesterol		82465
	Significant, separate service	-25	-25		ECG, rhythm strip		93040		Hemoccult, guaiac		82270
	Well visit	New	Est		Endometrial biopsy		58100		Hemoccult, immunoassay		82274
	< 1 y	99381	99391		Flexible sigmoidoscopy		45330		Hemoglobin A1C		85018
	1-4 y	99382	99392		Flexible sigmoidoscopy w/biopsy		45331		Lipid panel		80061
	5-11 y	99383	99393		Fracture care, cast/splint	29___			Liver panel		80076
	12-17 y	99384	99394		Site: _____				KOH prep (skin, hair, nails)		87220
	18-39 y	99385	99395		Nebulizer		94640		Metabolic panel, basic		80048
	40-64 y	99386	99396		Nebulizer demo		94664		Metabolic panel, comprehensive		80053
	65 y +	99387	99397		Spirometry		94010		Mononucleosis		86308
	Medicare preventive services				Spirometry, pre and post		94060		Pregnancy, blood		84703
	Pap		Q0091		Tympanometry		92567		Pregnancy, urine		81025
	Pelvic & breast		G0101		Vasectomy		55250		Renal panel		80069
	Prostate/PSA		G0103		Skin procedures		Units		Sedimentation rate		85651
	Tobacco counseling/3-10 min		99406		Burn care, initial	16000			Strep, rapid		86403
	Tobacco counseling/>10 min		99407		Foreign body, skin, simple	10120			Strep culture		87081
	Welcome to Medicare exam		G0344		Foreign body, skin, complex	10121			Strep A		87880
	ECG w/Welcome to Medicare exam		G0366		I&D, abscess	10060			TB		86580
	Flexible sigmoidoscopy		G0104		I&D, hematoma/seroma	10140			UA, complete, non-automated		81000
	Hemoccult, guaiac		G0107		Laceration repair, simple	120___			UA, w/o micro, non-automated		81002
	Flu shot		G0008		Site: _____ Size: ___				UA, w/ micro, non-automated		81003
	Pneumonia shot		G0009		Laceration repair, layered	120___			Urine colony count		87086
	Consultation/preop clearance				Site: _____ Size: ___				Urine culture, presumptive		87088
	Expanded problem focused		99242		Lesion, biopsy, one	11100			Wet mount/KOH		87210
	Detailed		99243		Lesion, biopsy, each add'l	11101			Vaccines		
	Comprehensive/mod complexity		99244		Lesion,destruct.,benign,1-14	17110			DT, <7 y		90702
	Comprehensive/high complexity		99245		Lesion,destruct.,premal.,single	17000			DTP		90701
	Other services				Lesion,destruct.,premal.,ea.add'l	17003			DtaP, <7 y		90700
	After posted hours		99050		Lesion, excision, benign	114___			Flu, 6-35 months		90657
	Evening/weekend appointment		99051		Site: _____ Size: ___				Flu, 3 y +		90658
	Home health certification		G0180		Lesion, excision, malignant	116___			Hep A, adult		90632
	Home health recertification		G0179		Site: _____ Size: ___				Hep A, ped/adol, 2 dose		90633
	Post-op follow-up		99024		Lesion, paring/cutting, one	11055			Hep B, adult		90746
	Prolonged/30-74 min		99354		Lesion, paring/cutting, 2-4	11056			Hep B, ped/adol 3 dose		90744
	Special reports/forms		99080		Lesion, shave	113___			Hep B-Hib		90748
	Disability/Workers comp		99455		Site: _____ Size: ___				Hib, 4 dose		90645
	Radiology				Nail removal, partial	11730			HPV		90649
					Nail removal, w/matrix	11750			IPV		90713
					Skin tag, 1-15	11200			MMR		90707
	Diagnoses				Medications		Units		Pneumonia, >2 y		90732
1	S91.301A				Ampicillin, up to 500mg	J0290			Pneumonia conjugate, <5 y		90669
2					B-12, up to 1,000 mcg	J3420			Td, >7 y		90718
3					Epinephrine, up to 1ml	J0170			Varicella		90716
4					Kenalog, 10mg	J3301			Immunizations & Injections		Units
	Next office visit				Lidocaine, 10mg	J2001			Allergen, one	95115	
	Recheck Prev (PRN) _____ D W M Y				Normal saline, 1000cc	J7030			Allergen, multiple	95117	
	Instructions:				Phenergan, up to 50mg	J2550			Imm admin, one	90471	
					Progesterone, 150mg	J1055			Imm admin, each add'l	90472	
					Rocephin, 250mg	J0696			Imm admin, intranasal, one	90473	
					Testosterone, 200mg	J1080			Imm admin,intranasal,each add'l	90474	
	Referral				Tigan, up to 200 mg	J3250			Injection, joint, small	20600	
	To:				Toradol, 15mg	J1885			Injection, joint, intermediate	20605	
	Instructions:				Miscellaneous services				Injection, joint, major	20610	
				✓	Tetanus Toxoid 20.00	90703			Injection, ther/proph/diag	90772	
									Injection, trigger point	20552	
	Physician signature								Supplies		
	X Horner Williams, MD										

Fig. 5.11 Encounter form for Adam Rogers.

APPLICATION EXERCISES

Health Insurance Professional's Notebook

A. Collect at least one each of the following documents from a local medical office or clinic. Label the various parts as to what information the area typically contains.
- Patient information form
- Insurance ID card (front and back)
- Ledger card
- Encounter form
- CMS-1500 claim form

B. Create a section in your Health Insurance Professional's Notebook under the title "Sample Documents" and file the documents collected in "A" of this section. This notebook is for your own personal use after you become employed, so include as much information as needed on these documents so that they can be a valuable reference tool on the job.

Chapter Checklist

Student Name: _____

Chapter Completion Date: _____

Evaluate your classroom performance. Complete the self-evaluation, and submit it to your instructor. When your instructor returns this form to you, compare your self-evaluation with the evaluation completed by your instructor.

1.	Record	Your start time and date: _____
2.	Read	The assigned chapter in the textbook
3.	View	PowerPoint slides (if available)
4.	Complete	Exercises in workbook as assigned
5.	Compare	Your answers to the answers posted on the bulletin board, website, or handout
5.	Correct	Your answers
7.	Complete	All tests and required activities
8.	Read	Assigned readings (if any)
9.	Complete	Chapter performance objectives (competencies), if any
10.	Evaluate	Your personal performance and submit it to your instructor
11.	Record	Your ending time and date: _____
12.	Move on	Begin next chapter as assigned

PERFORMANCE EVALUATION

Student Name: _____

Chapter Completion Date: _____

Evaluate your classroom performance. Compare this evaluation with the one provided by your instructor.

Skill	Student Self-Evaluation			Instructor Evaluation		
	Good	Average	Poor	Good	Average	Poor
Attendance/punctuality						
Personal appearance						
Applies effort						
Is self-motivated						
Is courteous						
Has positive attitude						
Completes assignments in timely manner						
Works well with others						

Student's Initials: _____

Date: _____

Points Possible: _____

Points Awarded: _____

Chapter Grade: _____

Instructor's Initials: _____

Date: _____

6 New and Traditional Reimbursement Models

Chapter 6 takes an in-depth look at both the older, more traditional models of reimbursement as well as the newer ones with emphasis on how healthcare reform has influenced how Americans are acquiring coverage through these new models. Chapter 6 focuses on one of the best-known third-party payers in the United States: Blue Cross and Blue Shield. The author has elected to include Blue Cross and Blue Shield under the broad umbrella of commercial insurance because it no longer operates as a national entity but as separate regional organizations. In this workbook chapter, numerous opportunities are presented to explore the national Blue Cross and Blue Shield Association and the regional company that serves the area in which the student resides. Chapter 6 also discusses filing claims, the explanation of benefits document (EOB), electronic remittance advice (ERA), and other pertinent topics associated with reimbursement.

WORKBOOK CHAPTER OBJECTIVES

After completing the workbook activities for Chapter 6, the student should be able to:
1. Define the terms used in the chapter.
2. Answer the review questions according to the evaluation criteria set by the instructor.
3. Analyze, apply, and evaluate information given in "real-world" situations, applying logical concepts for rational decision-making to current health insurance issues.
4. Apply systematic processes that focus on analyzing situations (including decision-making steps) to arrive at reasonable solutions in problem-solving scenarios and case studies.
5. Conduct Internet research to become more knowledgeable about the best-known healthcare insurer in the United States—Blue Cross and Blue Shield.
6. Abstract applicable information from healthcare documents necessary for completion of various forms used in healthcare billing and the claims process.
7. Generate information and documents for inclusion in the student's personal Health Insurance Professional's Notebook.
8. Create appropriate correspondence to a patient explaining professional fees.
9. Perform self-evaluation on successful content mastery of Chapter 6.

DEFINING CHAPTER TERMS

Using the computer, students should write an accurate definition for each of the chapter terms listed. These definitions should be in the students' own words. When finished, students should compare their definitions with those listed in the glossary at the back of the textbook and correct any inaccuracies.

Accountable Care Organization (ACO)
administrative services organization (ASO)
BlueCard Program
BlueCard Worldwide
Blue Cross and Blue Shield Federal Employee Program (FEP)
carrier
carve-out
coinsurance
commercial health insurance
copayment
covered expenses
credible coverage
deductible
electronic remittance advice (ERA)

Employee Retirement Income Security Act (ERISA) of 1974
employer coverage mandate
episode of care/bundled payment
ERISA plans
explanation of benefits (EOB)
Federal Employees Health Benefits (FEHB) Program
fee-for-service (FFS), or indemnity, insurance
fee schedule
fiscal intermediary (FI)
grandfathered
group insurance
healthcare service plans
health insurance exchange
health savings account (HSA)

high-deductible health plan (HDHP)
high-risk pools
individual market
integrated delivery system (IDS)
Medicare administrative contractor (MAC)
Medicare supplement plan
minimum essential coverage
partial (blended) capitation
participating provider (PAR)
patient-centered medical home (PCMH)
pay for performance policyholder

preexisting conditions
preferred provider organization (PPO)
premium
reasonable and customary fee
resource-based relative value system (RBRVS)
self-insured
single or specialty service plans
supplemental coverage
third-party administrator (TPA)
third-party payer
usual customary and reasonable (UCR)

ASSESSMENT

Multiple Choice

Directions: In the questions and statements presented, choose the response that **best** answers or completes the stem and circle the letter that precedes it.

1. The type of health insurance that offers the most choices of physicians and hospitals, in which patients can choose any provider they want and can change providers at any time, is a(n):
   a. Managed care plan
   b. Indemnity plan
   c. FFS plan
   d. Both b or c

2. An example of a third-party payer is:
   a. A commercial insurance company
   b. Blue Cross and Blue Shield
   c. Medicare/Medicaid
   d. All of the above

3. Group insurance is typically:
   a. The most expensive kind
   b. Paid entirely by the employer
   c. A contract between an insurance company and an employer
   d. Mandated by the federal government

4. People who were covered under an employer-sponsored group plan before the enforcement of the Affordable Care Act can usually keep their group coverage as long as the plan meets the:
   a. Minimum essential coverage (MEC) rule
   b. Third-party payer rule
   c. Managed care rule
   d. Both b or c

5. The best type of healthcare plan is a(n):
   a. HMO
   b. Indemnity plan
   c. PPO
   d. No one type is universally best

6. Standard costs associated with healthcare plans include the patient paying:
   a. A periodic payment (premium)
   b. A yearly deductible
   c. Per-visit coinsurance
   d. All of the above

7. Identify which of these is **not true** under the Patient Protection and Affordable Care Act of 2009 (PPACA):
   a. Everyone who enrolls in a plan under PPACA pays the same premium.
   b. Limits have been placed on the maximum out-of-pocket costs.
   c. The PPACA has set minimum essential coverage for certain plan types.
   d. No plan can apply a deductible or charge for specified preventive health services.

8. A comprehensive listing of medical charges is commonly referred to as a:
   a. Government payer schedule
   b. Fee schedule
   c. Commercial payer schedule
   d. Reimbursement schedule

9. For Americans today, accessibility to healthcare is viewed as a:
   a. Right
   b. Privilege
   c. Benefit
   d. Concession

10. When the fee charged by a provider falls within the parameters of the fee commonly charged for that particular service within a specific geographical area, it is said to be:
    a. Medically necessary
    b. A participating fee
    c. Reasonable and customary
    d. Medicare approved

11. A provider who signs a contractual arrangement with a third-party insurance contractor and agrees to accept the amount paid by the carrier as payment in full is referred to as a:
    a. Participating provider (PAR)
    b. Nonparticipating provider (nonPAR)
    c. Primary care provider (PCP)
    d. Principal attending physician (PAP)

12. The government health insurance program that provides coverage for its own civilian employees is called:
    a. Medicare
    b. Medicaid
    c. Federal Employees Health Benefits (FEHB) Program
    d. Blue Cross and Blue Shield

13. When the employer—not an insurance company—is responsible for the cost of its employees' medical services, the employer has a:
    a. Workers' compensation program
    b. Third-party group plan
    c. Self-insured program
    d. Disability benefits plan

14. The federal law designed to protect the rights of beneficiaries of employee benefit plans offered by employers and that sets minimum standards for pension plans in private industry is called:
    a. Social Security
    b. Workers' compensation
    c. Employee Retirement Income Security Act (ERISA)
    d. Consolidated Omnibus Budget Reconciliation Act (COBRA)

15. A person or organization that processes claims and performs other contractual administrative services is commonly referred to as a:
    a. Third-party administrator (TPA)
    b. Management commissioner (MC)
    c. Fiscal intermediary
    d. Third-party payer

16. The legislation that includes a mandate that insurance companies must cover certain preventive services for those who purchased or joined a new plan on or after September 23, 2010, without charging out-of-pocket costs is:
    a. ERISA
    b. COBRA
    c. Health Insurance Privacy and Portability Act
    d. Patient Protection and Affordable Care Act

17. Before the Affordable Care Act, a person's health insurance coverage that has been in effect for a specific number of days before enrolling in a new health plan is called:
    a. Credible coverage
    b. Group coverage
    c. Lifetime coverage
    d. Major medical coverage

18. Before the Affordable Care Act was signed into law, individuals who had been denied coverage because of a pre-existing condition and had been without coverage for at least 6 months could acquire healthcare insurance through a(n):
    a. Actuarial value pool
    b. Self-sponsored pool
    c. Indemnity pool
    d. High-risk pool

19. The Affordable Care Act states that by 2014, everyone in the United States should have access to a comprehensive set of healthcare benefits, which is referred to as:
    a. Minimum essential coverage
    b. Major medical coverage
    c. Essential benefits package
    d. Both a or c

20. A set of state-regulated and standardized healthcare plans from which individuals may purchase coverage that is eligible for federal subsidies are called:
    a. High-risk pools
    b. Health insurance exchanges
    c. Health savings accounts (HSAs)
    d. Self-insured accounts

True/False

Directions: Place a "T" in the blank preceding the statement if it is true; place an "F" if it is false.

_____ 1. With fee-for-service plans, patients can choose any physician they want and change physicians at any time.

_____ 2. A third-party payer is any organization that provides payment for specified coverage provided under a health plan.

_____ 3. Group insurance is generally more expensive because it covers more individuals.

_____ 4. BCBS offers only fee-for-service plans.

_____ 5. With FFS insurance, the policyholder controls the choice of physician and facility.

_____ 6. FFS plans all have the same deductible amount.

_____ 7. "Reasonable and customary" is a term used to refer to the commonly charged or prevailing fees for health services within a geographical area.

_____ 8. Commercial health insurance is standard in price and the kinds of benefits that the policy covers.

_____ 9. Most organizations that are self-insured are large entities, which can draw from hundreds or thousands of enrollees.

_____ 10. A health savings account (HSA) is a tax-advantaged account in which money can be set aside to pay for future medical expenses.

_____ 11. Blue Cross policies cover inpatient hospital care; Blue Shield covers physicians' services.

_____ 12. A high-deductible health plan (HDHP) is a health insurance plan with lower premiums and higher deductibles than a traditional health plan.

_____ 13. If an individual belongs to a BlueCard PPO, the initials PPO appear inside a blue globe.

_____ 14. Blue Cross and Blue Shield organizations are no longer governed at a national level, and each has its own specific guidelines for completing the CMS-1500 claim form.

_____ 15. It is important to consult all types of insurance plans for their specific guidelines to avoid claim delays and rejections.

_____ 16. Normally, when husband and wife are covered under separate policies, primary coverage follows the patient.

_____ 17. An explanation of benefits (EOB) is a document prepared by the carrier that gives details of how the claim was adjudicated.

_____ 18. The time limit for filing claims is the same for all third-party payers—1 year.

_____ 19. Filing CMS-1500 paper claims for commercial carriers is much the same as with all other carriers.

_____ 20. HIPAA mandates that all commercial claims be submitted electronically.

_____ 21. Today, insurers are encouraged to structure their reimbursement models based on the quality and utility of care provided rather than the sheer volume of services.

_____ 22. One objective of an Integrated Delivery System is (IDS) improving quality of care while lowering patient cost.

_____ 23. A model of care in which a primary provider manages and coordinates the care of all elements of a patient's health with a team of healthcare providers is called patient-centered facility care.

_____ 24. Medicare fiscal intermediaries (FIs) and carriers are now more commonly referred to as Medicare administrative contractors (MACs).

_____ 25. A consumer-directed health plan (CDHP) often involves pairing a high-deductible PPO plan with a tax-advantaged account, such as a health savings account (HSA).

Short Answer/Fill-in-the-Blank

Note: If space provided is not adequate, use a separate piece of blank paper.

1. Name four new models of healthcare delivery.

_____

_____

_____

_____

2. List three out-of-pocket costs that are standard for patients to pay with FFS plans.

_____

_____

_____

3. List four functions commonly performed by TPAs and administrative services organizations.

_____

_____

_____

_____

4. Explain what a "carve out" is and give an example.

_____

5. Explain (in your own words) the difference between a PAR and a nonPAR provider.

_____

6. What is a fiscal intermediary, and what functions does it perform?

_____

7. Explain what is meant by "timely filing" as it relates to claims.

_____

8. Timely filing for Blue Cross and Blue Shield claims is normally _____ days.

9. Provide a brief explanation of the process for submitting claims when a person is covered under two commercial policies or secondary coverage.

_____

_____

_____

_____

10. A report that carriers normally send to providers after each electronic claims transmission is called a(n):

_____

CRITICAL THINKING ACTIVITIES

A. You are working as a health insurance professional at Silverstone Mental Health Clinic. Patient Philippe Sanchez comes in for an appointment with Dr. Gerald T. Field, a psychiatrist. This is Mr. Sanchez's first visit to the clinic. Fig. 6.1 shows Mr. Sanchez's completed patient information form. Two insurance companies are listed, with Sunset Assurance, a family policy in his wife's name, listed first. The second one is a single policy in the patient's name. Mr. Sanchez explains that the family policy is in Maria's name through her employer, but it does not cover treatment for mental health. "Send my bill to the packing plant," he states. "They will take care of it." Further questions only confuse Mr. Sanchez, and it is apparent that he knows little about the two policies. How can you, the health insurance professional, determine:
- Which carrier is actually primary?
- Do both policies cover mental health treatment?
- Should you send a claim to both third-party payers?
- Where would you find out more information about the coverage of the American Indemnity policy and the Sunset Assurance policy?

Registration Data

1. Your Name ___Sanchez Philippe M___ Sex ☒ Male ☐ Female   Date of Birth ___06/16/1969___
   (Last)   (First)   (Middle)

2. Social Security #: ___111-22-3333___   Marital Status: S Ⓜ D Se W

3. Address: ___811 46th St.___
   (Street)
   ___Milton___   ___XY___   ___12345___
   (City)   (State)   (Zip)

4. ___SSS-621-8765___
   (Phone)

5. Employer: ___Southwest Packers Inc___   Occupation: ___Inspector___
   Employer Address: ___Hwy 409 West, Milton___   ___SSS-621-5432___
   (Work Phone)
   Spouse: ___Maria___   Employer: ___Milton Comm. Schools___ Occupation: ___Teacher Aide___
   Employer Address: ___1667 Parkway, Milton___   ___SSS-621-8864___
   (Work Phone)

6.

Other Household Members	Date of Birth	Relationship
Emilio	05/03/1995	Son
Rita	01/24/1998	daughter
	/ /	
	/ /	
	/ /	

7. Medical Insurance Information

	Ins. Company Name	Policy No.	Policy Holder	Sgl.	Fmly.	Primary	Sec.
(1)	Sunset Assurance	001-445678	Maria	☐	☒	☐	☐
(2)	American Indemnity	046911FML	Philippe	☒	☐	☐	☐
( )				☐	☐	☐	☐

(Type of Coverage)

Note: Both insurance policies are group policies.

8. Person to Contact in an Emergency ___Maria___ Relationship to you ___wife___
   Their Work Phone ___SSS-621-8864___ Their Home Phone ___SSS-621-8765___   DOB 03/18/1972

9. Party with primary responsibility for payment: ☒ Self ☐ Other
   Name _____   Relationship to you _____
   Address _____   Home Phone _____

For Office Use Only

Date Completed _____   Account No. _____   Patient No. _____

Household Status   ☐ Head of Household

☐ Spouse   ☐ Child   ☐ Other: _____

Head of Household Name _____

Fig. 6.1 Registration data sheet for Philippe Sanchez.

B. Eloise Stout comes to the orthopedic clinic where you work for treatment of a Colles fracture. She informs you that she lives out of state and is here on vacation visiting her daughter. Fig. 6.2 shows a facsimile of her insurance ID card. From the information on the ID card, answer these questions:
- What Blue Cross and Blue Shield plan does the patient have?
- What does the alpha prefix signify?
- If a "suitcase logo" appeared in the upper right-hand corner of this card (as it normally does with this specific program), what would it indicate?
- Will the patient be able to receive the same benefits as she would at home?
- What form will you use to submit the claim?
- Where will you send the completed claim?

```
┌──────────────────────────────────────────────────┐
│                                                    │
│        BlueCross BlueShield                        │
│           of Iowa          Preferred Blue          │
│                                                    │
│                                                    │
│   Eloise Stout                                     │
│   XQB 918 89 2910                                  │
│   Sarah Smith                                      │
│   PCP Eff Date: 01/01/99                           │
│   Copay $10 Office/$50 ER/$100 Hosp                │
│                                                    │
│                                                    │
│                                            PPO     │
│    BS Plan Code - 640     BC Plan Code - 140       │
└──────────────────────────────────────────────────┘
```

Fig. 6.2 Sample of a Blue Cross and Blue Shield ID card.

Note: You may have to go to a website for some answers. Use "Blue Card Program" as search words.
Note: Blue Cross and Blue Shield's address is 2604 West 32nd, Des Moines, IA 52230.

C. Many health insurance professional students have difficulty understanding the differences between Blue Cross and Blue Shield's Federal Employee Program (FEP) and the Federal Employees Health Benefits (FEHB) Program. Write a critical thinking paragraph briefly explaining each program and highlight the differences.

D. Two patient scenarios follow. Using the criteria given, calculate the total amount each patient will have to pay out of pocket, including the coinsurance and deductible. Assume in both cases that Blue Cross and Blue Shield's usual, customary, and reasonable fee for this procedure is $4250, and none of the yearly deductible has been met.

Patient 1

Steven Barnes	Provider is PAR
Cholecystectomy	Charge: $5000
Deductible: $500	Coinsurance 80/20
Total patient responsibility	

Patient 2

Sylvia Manley	Provider is nonPAR
Hysterectomy	Charge: $5000
Deductible: $250	Coinsurance 90/10
Total patient responsibility	

Illustrate on the portions of the following ledger cards how these charges and payments should be posted. The amount in the current balance column should reflect the total out-of-pocket amount the patient owes.

Note: When posting services and payments, make sure you include the date the insurance claim was submitted (1 day after service) and the date the claim was paid (3/13/20XX).

Patient 1 (Steven Barnes)

Date of Service	Procedure/Service	Amount Charged	Amount Paid	Adjustments	Current Balance
02/13/20XX	Cholecystectomy	5000.00			5000.00
03/13/20XX	Cholecystectomy	5000.00	4500.00	4.00	4496.00

Patient No. 2 (Sylvia Manley)

Date of Service	Procedure/Service	Amount Charged	Amount Paid	Adjustments	Current Balance
02/13/20XX	Hysterectomy	5000.00			5000.00
03/13/20XX	Hysterectomy	5000.00	4750.00	9.00	4741.00

PROJECTS/DISCUSSION TOPICS

A. Research and prepare for an in-class discussion on the process involved in a commercial insurer (e.g., Blue Cross) becoming a fiscal intermediary.

B. Research the Blue Cross and Blue Shield carrier in your state or region. Prepare a presentation or create a bulletin board display depicting the various plans, options, and programs your local Blue Cross and Blue Shield organization offers health insurance consumers in your community. (**Hint:** Go to http://www.bcbs.com and enter your zip code.)

C. Several topics are listed under "National Programs" on the Blue Cross and Blue Shield Association home page. Choose one of these topics, read the entire item, and write a critical thinking paragraph focusing on the main points of the article.

CASE STUDIES

Note: *In these case studies, unless your instructor tells you differently, assume that these are the patients' initial visits, so use qualifier 454 in Block 14 if an entry in this block is required by the carrier. In Block 17, use qualifier DK (ordering provider); Block 17a can be left blank.*

A. Review the Patient Information Form for Philippe Sanchez (see Fig. 6.1). Assume you have contacted American Indemnity and learned that they are primary and will accept claims submitted on the universal form (CMS-1500). Complete the top portion of the claim form (Fig. 6.3) or use the electronic file on the Evolve website, using the information from his registration data. (American Indemnity's address is 2345 West Palm Avenue, Petaluma, CA, 99001.) (Patient has an up-to-date release of information and assignment of benefits on file.)

HEALTH INSURANCE CLAIM FORM

APPROVED BY NATIONAL UNIFORM CLAIM COMMITTEE (NUCC) 02/12

CARRIER

| PICA | | PICA |

1. MEDICARE (Medicare#) MEDICAID (Medicaid#) TRICARE (ID#DoD#) CHAMPVA (Member ID#) GROUP HEALTH PLAN (ID#) FECA BLK LUNG (ID#) OTHER ☑ (ID#)

1a. INSURED'S I.D. NUMBER (For Program in Item 1)

2. PATIENT'S NAME (Last Name, First Name, Middle Initial)
Sanchez, Philippe

3. PATIENT'S BIRTH DATE MM DD YY   SEX M ☑ F

4. INSURED'S NAME (Last Name, First Name, Middle Initial)
Sanchez, Philippe

5. PATIENT'S ADDRESS (No., Street)
2346 West Palm Ave.

6. PATIENT RELATIONSHIP TO INSURED
Self ☑ Spouse Child Other

7. INSURED'S ADDRESS (No., Street)
2346 West Palm Ave.

CITY *Petaluma* STATE *CA*

8. RESERVED FOR NUCC USE

CITY *Petaluma* STATE *CA*

ZIP CODE *99001* TELEPHONE (Include Area Code) ( )

ZIP CODE *99001* TELEPHONE (Include Area Code) ( )

9. OTHER INSURED'S NAME (Last Name, First Name, Middle Initial)

10. IS PATIENT'S CONDITION RELATED TO:

11. INSURED'S POLICY GROUP OR FECA NUMBER
American Indemnity

a. OTHER INSURED'S POLICY OR GROUP NUMBER

a. EMPLOYMENT? (Current or Previous) YES ☑ NO

a. INSURED'S DATE OF BIRTH MM DD YY   SEX M F

b. RESERVED FOR NUCC USE

b. AUTO ACCIDENT? YES ☑ NO PLACE (State)

b. OTHER CLAIM ID (Designated by NUCC)

c. RESERVED FOR NUCC USE

c. OTHER ACCIDENT? YES ☑ NO

c. INSURANCE PLAN NAME OR PROGRAM NAME
American Indemnity

d. INSURANCE PLAN NAME OR PROGRAM NAME

10d. CLAIM CODES (Designated by NUCC)

d. IS THERE ANOTHER HEALTH BENEFIT PLAN? YES ☑ NO **If yes**, complete items 9, 9a, and 9d.

READ BACK OF FORM BEFORE COMPLETING & SIGNING THIS FORM.

12. PATIENT'S OR AUTHORIZED PERSON'S SIGNATURE I authorize the release of any medical or other information necessary to process this claim. I also request payment of government benefits either to myself or to the party who accepts assignment below.

SIGNED _____ DATE _____

13. INSURED'S OR AUTHORIZED PERSON'S SIGNATURE I authorize payment of medical benefits to the undersigned physician or supplier for services described below.

SIGNED _____

PATIENT AND INSURED INFORMATION

Fig. 6.3 Top half of CMS-1500 form for Philippe Sanchez.

B. The encounter form in Fig. 6.4 documents procedures, services, and a diagnosis for Susan Martin, a 9-year-old girl. Fig. 6.5 shows her completed patient information sheet. Using these two documents, complete these tasks:
1. Complete the patient ledger card in Fig. 6.6 or the electronic file on the Evolve website for this patient.
2. Using the information on the encounter form (see Fig. 6.4) and the completed ledger card (see Fig. 6.6), complete the bottom half (provider/supplier section) of the claim form in Fig. 6.7 or use the electronic file on the Evolve website.

Broadmoor Medical Clinic

Date of service: 12/04/20XX	Waiver? ☐
Patient name: Susan A. Martin	Insurance: BCBS
	Subscriber name: Anna Costello
Address: 603 Maplelawn, Milton, XY 12345	Group #: ... Previous balance: 0
	Copay: ... Today's charges: 80.00
Phone: 555-621-1111	Account #: X4Z 911999000 ... Today's payment: check# 10.00 (cash)
DOB: 6/1/19XX Age: 9 Sex: F	Physician name: Dr. Marilou Lucero ... Balance due: 70.00

RANK	Office visit		New	Est	RANK	Office procedures			RANK	Laboratory	
	Minimal			99211		Anoscopy		46600		Venipuncture	36415
✓	Problem focused	80.00	99201	99212		Audiometry		92551		Blood glucose, monitoring device	82962
	Expanded problem focused		99202	99213		Cerumen removal		69210		Blood glucose, visual dipstick	82948
	Detailed		99203	99214		Colposcopy		57452		CBC, w/ auto differential	85025
	Comprehensive		99204	99215		Colposcopy w/biopsy		57455		CBC, w/o auto differential	85027
	Comprehensive (new patient)		99205			ECG, w/interpretation		93000		Cholesterol	82465
	Significant, separate service		-25	-25		ECG, rhythm strip		93040		Hemoccult, guaiac	82270
	Well visit		New	Est		Endometrial biopsy		58100		Hemoccult, immunoassay	82274
	< 1 y		99381	99391		Flexible sigmoidoscopy		45330		Hemoglobin A1C	85018
	1-4 y		99382	99392		Flexible sigmoidoscopy w/biopsy		45331		Lipid panel	80061
	5-11 y		99383	99393		Fracture care, cast/splint		29___		Liver panel	80076
	12-17 y		99384	99394		Site: ___				KOH prep (skin, hair, nails)	87220
	18-39 y		99385	99395		Nebulizer		94640		Metabolic panel, basic	80048
	40-64 y		99386	99396		Nebulizer demo		94664		Metabolic panel, comprehensive	80053
	65 y +		99387	99397		Spirometry		94010		Mononucleosis	86308
	Medicare preventive services					Spirometry, pre and post		94060		Pregnancy, blood	84703
	Pap			Q0091		Tympanometry		92567		Pregnancy, urine	81025
	Pelvic & breast			G0101		Vasectomy		55250		Renal panel	80069
	Prostate/PSA			G0103		Skin procedures		Units		Sedimentation rate	85651
	Tobacco counseling/3-10 min			99406		Burn care, initial	16000			Strep, rapid	86403
	Tobacco counseling/>10 min			99407		Foreign body, skin, simple	10120			Strep culture	87081
	Welcome to Medicare exam			G0344		Foreign body, skin, complex	10121			Strep A	87880
	ECG w/Welcome to Medicare exam			G0366		I&D, abscess	10060			TB	86580
	Flexible sigmoidoscopy			G0104		I&D, hematoma/seroma	10140			UA, complete, non-automated	81000
	Hemoccult, guaiac			G0107		Laceration repair, simple	120___			UA, w/o micro, non-automated	81002
	Flu shot			G0008		Site: ___ Size: ___				UA, w/ micro, non-automated	81003
	Pneumonia shot			G0009		Laceration repair, layered	120___			Urine colony count	87086
	Consultation/preop clearance					Site: ___ Size: ___				Urine culture, presumptive	87088
	Expanded problem focused			99242		Lesion, biopsy, one	11100			Wet mount/KOH	87210
	Detailed			99243		Lesion, biopsy, each add'l	11101			Vaccines	
	Comprehensive/mod complexity			99244		Lesion,destruct.,benign,1-14	17110			DT, <7 y	90702
	Comprehensive/high complexity			99245		Lesion,destruct.,premal.,single	17000			DTP	90701
	Other services					Lesion,destruct.,premal.,ea.add'l	17003			DtaP, <7 y	90700
	After posted hours			99050		Lesion, excision, benign	114___			Flu, 6-35 months	90657
	Evening/weekend appointment			99051		Site: ___ Size: ___				Flu, 3 y +	90658
	Home health certification			G0180		Lesion, excision, malignant	116___			Hep A, adult	90632
	Home health recertification			G0179		Site: ___ Size: ___				Hep A, ped/adol, 2 dose	90633
	Post-op follow-up			99024		Lesion, paring/cutting, one	11055			Hep B, adult	90746
	Prolonged/30-74 min			99354		Lesion, paring/cutting, 2-4	11056			Hep B, ped/adol 3 dose	90744
	Special reports/forms			99080		Lesion, shave	113___			Hep B-Hib	90748
	Disability/Workers comp			99455		Site: ___ Size: ___				Hib, 4 dose	90645
	Radiology					Nail removal, partial	11730			HPV	90649
						Nail removal, w/matrix	11750			IPV	90713
						Skin tag, 1-15	11200			MMR	90707
	Diagnoses					Medications		Units		Pneumonia, >2 y	90732
1	R11.2/R50.9					Ampicillin, up to 500mg	J0290			Pneumonia conjugate, <5 y	90669
2						B-12, up to 1,000 mcg	J3420			Td, >7 y	90718
3						Epinephrine, up to 1ml	J0170			Varicella	90716
4						Kenalog, 10mg	J3301			Immunizations & Injections	Units
	Next office visit					Lidocaine, 10mg	J2001			Allergen, one	95115
	Recheck Prev (PRN) ___ D W M Y					Normal saline, 1000cc	J7030			Allergen, multiple	95117
	Instructions:					Phenergan, up to 50mg	J2550			Imm admin, one	90471
	Fluids and rest					Progesterone, 150mg	J1055			Imm admin, each add'l	90472
	OTC acetaminophen for fever					Rocephin, 250mg	J0696			Imm admin, intranasal, one	90473
	No Rx at this time					Testosterone, 200mg	J1080			Imm admin,intranasal,each add'l	90474
	Referral					Tigan, up to 200 mg	J3250			Injection, joint, small	20600
	To:					Toradol, 15mg	J1885			Injection, joint, intermediate	20605
						Miscellaneous services				Injection, joint, major	20610
	Instructions:									Injection, ther/proph/diag	90772
										Injection, trigger point	20552
	Physician signature									Supplies	
	x Dr. Marilou Lucero, MD										

Fig. 6.4 Encounter form for Susan Martin.

Chapter **6** **New and Traditional Reimbursement Models**

PATIENT INFORMATION SHEET

Today's date: 12/04/20XX

HEAD OF HOUSEHOLD

Head of household: Anna P. Costello

Social Security # 333-00-1111

Sex: F   Date of birth 4/2/76

Address: 603 Maplelawn

City, St: Milton, XY   Zip 12345

Home phone # SSS-621-1111

Occupation: seamstress

Employer's name: Apex Mattress Factory

Employer's address: North Ft. Gaslight Rd.

Employer's City, St: Milton, XY   Zip 12345

Employer's phone # SSS-621-2330

PATIENT INFORMATION

Patient's legal name: Susan Ann Martin

Nickname _____   Relationship to head of household: daughter

Date of birth 6/1/19XX   Age 9   Sex F   Marital Status _____

Employer name: student

Social Security # 911-999-0000

Employer address: _____

Employer phone # _____

City, St: _____   Zip _____

Workers' Compensation Carrier (If applicable) _____

Referring Physician _____

Allergies: penicillin

EMERGENCY INFORMATION

Other contact not living with you: Patsy Evans

Home phone# SSS-654-3210   Work phone# _____

Address 26 Fox Ct, #152   City Milton   St XY   Zip 12345

Patient relationship to other contact: grandmother

If patient is a child, parent name: Anna Costello

INSURANCE INFORMATION

Primary insurance BCBS   Subscriber Anna Costello

ID # XYZ911999000   Relationship to subscriber daughter

Secondary insurance: _____   Subscriber _____

ID # _____   Relationship to subscriber _____

OTHER FAMILY MEMBERS:

Name _____   Date of birth: _____

Name _____   Date of birth: _____

Name _____   Date of birth: _____

Name _____   Date of birth: _____

I understand that it is my responsibility that any incurred charges are paid.

To the extent necessary to determine liability for payment to obtain reimbursement, process claim forms, I authorize the release of any medical information necessary to process claims.

I here by assign all medical and/or surgical benefits, to include major medical benefits to which I am entitled, including Medicare, private insurance, and other health plans to Family Medicine of Mt. Pleasant, P.C.

This assignment will remain in effect until revoked by me in writing, a photocopy of this assignment is to be considered as valid as an original. I hereby authorize said assignee to release all information necessary to secure the payment.

Signed Anna P. Costello   Date 12/04/20XX

If patient is a minor, parent or guardian signature.

Fig. 6.5 Patient information sheet for Susan Martin.

STATEMENT

BROADMOOR MEDICAL CLINIC
4353 Pine Ridge Drive
Milton, XY 12345-0001
Telephone: 555-656-7890

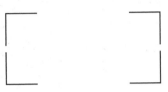

DATE	PROFESSIONAL SERVICE DESCRIPTION	CHARGE		CREDITS			CURRENT BALANCE	
				PAYMENTS	ADJUSTMENTS			

Due and payable within 10 days.   **Pay last amount in balance column** ⇧

Fig. 6.6 Blank patient ledger card for Susan Martin.

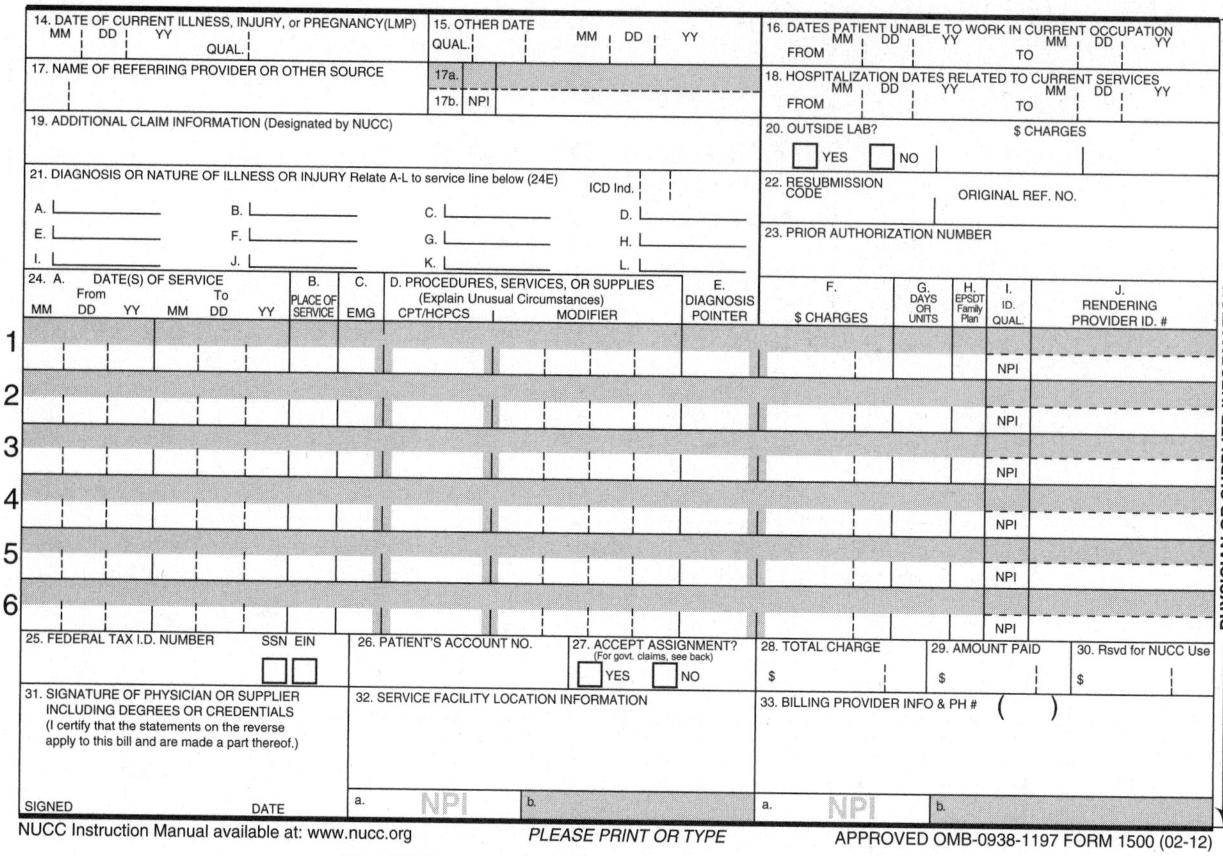
14. DATE OF CURRENT ILLNESS, INJURY, or PREGNANCY(LMP) MM DD YY QUAL.
15. OTHER DATE QUAL. MM DD YY
16. DATES PATIENT UNABLE TO WORK IN CURRENT OCCUPATION MM DD YY FROM MM DD YY TO
17. NAME OF REFERRING PROVIDER OR OTHER SOURCE
17a.
17b. NPI
18. HOSPITALIZATION DATES RELATED TO CURRENT SERVICES MM DD YY FROM MM DD YY TO
19. ADDITIONAL CLAIM INFORMATION (Designated by NUCC)
20. OUTSIDE LAB? YES NO $ CHARGES
21. DIAGNOSIS OR NATURE OF ILLNESS OR INJURY Relate A-L to service line below (24E) ICD Ind.
A. B. C. D.
E. F. G. H.
I. J. K. L.
22. RESUBMISSION CODE ORIGINAL REF. NO.
23. PRIOR AUTHORIZATION NUMBER
24. A. DATE(S) OF SERVICE From MM DD YY To MM DD YY
B. PLACE OF SERVICE
C. EMG
D. PROCEDURES, SERVICES, OR SUPPLIES (Explain Unusual Circumstances) CPT/HCPCS MODIFIER
E. DIAGNOSIS POINTER
F. $ CHARGES
G. DAYS OR UNITS
H. EPSDT Family Plan
I. ID. QUAL.
J. RENDERING PROVIDER ID. #
1 NPI
2 NPI
3 NPI
4 NPI
5 NPI
6 NPI
PHYSICIAN OR SUPPLIER INFORMATION
25. FEDERAL TAX I.D. NUMBER SSN EIN
26. PATIENT'S ACCOUNT NO.
27. ACCEPT ASSIGNMENT? (For govt. claims, see back) YES NO
28. TOTAL CHARGE $
29. AMOUNT PAID $
30. Rsvd for NUCC Use $
31. SIGNATURE OF PHYSICIAN OR SUPPLIER INCLUDING DEGREES OR CREDENTIALS (I certify that the statements on the reverse apply to this bill and are made a part thereof.)
SIGNED DATE
32. SERVICE FACILITY LOCATION INFORMATION
a. NPI b.
33. BILLING PROVIDER INFO & PH # ( )
a. NPI b.
NUCC Instruction Manual available at: www.nucc.org PLEASE PRINT OR TYPE APPROVED OMB-0938-1197 FORM 1500 (02-12)

Fig. 6.7 Bottom half of CMS-1500 form for Susan Martin.

C. Let's assume that in Case Study A, Mr. Sanchez's mental health treatment is covered under both of the policies he listed on his new patient registration form. You have determined that Maria's family policy through Wilton Community Schools is primary. Explain the procedure for filing dual claims when the patient is covered under a secondary policy.

Broadmoor Medical Clinic	Clinic EIN # 42-1898989
4353 Pine Ridge Drive	Dr. Robert L. Jones NPI 1234567890
Milton, XY 12345-0001	Dr. Marilou Lucero NPI 2907511822
Clinic NPI X100XX1000	
	Referring provider = DN Ordering provider = DK Supervising provider = DQ
Telephone: 555-656-7890	Date claim 1 day after examination

Note: Students should use the information in this provider block when completing the CMS-1500

D. Examine the EOB form shown in Fig. 6.8; then match each column number with the correct written explanation by placing the correct column number in the blank space preceding the written explanation.

_____ Amount applied to coinsurance

_____ Amount patient is responsible for paying

_____ Amount the provider charged for each service

_____ Amount(s) applied to copay, deductible, or not covered

_____ Balance the insurer will apply to benefits

_____ Coordination of benefits adjustment

_____ Date(s) patient received services

_____ Description of services rendered

_____ Fee adjustment

_____ Percentage of coverage

_____ Total amount paid by insurance plan

EXPLANATION OF BENEFITS

(This is NOT a bill)

July 1, 20XX

Group number:	0000123		
Member:	Jane M Sample		
Member's ID:	123456789 02		
Claim number:	8000000001		
Provider:	Smith, Robert		
Payment Reference ID:	2002062510100013		

1	2	3	4	5	6	7	8	9	10	11
Service/ product description	Dates you received service/product (m/d/y to m/d/y)	Charges billed by provider	Minus provider's fee adjustment	Minus your copay (C), deductible (D) or amount not covered (*)	Total amount eligible for benefits	%	Minus your co-insurance amount	Plus or (minus) coordination of benefits adjustment	Total paid by your plan	Amount you're responsible for
OFFICE VISIT	06/15/XX 06/15/XX	75.00	12.00	15.00 C	48.00	100%			48.00	15.00
LAB	06/15/XX 06/15/XX	89.12	15.36	50.00 D	23.76	100%			23.76	50.00
X-RAY	06/15/XX 06/15/XX	100.00	20.00		80.00	80%	16.00		64.00	16.00
SURGERY	06/15/XX 06/15/XX	50.00		50.00 575	0.00	0%			0.00	$0.00
Totals		$314.12	$47.38	$115.00	$151.76		$16.00		$135.76	$131.00

Your 20XX medical deductible satisfied so far: $100.00
Your 20XX family medical deductible satisfied so far: $300.00

Amount we paid your provider: **$135.76**

Amount you're responsible for: **$131.00**

* Message Codes:

575   This procedure is considered cosmetic. Your plan does not cover cosmetic services.

Fig. 6.8 Explanation of benefits form.

A. Blue Cross and Blue Shield is one of the most popular insurers in the United States. Visit their website (http://www.bcbs.com/). Research the available information to answer these questions. (**Note:** You may have to type in specific key words in the search box.)
  1. Who should the health insurance professional contact when there is a billing question?
  2. List the various types of coverage Blue Cross and Blue Shield offers its enrollees.
  3. Blue Cross and Blue Shield has _____ member companies and covers approximately _____ (number) people.
  4. What is "Blueworks?"
  5. What type of coverage would you likely purchase if you were traveling outside of the United States?
  6. To submit a claim for medical care overseas, you complete a(n) _____ and send it to the _____.

B. Search your Blue Cross and Blue Shield Association or regional website and locate the current guidelines for completing the CMS-1500 form.

C. Enter the title "Guidelines for the Role of Participating Physicians in Health Plans." Read and study this article and be prepared for an in-class discussion: http://www.bcbst.com/providers/role_physician.shtml.

D. Using search words "PAR versus nonPAR providers," search the Internet for advantages and disadvantages of each. Then prepare for a debate or in-class discussion on this topic.

E. Visit http://www.bcbs.com, and click on one of the spotlight topics (e.g., "Blue News," "Spotlight on Issues," or "Healthcare Reform"). Choose a topic of interest to you and prepare a brief oral presentation to the class focusing on the highlights of the topic.

Note: Websites change frequently. If any of these links are no longer valid, use comparable wording in your search engine.

Performance Objective 6.1: Patient Case Study 6.1

Conditions: Complete an encounter form and ledger card using the information on the documents in Case Study 6.1.
Supplies/Equipment: Ledger form (paper or electronic), pen, patient information form (Fig. 6.9), ID card (Fig. 6.10), encounter form (Fig. 6.11), and ledger card (Fig. 6.12)
Time Allowed: 20 minutes
Accuracy Needed to Pass: 100%

Procedural Steps	Points Earned	Comments
Evaluator: Note time began: _____		
1. Carefully read and study the applicable documents.		
Encounter Form		
1. Calculate the total charge of all services checked and enter the amount under "Today's charges." (10)		
2. Still using the encounter form and assuming the patient paid the coinsurance, calculate the amount paid and enter it under "Today's payments." (10)		
Ledger Card		
3. Complete the ledger card by listing each procedure/service separately. Post today's payment and calculate the balance due. (30)		
Optional: May deduct points for taking more time than allowed.		

Total Points = 50

Student's Score: _____

Evaluator: _____

Comments: _____

_____

_____

_____

Registration Data

1. Your Name Ebers   Karen   S   Sex ☐ Male   Date of Birth 07/28/2002
              (Last)   (First) (Middle)   ☒ Female

2. Social Security #: 222-99-0000   Marital Status: Ⓢ M D Se W

3. Address: 14276 Valley View Lane   4. SSS-756-1234
            (Street)   (Phone)
            Hopkins ,   X Y   98765
            (City)   (State)   (Zip)

5. Employer: Sunrise Care Center (mother)   Occupation: dietician
   Employer Address: 189 West Elm St.   SSS-786-3321
                                          (Work Phone)
   Spouse: N/A   Employer: Hopkins, XZ 98765   Occupation: _____
   Employer Address: _____   _____
                                                    (Work Phone)

6.
Other Household Members	Date of Birth	Relationship
Tricia Lambert	03/18/72	mother
Adam Ebers	11/04/99	brother
	/ /	
	/ /	
	/ /	

7. Medical Insurance Information

Ins. Company Name	Policy No.	Policy Holder	Sgl.	Type of Coverage Fmly.	Primary	Sec.
BCBS (Group #640)	XYZSIHI-0022	mother	☐	☒	☐	☐
_____	_____	_____	☐	☐	☐	☐
_____	_____	_____	☐	☐	☐	☐

8. Person to Contact in an Emergency Tricia Lambert Relationship to pt you mother
   Their Work Phone 756-3321 Their Home Phone 756-1234

9. Party with primary responsibility for payment: ☐ Self   ☒ Other
   Name Tricia Lambert   Relationship to you mother
   Address (see above)   Home Phone _____

For Office Use Only

Date Completed _____   Account No. _____   Patient No. _____

Household Status   ☐ Head of Household

               ☐ Spouse   ☐ Child   ☐ Other: _____

               Head of Household Name _____

Fig. 6.9 Registration data sheet for Karen Ebers.

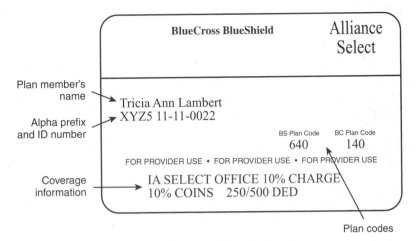

Fig. 6.10 ID card for Tricia Ann Lambert.

Broadmoor Medical Clinic

Date of service:	10/07/20XX		Waiver? ☐				
Patient name:	Karen S. Ebers		Insurance: BCBS				
			Subscriber name: Tricia Lambert				
Address:	14276 Valley View Lane		Group #:		Previous balance: Ø		
	Hopkins, XY 98765		Copay:		Today's charges:		
Phone: 555-756-1234			Account #: XYZ5 11-11-0022		Today's payment: check#		
DOB: 07/28/2002 Age:		Sex: F	Physician name: Dr. Marilou Lucero		Balance due:		

RANK	Office visit	New	Est	RANK	Office procedures			RANK	Laboratory	
	Minimal		99211		Anoscopy		46600		Venipuncture	36415
	Problem focused	99201	99212	✓	Audiometry	35.00	92551		Blood glucose, monitoring device	82962
	Expanded problem focused	99202	99213		Cerumen removal		69210		Blood glucose, visual dipstick	82948
	Detailed	99203	99214		Colposcopy		57452		CBC, w/ auto differential	85025
	Comprehensive	99204	99215		Colposcopy w/biopsy		57455		CBC, w/o auto differential	85027
	Comprehensive (new patient)	99205			ECG, w/interpretation		93000		Cholesterol	82465
	Significant, separate service	-25	-25		ECG, rhythm strip		93040		Hemoccult, guaiac	82270
	Well visit	New	Est		Endometrial biopsy		58100		Hemoccult, immunoassay	82274
	< 1 y	99381	99391		Flexible sigmoidoscopy		45330		Hemoglobin A1C	85018
	1-4 y	99382	99392		Flexible sigmoidoscopy w/biopsy		45331		Lipid panel	80061
✓	5-11 y	125.00 99383	99393		Fracture care, cast/splint	29___			Liver panel	80076
	12-17 y	99384	99394		Site:				KOH prep (skin, hair, nails)	87220
	18-39 y	99385	99395		Nebulizer		94640		Metabolic panel, basic	80048
	40-64 y	99386	99396		Nebulizer demo		94664		Metabolic panel, comprehensive	80053
	65 y +	99387	99397		Spirometry		94010		Mononucleosis	86308
	Medicare preventive services				Spirometry, pre and post		94060		Pregnancy, blood	84703
	Pap		Q0091		Tympanometry		92567		Pregnancy, urine	81025
	Pelvic & breast		G0101		Vasectomy		55250		Renal panel	80069
	Prostate/PSA		G0103		Skin procedures		Units		Sedimentation rate	85651
	Tobacco counseling/3-10 min		99406		Burn care, initial	16000			Strep, rapid	86403
	Tobacco counseling/>10 min		99407		Foreign body, skin, simple	10120			Strep culture	87081
	Welcome to Medicare exam		G0344		Foreign body, skin, complex	10121			Strep A	87880
	ECG w/Welcome to Medicare exam		G0366		I&D, abscess	10060			TB	86580
	Flexible sigmoidoscopy		G0104		I&D, hematoma/seroma	10140			UA, complete, non-automated	81000
	Hemoccult, guaiac		G0107		Laceration repair, simple	120___			UA, w/o micro, non-automated	81002
	Flu shot		G0008		Site: _____ Size: ___				UA, w/ micro, non-automated	81003
	Pneumonia shot		G0009		Laceration repair, layered	120___			Urine colony count	87086
	Consultation/preop clearance				Site: _____ Size: ___				Urine culture, presumptive	87088
	Expanded problem focused		99242		Lesion, biopsy, one	11100			Wet mount/KOH	87210
	Detailed		99243		Lesion, biopsy, each add'l	11101			Vaccines	
	Comprehensive/mod complexity		99244		Lesion,destruct.,benign,1-14	17110			DT, <7 y	90702
	Comprehensive/high complexity		99245		Lesion,destruct.,premal.,single	17000			DTP	90701
	Other services				Lesion,destruct.,premal.,ea.addfl	17003			DtaP, <7 y	90700
	After posted hours		99050		Lesion, excision, benign	114___			Flu, 6-35 months	90657
	Evening/weekend appointment		99051		Site: _____ Size: ___				Flu, 3 y +	90658
	Home health certification		G0180		Lesion, excision, malignant	116___			Hep A, adult	90632
	Home health recertification		G0179		Site: _____ Size: ___				Hep A, ped/adol, 2 dose	90633
	Post-op follow-up		99024		Lesion, paring/cutting, one	11055			Hep B, adult	90746
	Prolonged/30-74 min		99354		Lesion, paring/cutting, 2-4	11056			Hep B, ped/adol 3 dose	90744
	Special reports/forms		99080		Lesion, shave	113___			Hep B-Hib	90748
	Disability/Workers comp		99455		Site: _____ Size: ___				Hib, 4 dose	90645
	Radiology				Nail removal, partial	11730			HPV	90649
					Nail removal, w/matrix	11750			IPV	90713
					Skin tag, 1-15	11200			MMR	90707
	Diagnoses				Medications		Units		Pneumonia, >2 y	90732
1	Z00.129				Ampicillin, up to 500mg	J0290			Pneumonia conjugate, <5 y	90669
2					B-12, up to 1,000 mcg	J3420			Td, >7 y	90718
3					Epinephrine, up to 1ml	J0170			Varicella	90716
4					Kenalog, 10mg	J3301			Immunizations & Injections	Units
	Next office visit				Lidocaine, 10mg	J2001			Allergen, one	95115
	Recheck Prev (PRN) _____ D W M (Y)				Normal saline, 1000cc	J7030			Allergen, multiple	95117
	Instructions:				Phenergan, up to 50mg	J2550			Imm admin, one	90471
					Progesterone, 150mg	J1055			Imm admin, each add'l	90472
					Rocephin, 250mg	J0696			Imm admin, intranasal, one	90473
					Testosterone, 200mg	J1080			Imm admin,intranasal,each add'l	90474
	Referral				Tigan, up to 200 mg	J3250			Injection, joint, small	20600
	To:				Toradol, 15mg	J1885			Injection, joint, intermediate	20605
					Miscellaneous services				Injection, joint, major	20610
	Instructions:			✓	Tetanus Toxoid	20.00	90703		Injection, ther/proph/diag	90772
				✓	Vision Screening	40.00	99173		Injection, trigger point	20552
	Physician signature								Supplies	
	x Dr. Marilou Lucero, MD									

Fig. 6.11 Encounter form for Karen Ebers.

BCBS XYZ 511110022
$250; 90/10 10% COINS
A/C #11122

STATEMENT

BROADMOOR MEDICAL CLINIC
4353 Pine Ridge Drive
Milton, XY 12345-0001
Telephone: 555-656-7890

Tricia   03/18/1972
Adam   11/04/1999
Karen 04/28/2002

```
┌─────────────────────────────┐
│ TRICIA LAMBERT              │
│ 14276 VALLEY VIEW LANE      │
│ HOPKINS, XY 98765           │
└─────────────────────────────┘
```

20XX

DATE	PROFESSIONAL SERVICE DESCRIPTION	CHARGE	CREDITS		CURRENT BALANCE
			PAYMENTS	ADJUSTMENTS	

Due and payable within 10 days. **Pay last amount in balance column** ⇧

Fig. 6.12 Ledger card for Tricia Ann Lambert.

Performance Objective 6.2: Patient Case Study 6.1

Conditions: Complete a CMS-1500 form using the information provided in Case Study 6.1.

Supplies/Equipment: CMS-1500 form (paper or electronic) (Fig. 6.13), pen, patient information form, ID card, encounter form (see Fig. 6.11), and ledger card (see Fig. 6.12)

Guided Completion: For this claim form exercise, you also can use the electronic form on the Evolve website to help you complete this CMS-1500 claim form.

Time Allowed: 50 minutes

Accuracy Needed to Pass: 80%

Broadmoor Medical Clinic	Clinic EIN # 42-1898989
4353 Pine Ridge Drive	Dr. Robert L. Jones NPI 1234567890
Milton, XY 12345-0001	Dr. Marilou Lucero NPI 2907511822
Clinic NPI X100XX1000	
	Referring provider = DN Ordering provider = DK Supervising provider = DQ
Telephone: 555-656-7890	Date claim 1 day after examination

Note: For this Performance Objective, use the qualifier Y4 and the identifier number 112233445566 in Block 11b unless instructed otherwise. Use qualifier 454 in Block 14; qualifier DK in Block 17.

Procedural Steps	Points Earned	Comments
Evaluator: Note time began: _____		
1. Carefully read and study the applicable documents.		
2. Using the Blue Cross and Blue Shield template from Fig. 6.13, generate a clean claim for Karen Ebers' office visit. (100)		
Optional: May deduct points for taking more time than allowed.		

Total Points = 100

Student's Score: _____

Evaluator: _____

Comments: _____

_____

_____

_____

_____

HEALTH INSURANCE CLAIM FORM

APPROVED BY NATIONAL UNIFORM CLAIM COMMITTEE (NUCC) 02/12

| | PICA | | | | | | | PICA | | |

1. MEDICARE ☐ (Medicare#) MEDICAID ☐ (Medicaid#) TRICARE ☐ (ID#DoD#) CHAMPVA ☐ (Member ID#) GROUP HEALTH PLAN ☐ (ID#) FECA BLK LUNG ☐ (ID#) OTHER ☐ (ID#)

1a. INSURED'S I.D. NUMBER   (For Program in Item 1)

2. PATIENT'S NAME (Last Name, First Name, Middle Initial)

3. PATIENT'S BIRTH DATE   SEX
MM ┊ DD ┊ YY   M ☐ F ☐

4. INSURED'S NAME (Last Name, First Name, Middle Initial)

5. PATIENT'S ADDRESS (No., Street)

6. PATIENT RELATIONSHIP TO INSURED
Self ☐ Spouse ☐ Child ☐ Other ☐

7. INSURED'S ADDRESS (No., Street)

CITY   STATE

8. RESERVED FOR NUCC USE

CITY   STATE

ZIP CODE   TELEPHONE (Include Area Code)
(   )

ZIP CODE   TELEPHONE (Include Area Code)
(   )

9. OTHER INSURED'S NAME (Last Name, First Name, Middle Initial)

10. IS PATIENT'S CONDITION RELATED TO:

11. INSURED'S POLICY GROUP OR FECA NUMBER

a. OTHER INSURED'S POLICY OR GROUP NUMBER

a. EMPLOYMENT? (Current or Previous)
YES ☐ NO ☐

a. INSURED'S DATE OF BIRTH   SEX
MM ┊ DD ┊ YY   M ☐ F ☐

b. RESERVED FOR NUCC USE

b. AUTO ACCIDENT?   PLACE (State)
YES ☐ NO ☐

b. OTHER CLAIM ID (Designated by NUCC)

c. RESERVED FOR NUCC USE

c. OTHER ACCIDENT?
YES ☐ NO ☐

c. INSURANCE PLAN NAME OR PROGRAM NAME

d. INSURANCE PLAN NAME OR PROGRAM NAME

10d. CLAIM CODES (Designated by NUCC)

d. IS THERE ANOTHER HEALTH BENEFIT PLAN?
YES ☐ NO ☐ *If yes*, complete items 9, 9a, and 9d.

READ BACK OF FORM BEFORE COMPLETING & SIGNING THIS FORM.

12. PATIENT'S OR AUTHORIZED PERSON'S SIGNATURE I authorize the release of any medical or other information necessary to process this claim. I also request payment of government benefits either to myself or to the party who accepts assignment below.

SIGNED _____   DATE _____

13. INSURED'S OR AUTHORIZED PERSON'S SIGNATURE I authorize payment of medical benefits to the undersigned physician or supplier for services described below.

SIGNED _____

14. DATE OF CURRENT ILLNESS, INJURY, or PREGNANCY(LMP)
MM ┊ DD ┊ YY   QUAL. ┊

15. OTHER DATE
QUAL. ┊   MM ┊ DD ┊ YY

16. DATES PATIENT UNABLE TO WORK IN CURRENT OCCUPATION
FROM MM ┊ DD ┊ YY   TO MM ┊ DD ┊ YY

17. NAME OF REFERRING PROVIDER OR OTHER SOURCE
17a.
17b. NPI

18. HOSPITALIZATION DATES RELATED TO CURRENT SERVICES
FROM MM ┊ DD ┊ YY   TO MM ┊ DD ┊ YY

19. ADDITIONAL CLAIM INFORMATION (Designated by NUCC)

20. OUTSIDE LAB? $ CHARGES
YES ☐ NO ☐

21. DIAGNOSIS OR NATURE OF ILLNESS OR INJURY Relate A-L to service line below (24E)   ICD Ind. ┊
A. ┊_____ B. ┊_____ C. ┊_____ D. ┊_____
E. ┊_____ F. ┊_____ G. ┊_____ H. ┊_____
I. ┊_____ J. ┊_____ K. ┊_____ L. ┊_____

22. RESUBMISSION CODE   ORIGINAL REF. NO.

23. PRIOR AUTHORIZATION NUMBER

24. A. DATE(S) OF SERVICE						B. PLACE OF SERVICE	C. EMG	D. PROCEDURES, SERVICES, OR SUPPLIES (Explain Unusual Circumstances)		E. DIAGNOSIS POINTER	F. $ CHARGES	G. DAYS OR UNITS	H. EPSDT Family Plan	I. ID. QUAL.	J. RENDERING PROVIDER ID. #
From MM	DD	YY	To MM	DD	YY			CPT/HCPCS	MODIFIER						
1														NPI	
2														NPI	
3														NPI	
4														NPI	
5														NPI	
6														NPI	

25. FEDERAL TAX I.D. NUMBER   SSN ☐ EIN ☐

26. PATIENT'S ACCOUNT NO.

27. ACCEPT ASSIGNMENT? (For govt. claims, see back)
YES ☐ NO ☐

28. TOTAL CHARGE
$

29. AMOUNT PAID
$

30. Rsvd for NUCC Use
$

31. SIGNATURE OF PHYSICIAN OR SUPPLIER INCLUDING DEGREES OR CREDENTIALS
(I certify that the statements on the reverse apply to this bill and are made a part thereof.)

SIGNED _____   DATE _____

32. SERVICE FACILITY LOCATION INFORMATION

a. NPI   b.

33. BILLING PROVIDER INFO & PH # (   )

a. NPI   b.

NUCC Instruction Manual available at: www.nucc.org   PLEASE PRINT OR TYPE   APPROVED OMB-0938-1197 FORM 1500 (02-12)

Fig. 6.13 Blank CMS-1500 form for Karen Ebers.

Chapter **6 New and Traditional Reimbursement Models**

Scoring Rubric for CMS-1500 Performance Objective

Block No.	Points Allowed	Student's Score	Comments
1	1		
1a	2		
2	5		
3	1		
4	2		
5	5		
6	1		
7	3		
8	2		
9	5		
10	3		
11d	1		
14	1		
17	2		
17b	2		
21	5		
24a	2×4		
24b	1×4		
24d	2×4		
24e	1×4		
24f	1×4		
24g	1×4		
24j	1×4		
25	2		
26	1		
27	1		
28	4		
31	3		
32	4		
32a	1		
33	5		
33a	1		
33b	1		
TOTAL	100		

Performance Objective 6.3: Interpreting an Explanation of Benefits

Conditions: Student will interpret an EOB generated from Case Study 6.1.
Supplies/Equipment: Pen and EOB form from Blue Cross and Blue Shield claim (Fig. 6.14)
Time Allowed: 20 minutes
Accuracy Needed to Pass: 100%

Procedural Steps	Points Earned	Comments
Evaluator: Note time began: _____		
1. Carefully read and study the EOB document provided in Fig. 6.14.		
2. Using the ledger card generated in Performance Objective 6.1, post the insurance payment rec'd 10/30. (10)		
3. Calculate the amount that must be adjusted off. (10)		
4. Calculate the amount still owed by the patient (the last figure in the column "Current Balance" should reflect the amount the patient owes). (10)		
Optional: May deduct points for taking more time than allowed.		

Total Points = 30

Student's Score: _____

Evaluator: _____

Comments: _____

_____

_____

_____

_____

EXPLANATION OF BENEFITS

(THIS IS NOT A BILL)

This is your Explanation of HealthCare Benefits. This statement shows how we applied your coverage to claim(s) submitted to us. If you have any questions, please call our Customer Service Department at 555-666-0000 or 800-222-1111 weekdays between the hours of 8 a.m. and 5 p.m.

Insured Name: Tricia Ann Lambert
14276 Valley View Lane
Hopkins, XY 98765

ID # XYZ511110022

Patient: Karen S. Ebers

Service Date(s): 10-07-20XX

Provider: Broadmoor Medical Clinic

Billed Charges	Provider Savings	Amount Insurance Paid	Amount Patient Owes
$220.00	$28.50	$136.45	$55.05

CLAIM DETAILS

Billed Charge	125.00	20.00	35.00	40.00
Allowed Charge	111.00	17.50	23.00	-- *
Copayment (−)	11.00	1.75	2.30	-- *
Deductible (−)	-- **	-- **	-- **	-- **
Sub-Total	100.00	15.75	20.70	40.00
Insurance Paid	100.00	15.75	20.70	--

Group Number	Claim Number	Account Number	Provider Number	Date Received	Date Processed
000GRW0000	000050505011	1818181XZ	00234543	10-10-20XX	10-11-20XX

NOTES:

*D – Patient has met yearly deductible

**L – Contract Limitation(s)

A check in the amount of __$136.45__ **has been mailed to your provider.**

Fig. 6.14 Explanation of benefits for Tricia Lambert.

Composing a Patient Letter

You have received a letter from Tricia Lambert inquiring why there is a balance owing on Karen Ebers' account. Compose a letter of explanation. (*Instructor's hint:* The insurance policy does not cover routine eye examinations.)

Health Insurance Professional's Notebook

Locate your local or regional Blue Cross Blue Shield website on the Internet. Using a blank CMS-1500 claim form, generate a template illustrating the information required for each block. Incorporate this template under the "commercial claims" section in your notebook.

Chapter Checklist

Student Name: _____

Chapter Completion Date: _____

Evaluate your classroom performance. Complete the self-evaluation and submit it to your instructor. When your instructor returns this form to you, compare your self-evaluation with the evaluation completed by your instructor.

1.	Record	Your start time and date: _____
2.	Read	The assigned chapter in the textbook
3.	View	PowerPoint slides (if available)
4.	Complete	Exercises in workbook as assigned
5.	Compare	Your answers to the answers posted on the bulletin board, website, or handout
5.	Correct	Your answers
7.	Complete	All tests and required activities
8.	Read	Assigned readings (if any)
9.	Complete	Chapter performance objectives (competencies), if any
10.	Evaluate	Your personal performance and submit it to your instructor
11.	Record	Your ending time and date: _____
12.	Move on	Begin next chapter as assigned

PERFORMANCE EVALUATION

Student Name: _____

Chapter Completion Date: _____

Evaluate your classroom performance. Compare this evaluation with the one provided by your instructor.

Skill	Student Self-Evaluation			Instructor Evaluation		
	Good	Average	Poor	Good	Average	Poor
Attendance/punctuality						
Personal appearance						
Applies effort						
Is self-motivated						
Is courteous						
Has positive attitude						
Completes assignments in timely manner						
Works well with others						

Student's Initials: _____   **Instructor's Initials:** _____

Date: _____   **Date:** _____

Points Possible: _____

Points Awarded: _____

Chapter Grade: _____

7 The Changing Face of Managed Care

Chapter 7 deals with how managed care is changing. Because managed care can present a greater challenge than some of the other topics in the textbook, the activities in this chapter of the student workbook focus on helping the student "unravel" the mysteries and, in doing so, gain a better understanding of how managed care functions, how it differs from fee-for-service, and how to identify ways managed care is adapting to changes in healthcare.

Managed care includes medical plans in which access to healthcare services is structured in such a way as to provide quality medical care as it attempts to limit healthcare costs. Premiums are typically lower with managed care policies than for traditional fee-for-service healthcare plans, and the charge for each provider visit is comparatively small. As we learned from Chapter 7 in the textbook, a common form of managed care is the health maintenance organization (HMO), which restricts patients to the HMO's own group of medical professionals. Other forms of managed care include point of service (POS) and preferred provider organization (PPO) plans. Although these plans typically charge the low per-visit fee of an HMO for treatment by healthcare professionals within the plan's network, they also allow out-of-network treatment at a lower reimbursement rate.

WORKBOOK CHAPTER OBJECTIVES

After completing the workbook activities for Chapter 7, the student should be able to:
1. Define the terms used in the chapter.
2. Answer the review questions according to the evaluation criteria set by the instructor.
3. Demonstrate higher-order thinking (e.g., the ability to synthesize and critically evaluate new information).
4. Integrate knowledge and transfer it from one document to another.
5. Access the information needed from the Internet to complete workbook activities.
6. Perform basic math calculations for billing purposes.
7. Abstract applicable information from healthcare documents necessary for completion of various forms used in healthcare billing and the claims process.
8. Complete specific forms common to managed care organizations (MCOs).
9. Generate information and documents for inclusion in the student's personal Health Insurance Professional's Notebook.
10. Undertake self-criticism and evaluation, including seeking and responding to feedback and comments and setting realistic targets.

DEFINING CHAPTER TERMS

Using the computer, students should write an accurate definition for each of the chapter terms listed. These definitions should be in the students' own words. When finished, students should compare their definitions with those listed in the glossary at the back of the textbook and correct any inaccuracies.

capitation
closed-panel HMO
consultation
copayment
covered entities
direct contract model
enrollees
Exclusive Provider Organization (EPO)
full-service HMO
gatekeepers
group model
health information exchange (HIE)

health maintenance organization (HMO)
high deductible plans (HDPs)
iatrogenic effects
independent practice association (IPA)
insurance marketplace
integrated delivery systems (IDSs)
The Joint Commission
managed behavioral healthcare organization (MBHO)
managed care
meaningful use
mixed model
National Committee for Quality Assurance (NCQA)

97

network
network model
open-panel plan
point-of-service (POS)
preauthorization
precertification
predetermination of benefits
preferred provider organization (PPO)

primary care physician (PCP)
primary care preferred provider organizations
provider sponsored organization (PSO)
referral
specialist
staff model
utilization review
Utilization Review Accreditation Commission (URAC)

ASSESSMENT

Multiple Choice

Directions: In the questions and statements presented, choose the response that **best** answers or completes the stem and circle the letter that precedes it.

1. An organized, interrelated system of people and facilities that communicate with one another and work together as a unit is commonly referred to as a(n):
   a. Network
   b. Community
   c. Demographic
   d. Organizational unit

2. Individuals belonging to a managed healthcare plan are commonly referred to as:
   a. Beneficiaries
   b. Enrollees
   c. Receivers
   d. Entities

3. The two most common types of MCOs are:
   a. PPOs and individual practice associations (IPAs)
   b. IPAs and HMOs
   c. HMOs and PPOs
   d. PPOs and POSs

4. A specific provider who oversees an HMO member's total healthcare treatment is called a(n):
   a. Specific provider
   b. Attending physician
   c. Complete care provider
   d. Primary care physician (PCP)

5. The amount of money a patient has to pay out of pocket per visit is referred to as a(n):
   a. Copayment
   b. Deductible
   c. Premium
   d. Allowable fee

6. When an individual first enrolls in an HMO, he or she chooses a(n):
   a. Specialist
   b. Insurance carrier
   c. Fiscal intermediary
   d. Primary care physician (PCP)

7. Most managed healthcare plans emphasize:
   a. Small copayments
   b. Frequent physician visits
   c. Preventive healthcare
   d. Paying premiums on time

8. A multispecialty group practice in which all healthcare services are provided within the building(s) owned by the HMO is called a:
   a. Staff model
   b. Group model
   c. Network model
   d. Direct contact model

9. A reimbursement system in which healthcare providers receive a fixed fee for every patient enrolled in the plan, regardless of how many or few services the patient uses, is called a(n) _____ system.
   a. Usual, customary, and reasonable
   b. Capitation
   c. Misallocation
   d. Allowed fee

10. A managed care system composed of individual healthcare providers who offer healthcare services for HMO and non-HMO patients but maintain their own offices and identities is called a(n):
    a. Network model
    b. Open-panel IPA
    c. Direct-contact model
    d. POS plan

11. A plan that allows patients to use the HMO provider or go outside the plan and pay a higher copayment and deductible is a(n):
    a. Network model
    b. Open-end HMO
    c. Direct-contact model
    d. Full-service PSO

12. Most commercial healthcare organizations and MCOs request that they be made aware of and consent to certain procedures and services before their enrollees undergo them, a process called:
    a. Accreditation
    b. Precertification
    c. Utilization review
    d. Endorsement determination

13. The _____ process can help prevent situations in which the patient may be forced to pay significant out-of-pocket costs.
    a. Capitation
    b. Referral
    c. Predetermination of benefits
    d. Adjudication

14. A procedure required by third-party payers that requires permission before a provider can carry out specific procedures and treatments is a(n):
    a. A referral
    b. Certification
    c. Preauthorization
    d. A "medical right to know"

15. A type of managed care organization that provides Medicare beneficiaries with alternatives to original Medicare is a(n):
    a. HMO
    b. POS
    c. PSO
    d. IPA

99

Copyright © 2018, Elsevier Inc. All rights reserved.

Chapter **7** The Changing Face of Managed Care

16. It is predicted that under the Affordable Care Act, managed care organizations will increase rapidly, particularly with the expansion of:
    a. Private for-profit insurers
    b. Workers' compensation
    c. Medicaid
    d. Medicare

17. Which of these is affected by HIPAA regulations?
    a. Patient confidentiality
    b. Electronic transmission of transactions and code sets
    c. NPIs and EINs
    d. All of the above

18. Most MCOs are regulated from three areas. Which of these *is not* one of these areas?
    a. States
    b. Local government agencies
    c. Federal government
    d. Voluntary accreditation

19. To provide quality, affordable care for all Americans and to promote wellness, prevention of disease, and early intervention are the goals of:
    a. HIPAA
    b. NCQA
    c. The Affordable Care Act
    d. The Joint Commission

20. An independent nonprofit organization that measures, assesses, and reports on the quality of care and service in MCOs is the:
    a. NCQA
    b. URAC
    c. AHCPR
    d. CMA

True/False

Directions: Place a "T" in the blank preceding the sentence if it is true; place an "F" if it is false.

_____ 1. An HMO provides its members with basic healthcare services for a fixed price and for a given period.

_____ 2. PPOs typically do not require authorization from a PCP for a referral to a specialist.

_____ 3. PPOs are more tightly controlled by government regulations than HMOs.

_____ 4. HMOs typically have no deductibles or plan limits.

_____ 5. The federal government requires that HMOs operate their own facilities, staffed with salaried physicians.

_____ 6. HMOs are neither accredited nor certified.

_____ 7. Preauthorization pertains to medical necessity and appropriateness and guarantees payment.

_____ 8. Precertification involves collecting information before inpatient admissions or performance of selected ambulatory procedures and services.

_____ 9. A referral is a request by a healthcare provider for a patient under his or her care to be evaluated or treated or both by another provider.

_____ 10. In all managed care situations, for the healthcare plan to recognize the referral, it must come from the patient's designated PCP.

_____ 11. HIPAA requires that employers offer healthcare coverage.

_____ 12. Healthcare reform will likely eliminate most managed care arrangements.

100

Fill-in-the-Blank

Directions: Select the word or word groups from the box on the next page to complete these statements correctly. (**Note:** Some word or word groups can be used more than once.)

1. _managed care_ describes types of health insurance that control the use of health services by their members so that they can contain healthcare costs, the quality of care, or both.

2. An interrelated system in which people and facilities communicate with one another and work together as a unit is referred to as a(n) _network_.

3. Individuals who are eligible for healthcare services and benefits under a specific managed care plan are called _enrollees_.

4. Two common types of MCOs are _PPOs_ and _HMOs_.

5. _PPOs_ are groups of healthcare providers who work under one umbrella to provide medical services at a discount to individuals who participate in the managed care plan.

6. A(n) _PCP_ is a specific provider who oversees an HMO member's total healthcare treatment.

7. When a patient's problem exceeds the expertise of his or her PCP, the PCP can arrange a(n) _referral_ to a specialist to take over the patient's care.

8. _HMO_ typically have no deductibles or plan limits.

9. Managed care plans emphasize _behavioral_ healthcare.

10. A(n) _staff model_ HMO is a multispecialty group practice in which all healthcare services are provided within the building(s) owned by the HMO.

11. In a(n) _group model_, the HMO contracts with independent, multispecialty physician groups who provide all healthcare services to its members.

12. _premium_ is a fixed fee per member per specified time period (usually monthly).

13. The staff model is a(n) _closed-panel_ HMO.

14. The _direct contract_ HMO is similar to an IPA except the HMO contracts directly with the individual physicians.

15. An IPA is a(n) _open-panel plan_.

16. The _network model_ HMO is one that has multiple provider arrangements, including staff, group, or IPA structures.

17. The _POS_ is a "hybrid" type of managed care (also referred to as an _open-ended HMO_) that allows patients to use the HMO provider or go outside the plan and use any provider they choose.

18. _Utilization review_ is a system designed to determine the medical necessity and appropriateness of a medical service, procedure, or hospital admission.

19. _preauthorization_ is a procedure required by most managed healthcare and indemnity plans before a provider is able to carry out specific procedures or treatments for a patient.

20. A(n) _referral_ is when the PCP requests another physician to provide his or her expert opinion regarding the patient's condition.

capitation	closed panel
consultation	direct contract model
enrollees	group model
health maintenance organizations (HMOs)	open-panel plan
managed care	preauthorization
network model	preventive
point of service (POS) model	referral
preferred provider organizations (PPOs)	utilization review
primary care physician (PCP)	network
staff model	

Short Answer

Note: If space provided is not adequate, use a separate piece of blank paper.

1. An MCO typically performs three main functions, which are:

   _____

   _____

   _____

2. Explain briefly in your own words each of these types of managed care systems:

   PPO: _____

   HMO: _____

   IPA: _____

   POS: _____

3. Under the Federal HMO Act, an entity must have three characteristics to call itself an HMO. List them.

   _____

   _____

   _____

4. List two advantages and three disadvantages of PPOs.

   _____

   _____

   _____

   _____

   _____

   _____

5. Provide a brief description of the National Committee for Quality Assurance (NCQA) and how it "measures" an MCO.

   _____

   _____

   _____

   _____

   _____

6. Explain how an MCO acquires accreditation from The Joint Commission.

   _____

   _____

   _____

   _____

102

7. Explain the difference between a referral and a consultation.

_____

8. How do the Health Insurance Portability and Accountability Act's (HIPAA's) regulations affect managed care?

_____

9. In your own opinion, what is the future of managed care?

_____

CRITICAL THINKING ACTIVITIES

A. New patient Dorothy Scoval comes to the medical facility with a knee injury. She informs you that she is a current enrollee of Envision, a local HMO. Would the procedure for gathering demographic and insurance information differ with this patient compared with one who is insured under a traditional commercial plan? Explain why or why not.

B. Examine the ID card shown in Fig. 7.1 and then answer these questions from the information printed on the card.
   1. What is the name of the insured individual?
   2. What is the name of the patient's PCP?
   3. What dollar amount should you collect from the patient for an office visit?
   4. What type of HMO is this?
   5. If the patient was seen on February 2, 2017, would the HMO pay for the visit?

ENVISION HMO		
Dorothy M. Scoval	10/19/1961	For Inpatient
Name	Date of Birth	Preauthorization
123456789 02/13/2017	**56XXZ**	Telephone: 800-223-0000
Member No. Effective Date	Grp Code	FAX 555-445-5555
Francis Tompkins, MD	**555-111-4443**	
Primary Care Physician	Telephone No.	
GHJKL Copays	Office Visit $5	
Pharmacy Code	ER $10	
	Inpatient $15	

Fig. 7.1 Health maintenance organization ID card (Scoval).

C. Established patient Dorothy Scoval telephones 1 week after her initial encounter complaining of chest pain and short-ness of breath. She asks if she can schedule an appointment with an Envision cardiologist. The scheduling receptionist refers the call to you, the health insurance professional. How should this request be handled?

D. The medical facility in which you work as a health insurance professional is part of Envision, a staff model HMO. The healthcare providers are employees of the HMO and see patients on a "capitated" (per patient) basis. How does this payment structure affect claims submission for the plan's enrollees?

E. Healthcare reform has been a popular topic in the United States for many years; however, not everyone has a clear picture of exactly what managed care is and how it functions. Following are several statements regarding managed care, particularly HMOs. Place a "T" in the blank preceding all true statements; place an "F" in the blank if the statement is false.

_____ 1. Most HMOs typically offer substandard healthcare to keep costs under control.

_____ 2. MCOs encourage members to take a proactive or "preventive" role in their own healthcare.

_____ 3. All HMOs are the same.

_____ 4. The primary differences among managed care plans are found in the type of plan, what benefits it covers, and the out-of-pocket costs members will pay for services.

_____ 5. The NCQA has developed standards to evaluate the medical and quality systems in HMOs.

_____ 6. The main role of the PCP in HMOs is to serve as a "gatekeeper," rationing treatment options simply to contain costs.

_____ 7. The best physicians do not participate in HMO networks; members cannot be sure they are getting quality medical care.

_____ 8. Most healthcare providers participate in some type of managed care plan.

_____ 9. Most HMO members are dissatisfied with their plans.

_____ 10. Managed care plans are able to keep costs low because of an emphasis on disease prevention and wellness.

PROBLEM-SOLVING/COLLABORATIVE (GROUP) ACTIVITIES

A. Create a page for an Office Procedures Manual outlining the course of action to follow for obtaining preauthorization for a managed care patient who is to be admitted to the hospital for a surgical procedure. Include an example of a typical preauthorization form.

B. Four main HIPAA regulations affect healthcare:
   1. Maintaining patient confidentiality
   2. Implementing standards for electronic transmission of transactions and code sets
   3. Establishing national provider and employer identifiers
   4. Resolving security and privacy issues arising from the storage and transmission of healthcare data

   Select one of the regulations listed and prepare a 5-minute group presentation, expanding it as follows:
   ■ Its effect on patients
   ■ Its effect on healthcare providers
   ■ Pros and cons

C. Group study topics:
   1. Compare benefit structures offered in managed care with benefits in traditional indemnity insurance.
   2. Explain how capitation might lead to underuse of healthcare services. (This topic may require additional research. To learn more visit this link: http://www.bluecrossma.com/visitor/pdf/alternative-quality-contract.pdf)

PROJECTS/DISCUSSION TOPICS

A. Several federal laws govern health insurance; you already have learned about three of them in other chapters:
   ERISA—places critical limitations on health plan liability
   COBRA—provides substantial protection for preserving an individual's insurance coverage after job or life changes
   HIPAA—protects an individual's privacy and his or her ability to maintain healthcare coverage
   The fourth is the **Federal HMO Act.** Conduct in-depth research to learn about this important act. Then write a brief synopsis explaining what this act involves and how it affects today's healthcare market.

B. The **Patient Protection and Affordable Care Act of 2010** is the most recent and probably the most debated federal act affecting healthcare. You can find a detailed summary of this act on the Web at http://www.dpc.senate.gov/healthreformbill/healthbill04.pdf. Study the important points of this Act and be prepared for a discussion. (Note: If this URL is outdated, use appropriate search words to locate a similar article.)

C. **Discussion forum:** Study and prepare for a discussion regarding one or more of these topics:
What is managed care?
What do "capitation" and other managed care systems involve?
What ethical concerns does managed care raise?
What specific effect does managed care have on physician–patient relationships?
What should providers consider when evaluating managed care contracts?

D. Generate a chart comparing managed care with traditional (indemnity) insurance.

CASE STUDIES

A. Eric Thomas has healthcare coverage with a PPO. His deductible is $500, which he has met for the current year. According to his policy, if he is treated by a PPO member physician, his coinsurance ratio is 90/10. If he is treated by a non-PPO physician, the coinsurance ratio is 80/20. Calculate the amount Eric would have to pay either of the two listed physicians.

PPO Member Physician	Non-PPO Physician
Benjamin P. Moore, M.D.	Lydia R. Davis, M.D.
Est. Pt. Level II (99212) OV = $90	Est. Pt. Level II (99212) OV = $65
Eric's payment: _____	Eric's payment: _____

B. This case study is for patient Judith Kelley. Read it thoroughly and complete the referral authorization form in Fig. 7.2.

Patient Name: Judith A. Kelley
DOB: 03/14/1955
Med. Record No.: 10445
Health Insurance: Zenith HMO
Member No.: 444661112

Judith Kelley visited Kayla Parsons, her PCP, on 08/22/20XX, complaining of nausea, loss of appetite, and unexplained weight loss, which began about 2 months before this visit after a bout of the flu. After taking a detailed history and performing a complete examination, including a urinalysis and complete blood count, Dr. Parsons suspects Mrs. Kelley's symptoms point to a serious underlying condition and warrants a referral to a specialist for evaluation and treatment. Dr. Marvel Sutton is an endocrinologist and practices within the patient's HMO system. Initially, Dr. Parsons has authorized two visits with Dr. Sutton, and the first appointment date is 08/30/20XX.

ICD-10 Diagnoses: (1) Loss of weight— R63.4; (2) Nausea— R11.0
Referral No.: 032425
Provider ID No.: 6544355
Dr. Parson's phone number: 555-876-2123; fax: 555-876-2110

Note: Students should use their own names as the contact persons.

Chapter **7** **The Changing Face of Managed Care**

HEALTH Referral Authorization Form

This facsimile transmission is private, confidential and intended only of the recipient named hereon. If you receive this transmission in error, please contact Iowa Health's Medical Management Dept. at (555) 333-XXXX or (800) 222-XXXX.

FAX THIS COMPLETED FORM TO: (555) 333-XXXX or (800) 222-XXXX

Referral #: _____   **ALL REFERRALS EXPIRE IN 60 DAYS**

Patient Information

Member Name	Member #	DOB	Refer to Provider	Specialty

Please check the requested services: ☐ Evaluation and recommendation   ☐ Evaluate and treat
☐ OPS   ☐ One follow-up visit   ☐ Send report to PCP

Number of Visits:	Appointment Date:

Medical Information

Diagnosis:	ICD Code:

Symptoms: _____
_____
_____
_____

Previous Treatment (if pertinent for referral): _____
_____

Lab/X-Ray Finding (if pertinent for referral): _____
_____

Medical Record #:

Authorization

PCP Name	Phone # (Include Area Code)
Contact Name	Fax #

For Office use only

PCP Provider #		Refer to Provider	
Member Effective Date	Auth Type		Extent of Care
Auth Start Date	Auth End Date		# of Visits Approved
Approved by:		Date:	
Entered by:		Date:	

This referral does not constitute a payment agreement. Coverage is based on the eligibility of the member at the time the service is rendered.

Fig. 7.2 Referral authorization form (Kelley).

C. This case study is for patient Fredric Basquez. From this information, complete the prior authorization request form in Fig. 7.3.

Patient Name: Fredric M. Basquez
DOB: 09/26/1972
Health Insurance Plan: OutReach Plus
Subscriber ID No.: QST99442
Med. Record No.: BA092662
Social Security No.: 222-00-9999

Fredric Basquez comes to see Dr. Eric Woods, an orthopedic surgeon, for complaints of head and neck pain accompanied by numbness and tingling in his right arm after an all-terrain vehicle (ATV) accident. The patient reports he was riding on the back of his brother's ATV when the vehicle came into contact with a concealed tree stump. He was subsequently thrown from the vehicle, landing on the right side of his head. A 2-cm laceration of the right cheek was sutured in the emergency department yesterday, and débridement of minor abrasions and contusions of the face and shoulder was performed. Radiographs of the head and neck, done at the time of the emergency department visit, were inconclusive. He was given a prescription for naproxen. An emergency department staff member scheduled an appointment with this office for follow-up. A detailed history was taken, and a complete physical examination was done. Dr. Woods suspects a herniated disk with progressive objective neurologic deficits.

Provider ID No.: 6577890113
Dr. Woods' phone number: 555-232-0987; fax: 555-232-0980

Dr. Woods asks you to arrange an MRI for Mr. Basquez. You note from the patient's insurance ID card that prior authorization must be obtained for any outside diagnostic testing. From the previous information, complete the Prior Authorization Request form for Mr. Basquez's MRI. (**Note:** You will be attaching a copy of the initial history and physical examination [H & P] with this form.)

Note: Do not complete the area below the heavy black line.

Prior Authorization Request for MRI/CT Scan of the Neck and Spine

To Be Completed By Ordering Provider / *Date:*

Patient Name:	Patient Subscriber ID:	Patient Date of Birth:
Provider Name:	Provider ID Number:	Provider Phone: Provider Fax:

Please Indicate the Study Ordered:	☐ MRI	☐ Neck ☐ Spine	☐ CT	☐ Neck ☐ Spine
Diagnosis Code:			Scheduled Date:	

MRI Indications		CT Indications
☐ Myelopathy ☐ Infection of spine/cord/disk ☐ Spinal trauma ☐ Grossly abnormal plain films ☐ Co-existing systemic illness	☐ Congenital anomalies of spine ☐ Spinal stenosis ☐ Post-op spinal surgery w/residua ☐ Where contrast is required ☐ Known malignancy/suspected mets	☐ Spinal fracture

Conditional Indications		
Suspected herniated disk with one or more of the following:	☐ Progressive objective neurological deficits (sensory/motor loss, reflex change, fasciculations, wasting) ☐ Cauda equina syndrome	☐ Serious systemic illness (malignancy, TB, etc.) ☐ Spinal cord compression
Uncomplicated back pain or sciatica only after 4–6 weeks of the conservative treatment with:	☐ Home self-care ☐ Analgesics ☐ PT or chiropractic care ☐ Spinal exercises	
If none of the above, rationale for exception (all exceptions must have supporting documentation):		

Supporting Documentation: ☐ Initial Evaluation (H & P) ☐ Treatment Plan ☐ Office Notes

To Be Completed By ☐ Approved ☐ Denied

Comments: _____

This notice is not a guarantee payment will be provided and only approves the medical necessity and appropriateness of the medical services requested and authorized. The determination on payment of claims will be made when the claim is received. The claim will be subject to the terms and limitations of the member's benefit plan, including applicable deductibles and copayments. Additionally, prior authorization will be honored only if the member is a covered member and dues are paid at the time the services are provided. Payment will not be allowed if the member is not covered at the time of service.

Reviewed by: _____ Date: _____

Fig. 7.3 Prior authorization request (Basquez).

INTERNET EXPLORATION

A. Use the Internet to search for the words "managed healthcare," and locate a website that provides current information regarding new managed healthcare issues. Prepare a one-page essay or a 3-minute oral presentation titled "What's New in Managed Healthcare." Your instructor will provide specific guidelines for this activity.

B. Research The Joint Commission's website (http://www.jointcommission.org) and identify current updates regarding HIPAA compliance standards. At The Joint Commission's home page, enter HIPAA in the search box located in the top right corner.

C. Explore Kaiser Permanente's website (https://healthy.kaiserpermanente.org/html/kaiser/index.shtml). Note the various informational areas. Click on "prospective members," choose a region of interest to you, and check out the various plan options.

PERFORMANCE OBJECTIVES

Performance Objective 7.1: Completing a Preauthorization Form

Conditions: Student will complete a preauthorization/admission form from the information provided on the forms illustrated in Fig. 7.4 and 7.5.

Supplies/Equipment: Pen or computer, Envision HMO preauthorization request form (see Fig. 7.4), patient registration data form (see Fig. 7.5), and blank preauthorization/admission form (Fig. 7.6)

Time Allowed: 20 minutes

Accuracy Needed to Pass: 90%

Procedural Steps	Points Earned	Comments
Evaluator: Note time began: _____		
1. Carefully read and study the previously named forms and then correctly complete the preauthorization form; 1 point is awarded for each correctly completed blank on the form.		
2. Patient information (3)		
3. Provider information (8)		
4. Physician information (6)		
5. Procedure information (10)		
6. Student used a pen/wrote legibly (3)		
Optional: May deduct points for taking more time than allowed.		

Total Points = 30

Student's Score: _____

Evaluator: _____

Comments: _____

_____

_____

_____

_____

ENVISION HMO

PREAUTHORIZATION REQUEST FORM

PATIENT INFORMATION

Last Name: Scoval   First Name: Dorothy M

DOB: 10/16/1961   Member #: 123456789   Group #: 36XX2

PREAUTHORIZATION REQUEST INFORMATION

Please list **both** procedure/product code <u>and</u> narrative description:

CPT/HCPCS Code(s): 27407   Durable Medical Equipment: ☐ Rental ☐ Purchase

Description: Repair, primary, torn anterior cruciate ligament (Ⓛ Knee) CPT 27407

Date of Service: 12-23-20XX   Length of Stay (if applicable): 24-48 hrs

Place of Service or Vendor Name: Broadmoor Medical Center

Assistant Surgeon Requested? ☐ Yes ☑ No   Please list the code <u>and</u> narrative description:

1. ICD Code: ICD-10: M23.612; ICD-9: 717.89

    Description: Sprain/tear anterior cruciate ligament Ⓛ knee

2. ICD Code: _____

    Description: _____

Ordering Physician/Provider: John Langley, MD   Office Location: Suite 416 So. Vine   SSS-988-6604

FIRST <u>AND</u> LAST NAMES PLEASE   Milton, XY 12345.

Referring Physician/Provider: Francis Tompkins, MD

FIRST <u>AND</u> LAST NAMES PLEASE; REQUIRED FOR PRIME PLANS   FAX SSS-987-6540

Date: 11-14-20XX   Contact Person: Celia Reeves   Phone: SSS-987-6543

> ***Please note: Incomplete forms will delay the preauthorization process.***
> ***Requests received after 3:00 PM are processed the next working day.***
>
> PacificSource responds to preauthorization requests within 2 working days.
> A determination notice will be mailed to the requesting provider, facility, and patient.
>
> Please attach pertinent chart notes as appropriate.

FOR INTERNAL OFFICE USE ONLY:

STATUS: APPROVED / DENIED / PENDING / EXPLANATION   ENVISION Phone No.

DATE: 11-15-20XX ACUITY: UKN INITIALS: JIB   800-223-0000

Reason/Status R Code 56   S Code 114   Px Auth #004X39SRM

Hosp Auth #HSP003111

Field 11 Notes See pt record   LOS Approved F.W. Samules

☑ Chart notes filed with preauthorization

Notes Authorization numbers expire after 60 days

Field 10 Facility Copy 416 Suite 9 Bldg 4

Fig. 7.4 Preauthorization request form (Scoval).

Registration Data

1. Your Name <u>Scoval Dorothy M</u> Sex ☐ Male Date of Birth <u>10/16/1961</u>
   (Last)   (First)   (Middle) ☒ Female
2. Social Security #: <u>123-45-6789</u> Marital Status: Ⓢ M D Se W
3. Address: <u>320 Pine Grove</u> 4. <u>SSS-342-1110</u>
   (Street) (Phone)
   <u>Milton</u> <u>XY</u> <u>12345</u>
   (City) (State) (Zip)
5. Employer: <u>Kemper Engineering Inc</u> Occupation: <u>Eng. Asst.</u>
   Employer Address: <u>63 Highway 6West</u> <u>SSS-342-6780</u>
   (Work Phone)
   Spouse: _____ Employer: _____ Occupation: _____
   Employer Address: _____
   (Work Phone)

6.   Other Household Members Date of Birth Relationship
   _____ ___/___/___ _____
   _____ ___/___/___ _____
   _____ ___/___/___ _____
   _____ ___/___/___ _____
   _____ ___/___/___ _____

7. Medical Insurance Information

Ins. Company Name	Policy No.	Policy Holder	Sgl.	Type of Coverage Fmly.	Primary	Sec.
( ) Envision HMO	123456789	Self	☒	☐	☐	☐
( ) _____	_____	_____	☐	☐	☐	☐
( ) _____	_____	_____	☐	☐	☐	☐

8. Person to Contact in an Emergency <u>Henry Barton</u> Relationship to you <u>brother</u>
   Their Work Phone _____ Their Home Phone <u>SSS-342-1177</u>

9. Party with primary responsibility for payment: ☒ Self ☐ Other
   Name _____ Relationship to you _____
   Address _____ Home Phone _____

For Office Use Only

Date Completed _____ Account No. _____ Patient No. _____

Household Status ☐ Head of Household

☐ Spouse ☐ Child ☐ Other: _____

Head of Household Name _____

Fig. 7.5 Registration data sheet (Scoval).

PREAUTHORIZATION/ADMISSION FORM

Orders must be faxed to appropriate department. History and Physicals are required on all invasive procedures with conscious sedation. **If you have any questions, please call 555-992-XXXX.**

PATIENT INFORMATION

Patient Name: _____ SSN: _____ DOB: _____

PROVIDER INFORMATION

Policy Holder's Name: _____ SSN: _____

Policy Holder's Employer: _____ Employer's Phone Number: _____

Name of Health Plan: _____ Health Plan Phone Number: _____

Policy/ID #: _____ Group #: _____

PHYSICIAN INFORMATION

Physician Contact Person: _____ Coordinator's Phone Number: _____

Fax Number: _____ Primary Care Physician: _____

Requesting Physician: _____ Requesting Physician's Phone Number: _____

PROCEDURE INFORMATION

Procedure: _____ CPT Code: _____

Diagnosis: _____

Department(s) Involved *(Please check all appropriate areas.)*

OR_____ GI _____ RAD _____ Cath _____ CP _____ Women's Center _____ Day Surgery _____

Date of Procedure: _____ Authorized by: _____

Physician's Authorization Number: _____ Expiration Date: _____
Hospital Authorization Number: _____ Expiration Date: _____
Inpatient: _____ Outpatient: _____ Approximate Length of Stay: _____

Comments: _____
_____
_____

Fig. 7.6 Preauthorization/admission form (Scoval).

Performance Objective 7.2: Completing a Precertification Form

Conditions: Student will complete a precertification form (Fig. 7.7) for the upper gastrointestinal series from the information provided in the case study in Fig. 7.8. This is an outpatient procedure (length of stay is less than 24 hours). H & P and laboratory reports are to be attachments submitted with the precertification form. (**Note:** Student will be the "office contact person.")

Supplies/Equipment: Pen, Envision HMO precertification request form (see Fig. 7.7) and case study (see Fig. 7.8)

Time Allowed: 20 minutes

Accuracy Needed to Pass: 90%

Procedural Steps	Points Earned	Comments
Evaluator: Note time began: _____		
1. Carefully read and study the information provided and then complete the precertification form; 1 point is awarded for each correctly completed blank on the form.		
2. Patient information (7)		
3. Hospital information (3)		
4. Physician information (4)		
5. Procedure information (8)		
6. Diagnostic information (3)		
7. Student used a pen/wrote legibly (3)		
Optional: May deduct points for taking more time than allowed.		

Total Points = 28

Student's Score: _____

Evaluator: _____

Comments: _____

_____

_____

_____

_____

ENVISION HMO

REQUEST FOR INITIAL PRECERTIFICATION REVIEW
PHONE: 555-992-XXXX/FAX: 555-992-XXXX

Date:_____ Outpatient:_____ Inpatient:_____

Patient's Name:_____ Member #:_____ Group #:_____

Patient's Address:_____ DOB:_____

Hospital Name:_____ Phone #:_____

Hospital Address:_____

Physician Name:_____ Phone #:_____

Physician Address:_____

Office Contact Person:_____

Admission Date:_____ Anticipated Length of Stay:_____

Admitting DX Code:_____

Surgery/CPT Code:_____ Date of Surgery:_____

Related HX/Current Signs/Symptoms:_____

_____

_____

_____

_____

Lab Findings:_____

X-Ray/Diagnostic Findings:_____

Current Medications/Freq.:_____

Plan of Treatment:_____

_____

_____

FOR ENVISION USE ONLY: Date Received _____ by (initials) Date Referred for Review _____

Rev. Initials _____ Reference ID # _____ Date of PX Notification _____ Office Contact _____

Fig. 7.7 Request for initial precertification review (Oliver).

Case Study: Before performing certain diagnostic tests, it is customary to contact the patient's insurance carrier to make sure the procedure/service will be covered under his or her policy. This is referred to as *precertification*, which differs from preauthorization. This case study involves notifying the patient's insurance carrier of a planned diagnostic procedure.

Date: 4/19/20XX

Patient Name: Justin C. Oliver   DOB: 7/22/67   Record # OL72267
                916 No. Court   SS # 666-77-8888
                Milton, XY 12345

Patient is in the office today with continuing complaints of severe heartburn. He has been seen in the office by me on several occasions prior to this for treatment of GERD. He is currently on Naprosyn 500 mg BID with food PRN and Prevacid 15 mg one daily. He was advised on his last visit that if his stomach keeps bothering him with this heartburn, we may need to do a UGI or other testing. He is back in the office today requesting this procedure. He will be going to Envision Laboratory tomorrow for a CBC, CMP, lipid panel, and possibly a TSH. We will request a UGI to be performed at Broadmoor Medical Center on 4/22 and will see him back in 1 week.

Diagnosis   GERD K21.9   CPT Code for Upper Gastrointestinal (UGI) Series 74246
code: ICD-10

(s) Dennis R. Mulligan, MD   Broadmoor Medical Center
4353 Pine Ridge Drive, Suite 233   4500 Pine Ridge Drive
Milton, XY 12345   Milton, XY 12345
                                             Phone: 555-876-5433
                                             Fax: 555-876-5400

ENVISION HMO

Justin C. Oliver	**07/22/1967**	For Inpatient Preauthorization
Name	Date of Birth	Telephone: 800-223-0000
123654998 **01/17/20XX**	**92LMQ**	FAX 555-445-5555
Member No. Effective Date	Grp Code	
Dennis R. Mulligan, MD	**555-544-6601**	
Primary Care Physician	Telephone No.	

GHJKL   Copays   Office Visit $5
Pharmacy Code   ER/Outpatient $10
                           Inpatient $15

Fig. 7.8 Case study (Oliver).

Generate a Document for a Nonroutine HMO Patient

Morris Bennett comes to Broadmoor Medical Clinic, where you are employed as a health insurance professional, complaining of severe pain in the right lower quadrant accompanied by cramping, mild fever, and constipation of 4 days' duration. Morris is employed by John Deere Health, an HMO in Illinois, and became ill when visiting relatives over the Thanksgiving holiday in the city where your office is located. You contact his insurance carrier, and they fax Mr. Bennett this instruction sheet for claims purposes:

If you need to pay for care because of an emergency or urgent (nonroutine) situation when traveling outside of our network or on vacation, send an itemized bill including the following information:
1. Member's name and member ID
2. Date of service or supplies provided
3. State or country in which services were rendered or supplies obtained
4. Description of services/supplies
5. The provider's name, address, and tax identification number
6. An interpretation of the claim, if in a foreign language (any information provided will assist in making the proper payment determination and prevent delays)
7. Accident details (if applicable)

The chart notes indicate that Mr. Bennett has been under the care of Dr. Edgar Billingham for treatment of diverticulosis for quite some time. Today, he was prescribed ampicillin, 500 mg TID #30, and was instructed to drink only clear fluids for 2 to 3 days for bowel rest. He was given instructions regarding prevention and control of this disorder and told to see his family physician on returning home.

The claim address is John Deere Health, 4000 16th Avenue, Moline, XY 61265.

Include patient name, patient ID, and a daytime phone number at which the patient can be reached. Payment is subject to the terms and conditions of the Plan Administrator's benefit plan.

From the information on Mr. Bennett's registration and encounter forms (Figs. 7.9 and 7.10), (1) generate an itemized bill (using the blank ledger card in Fig. 7.11) and (2) compose a brief explanatory cover letter to accompany the bill.

Registration Data

1. Your Name __Bennett Morris T.__   Sex ☒ Male   Date of Birth __10-21-46__
   (Last)   (First)   (Middle)   ☐ Female

2. Social Security #: __333-44-SSSS__   Marital Status: S (M) D Se W

3. Address: __2900 Sunnylawn__   4. __SSS-343-2222__
   (Street)   (Phone)
   __Moline__   __IL__   __SSS66__
   (City)   (State)   (Zip)

5. Employer: __John Deere Enterprises__   Occupation: __Inspector__
   Employer Address: __4910 John Deere Blvd. Moline, IL SSS66__   __SSS-343-8762__
   (Work Phone)
   Spouse: __Frieda__   Employer: __N/A__   Occupation: __Housewife__

   Employer Address: _____   _____
   (Work Phone)

6.

Other Household Members	Date of Birth	Relationship
	/ /	
	/ /	
	/ /	
	/ /	
	/ /	

7. Medical Insurance Information

Ins. Company Name	Policy No.	Policy Holder	Sgl.	Type of Coverage Fmly.	Primary	Sec.
( ) __John Deere Health__	__333XLM__	__Morris Bennett__	☐	☒	☐	☐
( )			☐	☐	☐	☐
( )			☐	☐	☐	☐

8. Person to Contact in an Emergency __Frieda Bennett__ Relationship to you __Spouse__
   Their Work Phone _____   Their Home Phone __SSS-343-2229__

9. Party with primary responsibility for payment: ☒ Self   ☐ Other
   Name _____   Relationship to you _____
   Address _____   Home Phone _____

For Office Use Only

Date Completed _____   Account No. _____   Patient No. _____

Household Status   ☐ Head of Household

☐ Spouse   ☐ Child   ☐ Other: _____

Head of Household Name _____

Fig. 7.9 Registration data sheet (Bennett).

Broadmoor Medical Clinic

Date of service: 11/26/XX	Waiver? ☐
Patient name: Morris T. Bennett	Insurance: John Deere Health
	Subscriber name: Morris Bennett
Address: 2900 Sunnylawn, Moline, IL 55566	Group #: Previous balance: 0
	Copay: Today's charges: 250.00
Phone: 555-343-2222	Account #: 333XLM Today's payment: check# 5.00
DOB: 10/21/46 Age: Sex: M	Physician name: R. L. Jones, MD Balance due: 245.00

RANK	Office visit	New	Est	RANK	Office procedures			RANK	Laboratory		
	Minimal		99211		Anoscopy	46600		✓	Venipuncture	10.00	36415
	Problem focused	99201	99212		Audiometry	92551			Blood glucose, monitoring device		82962
	Expanded problem focused	99202	99213		Cerumen removal	69210			Blood glucose, visual dipstick		82948
✓	Detailed 85.00	99203	99214		Colposcopy	57452			CBC, w/ auto differential		85025
	Comprehensive	99204	99215		Colposcopy w/biopsy	57455			CBC, w/o auto differential		85027
	Comprehensive (new patient)	99205			ECG, w/interpretation	93000			Cholesterol		82465
	Significant, separate service	-25	-25	✓	ECG, rhythm strip	93040			Hemocult, guaiac	30.00	82270
	Well visit	New	Est		Endometrial biopsy	58100			Hemocult, immunoassay		82274
	< 1 y	99381	99391		Flexible sigmoidoscopy	45330			Hemoglobin A1C		85018
	1-4 y	99382	99392		Flexible sigmoidoscopy w/biopsy	45331			Lipid panel		80061
	5-11 y	99383	99393		Fracture care, cast/splint	29____			Liver panel		80076
	12-17 y	99384	99394		Site: ____				KOH prep (skin, hair, nails)		87220
	18-39 y	99385	99395		Nebulizer	94640			Metabolic panel, basic		80048
	40-64 y	99386	99396		Nebulizer demo	94664			Metabolic panel, comprehensive		80053
	65 y +	99387	99397		Spirometry	94010			Mononucleosis		86308
	Medicare preventive services				Spirometry, pre and post	94060			Pregnancy, blood		84703
	Pap		Q0091		Tympanometry	92567			Pregnancy, urine		81025
	Pelvic & breast		G0101		Vasectomy	55250			Renal panel		80069
	Prostate/PSA		G0103		Skin procedures		Units		Sedimentation rate		85651
	Tobacco counseling/3-10 min		99406		Burn care, initial	16000			Strep, rapid		86403
	Tobacco counseling/>10 min		99407		Foreign body, skin, simple	10120			Strep culture		87081
	Welcome to Medicare exam		G0344		Foreign body, skin, complex	10121			Strep A		87880
	ECG w/Welcome to Medicare exam		G0366		I&D, abscess	10060			TB		86580
	Flexible sigmoidoscopy		G0104		I&D, hematoma/seroma	10140		✓	UA, complete, non-automated 15.00		81000
	Hemocult, guaiac		G0107		Laceration repair, simple	120___			UA, w/o micro, non-automated		81002
	Flu shot		G0008		Site: ____ Size: ____				UA, w/ micro, non-automated		81003
	Pneumonia shot		G0009		Laceration repair, layered	120___			Urine colony count		87086
	Consultation/preop clearance				Site: ____ Size: ____				Urine culture, presumptive		87088
	Expanded problem focused		99242		Lesion, biopsy, one	11100			Wet mount/KOH		87210
	Detailed		99243		Lesion, biopsy, each add'l	11101		✓	Handling 10.00		99000
	Comprehensive/mod complexity		99244		Lesion,destruct.,benign,1-14	17110			Vaccines		
	Comprehensive/high complexity		99245		Lesion,destruct.,premal.,single	17000			DT, <7 y		90702
	Other services				Lesion,destruct.,premal.,ea.add'l	17003			DTP		90701
	After posted hours		99050		Lesion, excision, benign	114___			Flu, 6-35 months		90700
	Evening/weekend appointment		99051		Site: ____ Size: ____				Flu, 3 y +		90657
	Home health certification		G0180		Lesion, excision, malignant	116___			Hep A, adult		90658
	Home health recertification		G0179		Site: ____ Size: ____				Hep A, ped/adol, 2 dose		90632
	Post-op follow-up		99024		Lesion, paring/cutting, one	11055			Hep B, adult		90633
	Prolonged/30-74 min		99354		Lesion, paring/cutting, 2-4	11056			Hep B, ped/adol 3 dose		90746
	Special reports/forms		99080		Lesion, shave	113___			Hep B-Hib		90744
	Disability/Workers comp		99455		Site: ____ Size: ____				Hib, 4 dose		90748
	Radiology				Nail removal, partial	11730			HPV		90645
					Nail removal, w/matrix	11750			IPV		90649
					Skin tag, 1-15	11200			MMR		90713
	Diagnoses				Medications		Units		Pneumonia, >2 y		90707
1	K57.10				Ampicillin, up to 500mg	J0290			Pneumonia conjugate, <5 y		90732
2					B-12, up to 1,000 mcg	J3420			Td, >7 y		90669
3					Epinephrine, up to 1ml	J0170			Varicella		90718
4					Kenalog, 10mg	J3301			Immunizations & Injections		90716
	Next office visit				Lidocaine, 10mg	J2001			Allergen, one	95115	Units
	Recheck Prev PRN D W M Y				Normal saline, 1000cc	J7030			Allergen, multiple	95117	
	Instructions: Make appt w/pcp upon returning home				Phenergan, up to 50mg	J2550			Imm admin, one	90471	
					Progesterone, 150mg	J1055			Imm admin, each add'l	90472	
					Rocephin, 250mg	J0696			Imm admin, intranasal, one	90473	
					Testosterone, 200mg	J1080			Imm admin,intranasal,each add'l	90474	
	Referral				Tigan, up to 200 mg	J3250			Injection, joint, small	20600	
	To:				Toradol, 15mg	J1885			Injection, joint, intermediate	20605	
	Instructions:				Miscellaneous services				Injection, joint, major	20610	
									Injection, ther/proph/diag	90772	
									Injection, trigger point	20552	
	Physician signature								Supplies		
	X R. L. Jones, MD										

Fig. 7.10 Encounter form (Bennett).

Insurance:
John Deere Health HMO
ID# 333XLM
DOB: 10/21/1946
A/C#32100

STATEMENT

BROADMOOR MEDICAL CLINIC
4353 Pine Ridge Drive
Milton, XY 12345-0001
Telephone: 555-656-7890

Spouse: Frieda

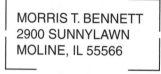

MORRIS T. BENNETT
2900 SUNNYLAWN
MOLINE, IL 55566

DATE 20XX	PROFESSIONAL SERVICE DESCRIPTION	CHARGE	CREDITS		CURRENT BALANCE
			PAYMENTS	ADJUSTMENTS	

Due and payable within 10 days.

Pay last amount in balance column ⇧

Fig. 7.11 Ledger card (Bennett).

Health Insurance Professional's Notebook

Continue construction of your notebook. In Chapter 7, you might want to include these items:

- A brief description of each of the HMO models
- An explanation of how HMOs in your area handle claims
- A description of how PPOs differ from HMOs
- A list of the PPOs in your area along with guidelines for completing CMS-1500 forms
- Examples of HMO and PPO cards with explanations of what each entry means (see Fig. 7.11)
- Examples of common forms used with managed care plans:
  - Preauthorization
  - Precertification
  - Referral
  - Request for consultation
  - Preadmission

ENRICHMENT ACTIVITIES

A. Contact an HMO or other managed care plan health insurance professional in your area. Interview the health insurance professional to determine (1) what benefits are offered and (2) how claims are handled. Request information brochures or fact sheets.

B. Visit a local medical facility that is a member of an HMO or other managed care plan. Interview the health insurance professional there to determine the differences in handling managed care cases compared with cases with traditional insurance. Request copies of any applicable office brochures and preauthorization/referral forms.

C. Generate a bulletin board collage of the various brochures, fact sheets, and forms you acquired from A and B.

Chapter Checklist

Student Name: _____

Chapter Completion Date: _____

Evaluate your classroom performance. Complete the self-evaluation and submit it to your instructor. When your instructor returns this form to you, compare your self-evaluation with the evaluation completed by your instructor.

1.	Record	Your start time and date: _____
2.	Read	The assigned chapter in the textbook
3.	View	PowerPoint slides (if available)
4.	Complete	Exercises in workbook as assigned
5.	Compare	Your answers to the answers posted on the bulletin board, website, or handout
5.	Correct	Your answers
7.	Complete	All tests and required activities
8.	Read	Assigned readings (if any)
9.	Complete	Chapter performance objectives (competencies), if any
10.	Evaluate	Your personal performance and submit it to your instructor
11.	Record	Your ending time and date: _____
12.	Move on	Begin next chapter as assigned

PERFORMANCE EVALUATION

Student Name: _____

Chapter Completion Date: _____

Evaluate your classroom performance. Compare this evaluation with the one provided by your instructor.

Skill	Student Self-Evaluation			Instructor Evaluation		
	Good	Average	Poor	Good	Average	Poor
Attendance/punctuality						
Personal appearance						
Applies effort						
Is self-motivated						
Is courteous						
Has positive attitude						
Completes assignments in timely manner						
Works well with others						

Student's Initials: _____

Date: _____

Points Possible: _____

Points Awarded: _____

Chapter Grade: _____

Instructor's Initials: _____

Date: _____

8 Understanding Medicaid

We learned in the textbook that Medicaid is a medical assistance program jointly financed by state and federal governments for low-income, blind, and disabled individuals. It was first enacted in 1965 as an amendment to the Social Security Act of 1935. Today, Medicaid is a major social welfare program and is administered by the Centers for Medicare and Medicaid Services (CMS) under the direction of the US Department of Health and Human Services (HHS).

The student workbook presents activities and work assignments to familiarize students with the structure of Medicaid and some of the more important issues and functions involved with the healthcare of Medicaid recipients. Because Medicaid health benefits differ from state to state, it is difficult to generate exercises that represent all states. The author uses a fictitious state—Xtra (XT)—and applies some of the more general rules to this state. It is important, however, for health insurance professionals to keep in mind that benefits, forms, and claims completion guidelines used herein are generic and may or may not apply to the Medicaid program in a particular state. On-the-job health insurance professionals should become familiar with the actual Medicaid guidelines in their area. Keep in mind that Medicaid is an ever-changing program, and it is important that health insurance professionals keep abreast of any changes.

WORKBOOK CHAPTER OBJECTIVES

After completing the workbook activities for Chapter 8, the student should be able to:
1. Define the terms used in the chapter.
2. Answer the review questions according to the evaluation criteria set by the instructor.
3. Demonstrate the ability to think logically and draw conclusions from facts and evidence.
4. Explore websites to acquire information needed to complete workbook activities.
5. Abstract applicable information from healthcare documents necessary for completion of various forms used in Medicaid claims.
6. Complete specific forms common to the health insurance professional's role in Medicaid claims.
7. Generate information and collect documents for inclusion in the student's personal Health Insurance Professional's Notebook relative to Medicaid.
8. Undertake self-analysis and evaluation in completed workbook activities.

DEFINING CHAPTER TERMS

Using the computer, students should write an accurate definition for each of the chapter terms listed. These definitions should be in the students' own words. When finished, students should compare their definitions with those listed in the glossary at the back of the textbook and correct any inaccuracies.

abuse	Emergency Medical Treatment and Labor Act (EMTALA)
adjudicated	fraud
Affordable Care Act (ACA)	HCBS Waivers programs
balance billing	mandated (or mandatory) services
capitation	Maternal and Child Health Services
categorically needy	Medicaid
Children's Health Insurance Program (CHIP)	Medicaid contractor
community call plan	Medicaid expansion
Community First Choice (CFC) Option	Medicaid Integrity Program (MIP)
cost avoid(ance)	Medicaid secondary claim
cost sharing	Medicaid "simple" claim
crossover claims	medically necessary
dual eligibility	medically needy
Early and Periodic Screening, Diagnosis, and Treatment (EPSDT)	Medicare-Medicaid (Medi-Medi)
	Medicare Savings Programs (MSPs)

125

modified adjusted gross income (MAGI)
participating provider
pay-and-chase claims
payer of last resort
Plan to Achieve Self-support (PASS)
preferred drug list
Program of All-Inclusive Care for the Elderly (PACE)
reciprocity
remittance advice (RA)

retroactive eligibility
spend down
subsidies
supplemental security income (SSI)
Temporary Assistance for Needy Families (TANF)
third-party liability (TPL)
Ticket to Work
urgent care centers

ASSESSMENT

Multiple Choice

Directions: In the questions and statements presented, choose the response that **best** answers or completes the stem and circle the letter that precedes it.

1. Title XIX of the Social Security Act of 1965 established:
   a. Social Security benefits to people older than 65
   b. Workers' compensation
   c. Medicare
   d. Medicaid

2. Medicaid is administered by:
   a. Congress
   b. The Centers for Medicare and Medicaid Services (CMS)
   c. The Social Security Administration
   d. The Federal Insurance Advisory Board

3. All Americans younger than age 65 with income at or lower than 133% of the Federal Poverty Level (FPL) were eligible for Medicaid beginning in the year:
   a. 2010
   b. 2012
   c. 2013
   d. 2014

4. SSI is a cash benefit program controlled by:
   a. The Social Security Administration
   b. The Centers for Medicare and Medicaid Services (CMS)
   c. Individual state governments
   d. The Federal Insurance Advisory Board

5. Categorically needy individuals typically include:
   a. Individuals receiving SSI
   b. Pregnant women and children
   c. Low income families
   d. All of the above

6. The term used for the process of depleting private or family finances to the point at which the individual or family becomes eligible for Medicaid assistance is:
   a. Cataloging
   b. Spend down
   c. Asset reduction
   d. Diminution

7. Identify which of these does *not* fall under the "mandatory" services that must be offered to categorically needy Medicaid beneficiaries:
   a. Inpatient hospital services
   b. Physician services
   c. Optometrist services and eyeglasses
   d. Laboratory and x-ray services

8. The optional services states can choose to provide to recipients of its Medicaid program include:
   a. Clinic services
   b. Physical and occupational therapy
   c. Dentures
   d. All of the above

9. A state option that provides individuals with disabilities who are eligible for nursing homes and other institutional settings with options to receive community-based services is called:
   a. Community First Choice Option
   b. Elderly Community Housing Program
   c. Medicaid Integrity Option
   d. Qualified Medicaid Beneficiary Option

10. Nearly all Medicaid contractors accept which type(s) of claims?
    a. Paper claims
    b. Telephone claims
    c. Electronic claims
    d. Both a and c

11. The program that provides comprehensive alternative care for noninstitutionalized elderly who otherwise would be in a nursing home is known as:
    a. SSI
    b. SSDI
    c. PACE
    d. Long-term care

12. An organization that Medicaid state programs typically contracts with that administer government healthcare programs, including claims processing, is called a(n):
    a. Third-party contractor
    b. Fiscal insurer
    c. Medicaid contractor
    d. Medicaid beneficiary

13. Cost-sharing cannot be charged for any of these *except:*
    a. Preventive services for children
    b. Pregnancy-related services
    c. Emergency services
    d. Cosmetic services

14. As a general rule, Medicaid only pays for services that are determined to be:
    a. Reciprocal
    b. Compulsory
    c. Preventive
    d. Medically necessary

15. Medicaid coverage should be verified:
    a. Every time a patient comes to the office
    b. At least once a month
    c. At least annually
    d. Biannually

16. Providers can reduce the number of denied claims by utilizing:
    a. Cost sharing
    b. Eligibility verification systems
    c. Paper claim forms
    d. Medicaid contractors

17. Aged or disabled individuals who are very poor are covered under the Medicaid and Medicare programs, commonly referred to as:
    a. Dual eligibles
    b. Medi-Medi
    c. Supplemental coverage
    d. Both a and b

18. All Medicare Savings Programs (MSPs), also known as Medicare buy-in programs, save the Medicare beneficiary money by paying for the:
    a. Part A premium
    b. Part B premium
    c. Part C premium
    d. All of the above

19. The differences between Medicare and Medicaid include all of these *except:*
    a. Medicare is a needs-based healthcare program.
    b. Medicaid requires mandatory contribution of all of a recipient's income in certain programs.
    c. Medicare is federally controlled and uniform across all states.
    d. Medicaid individuals do not have contributions deducted from wages.

20. It is good practice to file all Medicaid claims:
    a. In a timely manner
    b. Within 2 years of the date of services
    c. After the patient has been released from medical care
    d. Within 6 months

21. What kind of a claim is generated when the beneficiary has a second type of healthcare coverage?
    a. A Medicaid simple claim
    b. A Medicaid ancillary claim
    c. A Medicaid secondary claim
    d. A disproportionate share claim

22. When one state allows Medicaid beneficiaries from other states to be treated in its medical facilities, this exchange of privileges is referred to as:
    a. Reciprocity
    b. Medi-Medi
    c. Coinsurance
    d. Dual coverage

23. Every time a claim is sent to Medicaid, a document is generated explaining how the claim was adjudicated or how the payment was determined, which is called a:
    a. Crossover
    b. Documentation of services
    c. Payment resolution
    d. Remittance advice

24. Some Medicaid services require:
    a. A copayment
    b. Prior approval
    c. Preauthorization
    d. All of the above

128

25. When a healthcare provider engages in intentional misrepresentation or deception that could result in an unauthorized benefit to an individual, it is called:
    a. Fraud
    b. Abuse
    c. Negligence
    d. Malpractice

True/False

Directions: Place a "T" on the blank preceding the statement if it is true; place an "F" if the statement is false.

_F_ 1. Medicaid benefits are the same from state to state.

_T_ 2. All states have a Medicaid program.

_T_ 3. In 1972, federal law established the Supplemental Security Income (SSI) program, which provides federally funded cash assistance to unmarried pregnant women with dependent children.

_T_ 4. To be eligible for SSI, an individual must be at least 65 years old, blind, or disabled and must have limited resources.

_F_ 5. All states must cover the cost of prescription drugs for all categories of Medicaid recipients.

_T_ 6. In most states, SSI beneficiaries also can get medical assistance (Medicaid) to pay for hospital stays, doctor bills, prescription drugs, and other health costs.

_F_ 7. People who are eligible for SSI are not entitled to receive Social Security benefits.

_T_ 8. Eligibility for SSI benefits is based on an individual's employment record.

_T_ 9. States must cover categorically needy individuals, but they have options as to how to define "categorically needy."

_T_ 10. To be eligible for the PACE program, individuals must be 65 or older.

_F_ 11. Providers are never allowed to ask a Medicaid-eligible patient to make a copayment.

_T_ 12. Medicaid is allowed to impose cost-sharing charges and premiums on certain categories of Medicaid recipients.

_F_ 13. States cannot establish different copayment schedules for generic versus brand-name drugs.

_T_ 14. States have the option to charge higher copayments for people who visit a hospital emergency department for treatment of a nonemergency.

_T_ 15. All healthcare providers must accept and treat some categories of Medicaid patients.

_T_ 16. Healthcare providers have a choice whether or not to treat Medicaid patients.

_F_ 17. Providers must agree to accept what Medicaid pays as payment in full for covered services and are prohibited by law to "balance bill."

_T_ 18. With a point-of-sale device, the patient is issued an ID card that is similar in size and design to a credit card.

_F_ 19. Medicaid rarely pays all of the cost-sharing portions (deductibles and coinsurance) of Medicare Part A and B for dually eligible beneficiaries.

_F_ 20. Medicaid is always the "payer of last resort."

_F_ 21. Both federal and state governments discourage managed healthcare as an option for Medicaid benefits.

_F_ 22. The time limit for filing Medicaid claims in all states is 1 year.

_T_ 23. Assignment should be accepted on all Medicaid claims.

_T_ 24. Prior approval may be required for certain categories of Medicaid services.

_T_ 25. Fraud typically involves payment for items or services in which there was no intent to deceive or misrepresent.

Short Answer/Fill-in-the-Blank

Directions: Read the statements; then, using the textbook for review, insert the correct word or words that complete the sentence or answer the question.

1. Medicaid was originally created to give _____ access to healthcare.

2. The Medicaid program formerly referred to as Aid to Families with Dependent Children (AFDC) is now called _____ in many states.

3. List the groups that state programs must cover under broad federal guidelines.

4. The concept of the _____ process occurs when the state allows an individual to deduct the costs of his or her medical care in order to become eligible for Medicaid services in long-term care facilities, such as nursing homes.

5. As of January 1, 2006, full-benefit dual-eligible individuals began receiving drug coverage through what federal act?

   _____

6. List some of the mandatory services that Medicaid recipients must be provided with according to federal standards.

   _____

   _____

   _____

7. List some of the optional services that individual states can provide.

   _____

   _____

   _____

8. Define and explain the function of a Medicaid contractor.

   _____

9. List some common responsibilities of a Medicaid contractor.

   _____

   _____

   _____

10. List five ways to verify Medicaid eligibility.

   _____

   _____

   _____

   _____

   _____

11. Explain the basic differences between Medicare and Medicaid.

_____

_____

_____

_____

_____

12. List four examples of third-party liability (TPL).

_____

_____

_____

_____

_____

_____

CRITICAL THINKING ACTIVITIES

A. Explain the difference between "categorically needy" and "medically needy" and give examples of individuals who fall into each group.

B. You are a health insurance professional employed by Generic Family Practice. On September 7, 20XX, Emily Carson brought her 4-year-old son, Cory, to the office. Cory, who is complaining of ear pain and a sore throat, is new to the practice. Ms. Carson, a single mother, states that she and Cory are on Medicaid. After greeting Ms. Carson, what is the first thing you should do?

C. Brice Samuels, a 9-year-old girl, comes to Generic Family Practice on a monthly basis for follow-up treatment for a severe case of asthma. Gina Peters, a temp who is filling in for you during an absence, notes that Brice was eligible for Medicaid every month for the past 2 years. Assuming that Brice is eligible for Medicaid benefits on this visit, Gina neglects to verify current eligibility.
   1. What, if any, possible problems could result from Gina's failure to follow proper procedures?
   2. If Brice's visits have been covered by Medicaid for the past 2 years, what possible reasons might there be for Medicaid to discontinue benefits?

D. Lamont Frasier, the senior physician at Generic Family Practice and a Medicaid PAR, tells you that because he is getting close to retirement, he does not want you to accept any more Medicaid patients. "I have a total of 50 Medicaid patients, and that's enough," he tells you. What might be an appropriate response to Dr. Frasier's statement?

E. Dr. Frasier has several patients (65 or older) whom he sees periodically at the Sunshine Nursing Home. You do not see these patients, but you are responsible for the billing. Two of them are on Medicaid. How do you process Dr. Frasier's fees for these two Medicaid patients?

F. Dr. Alexandra Parsons, a psychiatrist, charges $250 for 1 hour of psychotherapy and $175 for a 30-minute session. She knows that Medicaid's allowable charge is $200 and $150, respectively, so she cuts the time she spends with her patients accordingly. When she counsels Wayne Gerber, she spends 40 minutes with him and charges Medicaid the full hour. She sees Tabitha Enrich for 20 minutes and charges Medicaid for the full 30 minutes. Dr. Parsons rationalizes that, by doing this, she does not lose so much money and really doesn't cheat the patient. You are Dr. Parsons' health insurance professional. Is this fraud? If so, what should you do?

PROBLEM-SOLVING/COLLABORATIVE (GROUP)

A. Beverly Franklin was driving her 8-year-old daughter Suzie to school on a foggy morning in April when her car was rear-ended by Tim Wright, father of another third-grade student. Suzie, who sustained cuts and bruises and complaining of neck pain, was brought to the Sunny Day Medical Clinic where you are employed as a health insurance professional. You verify that Suzie is eligible for Medicaid for the month of April, and after the encounter, you submit a claim to Medicaid.
1. Create a template for a Medicaid "simple" claim form by shading out all blocks that do not require completion. Use one of the blank universal CMS-1500 forms, provided in the back of the workbook, for this activity.
2. Using the top half of a blank CMS-1500 form, enter the correct information in all required blocks to generate a claim for Suzie Franklin. Use the information on the Medicaid ID card in Fig. 8.1. (Use ROBERT L JONES MD as the ordering provider in Block 17 preceded by qualifier DK. Enter Dr. Jones' NPI number [1234567890] in Block 17b.)

```
XTRA DEPARTMENT OF HUMAN SERVICES
MEDICAL ASSISTANCE ELIGIBILITY CARD

NOVEMBER  Month Valid                    20XX Year
30-8      Aid-Type      J35982000        29 County

PERSON ID        NAME          BIRTHDATE    OTHER
1300876G   BEVERLY FRANKLIN   12/10/1964    0002
2077200B    SUZIE FRANKLIN    02/05/2008    0000


   Client Address:  206 Elm Street     PH 555 666 8890
                    Middletown, XT 12345
```

Fig. 8.1 Medicaid ID card (Franklin).

B. A week after you submit the claim for Suzie Franklin, Medicaid denies the claim. Answer these questions for clarification and understanding of why Medicaid denied the claim.
1. In a situation such as this, why did Medicaid deny the claim, and what is the technical term for Medicaid's denial?
2. Who carries primary liability in this case?
3. What are your options for getting the claim paid?
4. If your state's policy allows Medicaid to "pay and chase," how will this affect payment of this claim?

C. Study the sample Medical Assistance ID (MAID) card in Fig. 8.2 and its accompanying key in Fig. 8.3. Then answer these questions (answers can be typed into a computer file and printed):
1. What are the name and address of the client, head of household, or guardian?
2. What are the dates of eligibility?
3. How can you determine whether this client is on Medicare?
4. What is the client's birth date?
5. Is this individual a client of the Division of Developmental Disabilities?
6. Is this individual covered under a private insurance plan?
7. Is this client restricted to one provider?
8. How would you know if this client has elected hospice care?
9. What do the alpha characters *CNP* indicate?

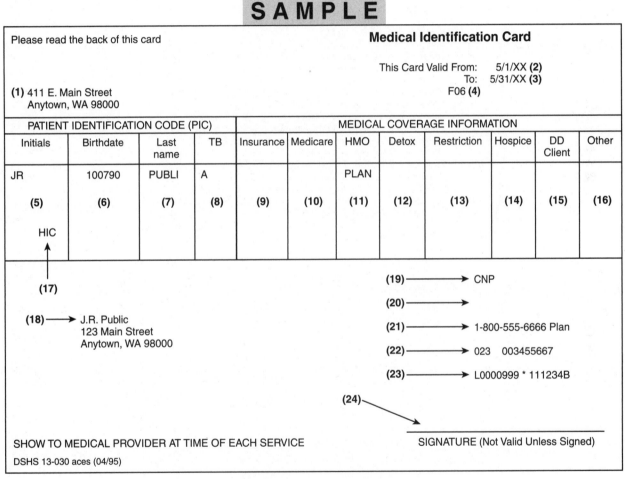

Fig. 8.2 Sample Medicaid ID card.

Key to Medical Assistance ID Card

Top Portion of the MAID Card:

1. Address of CSO
2. Date eligibility begins
3. Date eligibility ends
4. Medical coverage group

Patient Identification Code (PIC) Includes:

5. First and middle initials (or a dash [-] if the middle initial is not known)
6. Six-digit birth date, consisting of numerals only (MMDDYY)
7. First five letters of the last name (and spaces if the name is fewer than five letters)
8. Tie breaker (an alpha or numeric character)

Medical Coverage Information:

9. **Insurance carrier code:** A four-character alphanumeric code (insurance carrier code) in this area indicates the private insurance plan information
10. **Medicare:** An X indicates the Client has Medicare coverage
11. **HMO** (health maintenance organization): Alpha code indicates enrollment in an MAA Healthy Options managed healthcare plan. **Managed healthcare plan is the same as HMO.** This area may also contain the alpha code PCCM (Primary Care Case Manager)
12. **Detox:** An X indicates eligibility for a 3-day alcohol or a 5-day drug detoxification program
13. **Restriction:** An X indicates the Client is assigned to one provider and one pharmacist. The words "Client on review" in Field 20 will also indicate restricted Clients
14. **Hospice:** An X indicates the Client has elected hospice care
15. **DD Client:** An X indicates this person is a Client of the Division of Developmental Disabilities
16. **Other:** This area is not currently in use

Lower Portion of the MAID Card:

17. Alpha Code HIC indicates the Client is on Medicare
18. Indicates name and address of Client, head of household, or guardian
19. Indicates medical program and scope of care indicators
20. Space reserved for other messages (e.g., Client on review, delayed certification, emergency hospital only)
21. Indicates phone number and name of PCCM or Healthy Options plan
22. Indicates local field office (3 digits) and ACES assistance unit number (9 digits)
23. Internal control numbers for MAA use only
24. Client's signature may be used to verify identity of Client

Fig. 8.3 Key to Medicaid ID card.

PROJECTS/DISCUSSION TOPICS

A. The textbook discussed the terms *cost avoid* and *pay and chase*. These terms may be foreign to most health insurance students and may need further explanation for a better understanding. Research the meaning of these terms and prepare for an in-class discussion. Have examples to illustrate their meaning ready for presentation. **Note:** To research this topic, use the words "Medicaid cost avoid(ance)" and "Medicaid pay and chase" in your search engine.

B. Another term that may cause confusion is *adjudicated*. Prepare a clear and concise explanation of this term as it pertains to health insurance claims. Compare your definition with others in the class. With the help of your classmates, choose the five definitions you think are best. From this list, generate one final, all-inclusive definition.

C. Determine the statute of limitations regarding the retention of copies of Medicaid claims in your state by logging on to your state Medicaid website, contacting your local Medicaid contractor, or telephoning a medical facility in your area that provides services to Medicaid-eligible patients.

D. Fig. 8.4 in the workbook shows a sample Medicaid Identification Card for the state of Utah. Study it and be prepared for an in-class discussion regarding what information can be gathered from this document. (Disregard any illegible "coded" information.)

E. Prepare a one-page paper suitable for display in a medical facility's information library explaining the Qualified Medicare Beneficiary (QMB) and the Specified Low-Income Medicare Beneficiary (SLMB) programs.

1. Dates of Medicaid eligibility
2. Types of services covered
3. *Health Maintenance Organization indicator
4. Third Party Liability (insurance) indicator
5. Client name
6. Medicaid Identification Number
7. Sex is M or F: male/female
8. Date of birth
9. Age
10. *Medical Provider: HMO or Primary Care Provider
11. **Pharmacy provider
12. **Dental care provider
13. *Mental health services provider
14. Copayment/co-insurance indicators for certain types of services
15. TPL information
16. Additional Medicaid clients
17. (F) indicates a client entitled to the FULL scope of Medicaid services
18. Information for Medicaid client
19. Information for Medicaid Provider

*When a healthcare provider is identified for a service type, the client must use that provider.

**Managed care plans do not cover pharmacy, dental, or chiropractic services. Card states "A participating physician/pharmacist/dentist." The client may choose a provider who accepts Medicaid for the service needed.

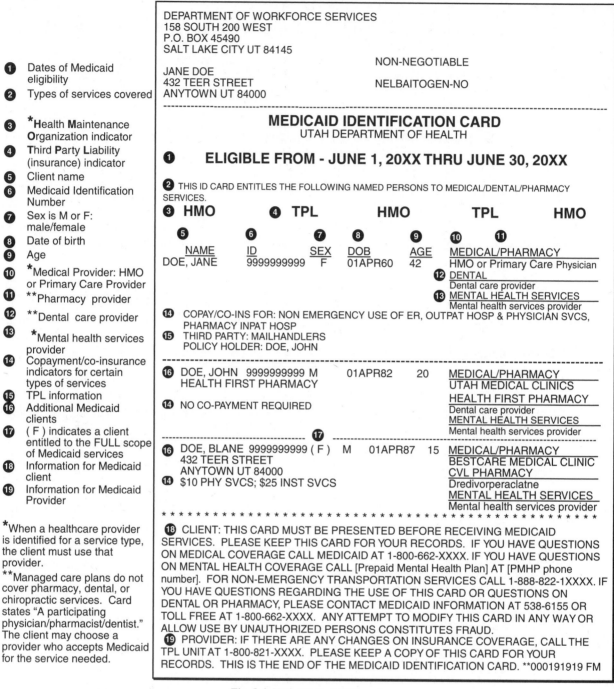

DEPARTMENT OF WORKFORCE SERVICES
158 SOUTH 200 WEST
P.O. BOX 45490
SALT LAKE CITY UT 84145

JANE DOE
432 TEER STREET
ANYTOWN UT 84000

NON-NEGOTIABLE

NELBAITOGEN-NO

MEDICAID IDENTIFICATION CARD
UTAH DEPARTMENT OF HEALTH

1 **ELIGIBLE FROM - JUNE 1, 20XX THRU JUNE 30, 20XX**

2 THIS ID CARD ENTITLES THE FOLLOWING NAMED PERSONS TO MEDICAL/DENTAL/PHARMACY SERVICES.

3 **HMO**   4 **TPL**   **HMO**   **TPL**   **HMO**

5 NAME	6 ID	7 SEX	8 DOB	9 AGE	10 11 MEDICAL/PHARMACY
DOE, JANE	9999999999	F	01APR60	42	HMO or Primary Care Physician

12 DENTAL
Dental care provider
13 MENTAL HEALTH SERVICES
Mental health services provider

14 COPAY/CO-INS FOR: NON EMERGENCY USE OF ER, OUTPAT HOSP & PHYSICIAN SVCS, PHARMACY INPAT HOSP
15 THIRD PARTY: MAILHANDLERS
POLICY HOLDER: DOE, JOHN

----

16 DOE, JOHN 9999999999 M   01APR82   20   MEDICAL/PHARMACY
HEALTH FIRST PHARMACY   UTAH MEDICAL CLINICS
                                                  HEALTH FIRST PHARMACY
14 NO CO-PAYMENT REQUIRED   Dental care provider
                                                  MENTAL HEALTH SERVICES
                                                  Mental health services provider

-- 17 --

16 DOE, BLANE 9999999999 (F)   M   01APR87   15   MEDICAL/PHARMACY
432 TEER STREET   BESTCARE MEDICAL CLINIC
ANYTOWN UT 84000   CVL PHARMACY
14 $10 PHY SVCS; $25 INST SVCS   Dredivorperaclatne
                                                        MENTAL HEALTH SERVICES
                                                        Mental health services provider

* *

18 CLIENT: THIS CARD MUST BE PRESENTED BEFORE RECEIVING MEDICAID SERVICES. PLEASE KEEP THIS CARD FOR YOUR RECORDS. IF YOU HAVE QUESTIONS ON MEDICAL COVERAGE CALL MEDICAID AT 1-800-662-XXXX. IF YOU HAVE QUESTIONS ON MENTAL HEALTH COVERAGE CALL [Prepaid Mental Health Plan] AT [PMHP phone number]. FOR NON-EMERGENCY TRANSPORTATION SERVICES CALL 1-888-822-1XXXX. IF YOU HAVE QUESTIONS REGARDING THE USE OF THIS CARD OR QUESTIONS ON DENTAL OR PHARMACY, PLEASE CONTACT MEDICAID INFORMATION AT 538-6155 OR TOLL FREE AT 1-800-662-XXXX. ANY ATTEMPT TO MODIFY THIS CARD IN ANY WAY OR ALLOW USE BY UNAUTHORIZED PERSONS CONSTITUTES FRAUD.
19 PROVIDER: IF THERE ARE ANY CHANGES ON INSURANCE COVERAGE, CALL THE TPL UNIT AT 1-800-821-XXXX. PLEASE KEEP A COPY OF THIS CARD FOR YOUR RECORDS. THIS IS THE END OF THE MEDICAID IDENTIFICATION CARD. **000191919 FM

Fig. 8.4 Utah Medicaid ID card.

CASE STUDIES

Complete a CMS-1500 for each of these case studies using the patient record, the Medicaid ID card, and the ledger card. Use a blank CMS-1500 form, located in the back of the workbook (or the practice management software, if available). Post the charges on the ledger card. (Date claim form submissions *1 day after encounter.*) Use the information in the Broadmoor Medical Clinic provider box for claims completion. The author has used eight-digit dates in all applicable blanks except Block 24A; however, follow your instructor's or your local Medicaid carrier's guidelines.

Provider Box	
Broadmoor Medical Clinic 4353 Pine Ridge Drive Milton, XY 12345-0001 Clinic NPI X100XX1000 Telephone: 555-656-7890	Clinic EIN No. 42-1898989 Robert L. Jones, MD; NPI 1234567890; Marilou Lucero, MD; NPI 2907511822; Date claims 1 day after examination Referring provider = DN Ordering provider = DK Supervising provider = DQ

Note: Unless specifically noted, assume that the provider signing the claim is the "ordering provider" of services. Completion of Blocks 14 through 17b is conditional on Medicaid claims. Some states require that Blocks 14, 15, and 16 be completed only if the provider is a chiropractor. Others require Blocks 17 through 17b be reported if the patient is a MediPASS recipient, and the MediPASS provider authorized the service. In such cases, the 10-digit NPI MediPASS authorization number is reported in Block 17a. In these workbook exercises, enter the name of the referring or ordering provider in Block 17 preceded by the two-letter code (see Provider Box) and report his or her NPI in Block 17b. **Acquire and follow your local Medicaid carrier's specific guidelines or use the Medicaid claims completion guidelines located in Appendix B in the back of the textbook.**

A. Medicaid patient Pricilla Atkins—Record No. 052541 (Figs. 8.5, 8.6, and 8.7).
   Guided Completion: For this exercise, you can use the CMS-1500 form or the practice management software, if available.

B. Medicaid patient Hattie Lawrence—Record No. 052544 (Figs. 8.8, 8.9, and 8.10).
   Guided Completion: For this exercise, you can also use the CMS-1500 claim form or the practice management software, if available.
   Note: This patient has both Medicare and Medicaid.

C. Using the Medicare/Medical Insurance Record Tracking Form (Fig. 8.11), post the two Medicaid claims generated in Case Studies A and B.
   Note: Remember to post the Medicaid claim filing notation on the ledger card.
   Note: If you are using the practice management software, enter the information for Atkins and Lawrence in the appropriate screens.

Patient Record No. 052541

Name: Pricilla Atkins   Birth Date: 06/15/99   Sex: F

Address: 456 Summer Street   City/State/Zip: Middletown, XT 12345

Employer/Occupation: _____

Employer Address/Phone No.: _____

Responsible Party (Spouse/Parent/Guardian): Sherril Atkins

Relationship to Patient: mother

Occupation/Employer: custodian at Silver Creek Shopping Center

Employer Address/Phone No.: 4500 Highway 406 W., Middletown, XT 12345

Primary Insurance: _____ Subscriber: _____

Policy No.: _____ Group No.: _____ Effective Date: _____

Other Insurance: _____ Subscriber: _____

Policy No.: _____ Group No.: _____ Effective Date: _____

Medicare No.: _____ Medicaid No.: 169426G   SSN: _____

Name/NPI of Referring Provider: _____

Referring Provider's Address/Phone No.: _____

PROGRESS NOTES

02/13/20XX   Pricilla returns to the office today for destruction of two flat warts on
                her left hand. The lesion that was removed from her right hand two
                weeks ago is healing nicely. RTN 2 wks.

DIAGNOSIS   Juvenile warts (B07.8) R. L. Jones, M.D.

CHARGES: 17110 Ex Les. x 2 (L) $80.00

Fig. 8.5 Patient record (Atkins).

**XTRA DEPARTMENT OF HUMAN SERVICES
MEDICAL ASSISTANCE ELIGIBILITY CARD**

| FEBRUARY Month Valid | | | 20XX Year |
| 30-8 Aid-Type | J35982000 | | 29 County |

PERSON ID	NAME	BIRTHDATE	OTHER
169426G	PRICILLA ATKINS	06/15/1999	0000
2899123B	JACOB ATKINS	11/22/2002	0000

Client Address: 456 Summer Street   PH 555 666 7377
Middletown, XT 12345

Fig. 8.6 Medicaid ID card (Atkins).

Ins: Medicaid
Ph # 555-666-7377

STATEMENT

169426G Pricilla 6/15/99
2899123B Jacob 11/22/02

BROADMOOR MEDICAL CLINIC
4353 Pine Ridge Drive
Milton, XY 12345-0001
Telephone: 555-656-7890

Mrs. Sherril Atkins
456 Summer Street
Middletown, XT 12345

DATE 20XX	PROFESSIONAL SERVICE DESCRIPTION	CHARGE	CREDITS		CURRENT BALANCE
			PAYMENTS	ADJUSTMENTS	
1/31	99212 OV EST (Pricilla)	65 00			65 00
1/31	17000 EX LES (RT)	45 00			110 00
2/3	Medicaid Claim	—			
2/10	Medicaid Ck#0317004		110 00		— 0 —

Due and payable within 10 days.   Pay last amount in balance column ⇧

Fig. 8.7 Ledger card (Atkins).

Patient Record No. 052544

Name: Hattie Lawrence   Birth Date: 06/02/1939   Sex: F

Address: 2925 Aspen Road   City/State/Zip: Milton, XT 12345

Employer/Occupation: unemployed

Employer Address/Phone No.: _____

Responsible Party (Spouse/Parent/Guardian): self

Relationship to Patient: _____

Occupation/Employer: _____

Employer Address/Phone No.: _____

Primary Insurance: _____ Subscriber: _____

Policy No.: _____ Group No.: _____ Effective Date: _____

Other Insurance: _____ Subscriber: _____

Policy No.: _____ Group No.: _____ Effective Date: _____

Medicare No.: 111223333A Medicaid No.: 788244F   SSN: 111-22-3333

Name/NPI of Referring Provider: Everette Barclay, MD 0045557111

Referring Provider's Address/Phone No.: 19 Royal Circle, Ste 440, Milton, XY 23456

PROGRESS NOTES

10/03/20XX   This elderly woman is in the office today complaining of mild pain in the R ear. This has been bothering her for about a week now. She has tried home remedies, which help some, but do not relieve the pain for more than a few hours. Today, she is having some associated dizziness. See H&P in health record.

Patient was given a prescription for E-Mycin and Benadryl OTC.

PLAN: Patient is to return in one week for recheck. If not improved, we will do a head CT scan and arrange for hearing test.

DX   Labyrinthitis (H83.01) *M. Lucero*

CHARGES: 99212 OV EST PT $60.00

Fig. 8.8 Patient record (Lawrence).

```
XTRA DEPARTMENT OF HUMAN SERVICES
MEDICAL ASSISTANCE ELIGIBILITY CARD

OCTOBER  Month Valid                              20XX Year
31-6      MM-Type        J35982000                29 County

PERSON ID        NAME           BIRTHDATE    OTHER
788244F      HATTIE LAWRENCE    06/02/1939   0003




Client Address: 2925 Aspen Road        PH 555 666 2244
                Middletown, XT 12345
```

Fig. 8.9 Medicaid ID card (Lawrence).

Medicaid 788244F
Medicare 111223333A
Ph # 555-666-2244

STATEMENT

BROADMOOR MEDICAL CLINIC
4353 Pine Ridge Drive
Milton, XY 12345-0001
Telephone: 555-656-7890

Ms. Hattie Lawrence
2925 Aspen Road
Middletown, XT 12345

| DATE 20XX | PROFESSIONAL SERVICE DESCRIPTION | CHARGE | CREDITS | | CURRENT BALANCE |
			PAYMENTS	ADJUSTMENTS	

Due and payable within 10 days.   Pay last amount in balance column ⇧

Fig. 8.10 Ledger card (Lawrence).

Name: Broadmoor Med. Clinic

Year: 20XX **Page:** 122

**Medical Insurance
Record Tracking Form**

Service Provided			Medicare/Medicaid						Private Insurance			Patient Responsibility	
Date of Service	Patient Name & ID Number	CPT Service Codes	Assigned Y or N	Amount Billed	Amount Approved	Applied To Deductible	Amount Paid Provider	Amount Paid Patient	Date Sent	Amount Paid Provider	Amount Paid Patient	Amount Patient Paid	Date Paid Check #

Fig. 8.11 Insurance tracking form.

A. Find the appropriate website for your state Medicaid program. (**Hint:** Enter your state's name and *Medicaid*—e.g., Iowa Medicaid or Iowa Department of Human Services.) Determine the:
- Current Medicaid contractor
- Optional covered benefits for your state
- List of programs your state offers
- Claim submission information

B. Some states provide a choice of Medicaid plans—fee for service or managed care. Visit your state's Medicaid website to see if your state offers both a fee-for-service and a managed care choice. If so, generate a chart comparing the two plans. If your state does not have a managed care plan, choose one that does.

C. Visit the CMS fraud and abuse website at http://www.cms.gov/Medicare-Medicaid-Coordination/Fraud-Prevention/ FraudAbuseforConsumers/Report_Fraud_and_Suspected_Fraud.html. Create a page for the Office Procedures Manual giving step-by-step instructions for reporting suspected fraud and abuse in your state. Include a list of pertinent names, addresses, and telephone numbers.

D. Visit the CMS website at https://www.medicaid.gov/chip/chip-program-information.html.
- Review the CHIP policy.
- Study how children qualify for coverage under CHIP.
- Determine any cost-sharing regulations.
- What is CHIPRA?

Note: If any of these websites are no longer valid links, use appropriate search words to locate related sites that provide similar information.

PERFORMANCE OBJECTIVES

Use the blank CMS-1500 forms and ledger cards (back of workbook) or the practice management software (if available) for the exercises in these performance objectives.

Important Note: The Medicaid patients in Broadmoor Medical Clinic must pay a 10% copayment for services and procedures rendered.

Performance Objective 8.1: Medicaid Simple Claim

Conditions: Student will complete a Medicaid "simple" claim and ledger card using the information in Patient Record No. 052547.

Supplies/Equipment: Patient Record No. 052547 (Fig. 8.12), CMS-1500 claim form (paper or electronic), and blank ledger card (paper or electronic)

Practice Management: To complete this exercise using practice management software, refer to the Evolve site to follow directions.

Time Allowed: 50 minutes

Accuracy Needed to Pass: 90%

Procedural Steps	Points Earned	Comments
Evaluator: Note time began: _____		
1. Carefully read and study Patient Record No. 052547.		
2. Complete ALL blocks required for a Medicaid simple claim. (30)		
3. Generate a ledger card; post date of OV, CPT code/description, fee, copayment, and balance. (14)		
4. Note Medicaid claim submission. (1)		
5. Proofread the claim for accuracy.		
Optional: May deduct points for taking more time than allowed.		

Total Points = 45

Student's Score: _____

Evaluator: _____

Comments: _____

_____

_____

_____

_____

Patient Record No. 052547

Name: Charles T. Brown   Birth Date: 07/30/2000   Sex: M

Address: 55 N. Winston Dr.   City/State/Zip: Middletown, XT 12345

Employer/Occupation: student

Employer Address/Phone No.: _____

Responsible Party (Spouse/Parent/Guardian): Marvel Brown   Phone: 555-334-3344

Relationship to Patient: father   (Same address)

Occupation/Employer: janitor – Washington Heights Apartments

Employer Address/Phone No.: 3939 Belview Ct., Middletown, XT 12345

Primary Insurance: BCBS**   Subscriber: Marvel Brown

Policy No.: _____ Group No.: _____ Effective Date: _____

Other Insurance: _____ Subscriber: _____

Policy No.: QKZ111006666   Group No.: _____ Effective Date: _____

Medicare No.: _____ Medicaid No.: 5748392   SSN: _____

Name/NPI of Referring Provider: _____

Referring Provider's Address/Phone No.: _____

PROGRESS NOTES

11/09/20XX

CC	Charles is a new patient in the office today with complaints of pain and swelling in the R ankle. Applying weight on the ankle causes the pain to increase. He reports that he "crashed into another player" during soccer practice at the YMCA today.
PX	See patient's health record. X-ray revealed no fracture.
ASSESSMENT	Sprain, R ankle (S93.401A)
PLAN	Charles was referred to Dr. Jamie Richards in the Orthopedic Clinic for treatment. *M. Lucero*

Charges: 99202   OV New PT $65.00
            73600   X-ray R ankle   40.00

**Pt not covered under father's BCBS plan.

Fig. 8.12 Medical record (Brown).

Performance Objective 8.2: Medicaid Secondary Claim

Conditions: Student will complete a Medicaid secondary claim and ledger card using the information in Patient Record No. 052545.

Supplies/Equipment: Patient Record No. 052545 (Fig. 8.13), CMS-1500 claim form (paper or electronic), and blank ledger card (paper or electronic)

Practice Management: To complete this exercise using practice management software, refer to the Evolve site to follow directions.

Time Allowed: 50 minutes

Accuracy Needed to Pass: 90%

Procedural Steps	Points Earned	Comments
Evaluator: Note time began: _____		
1. Carefully read and study Patient Record No. 052545.		
2. Complete ALL blocks required for a Medicaid secondary (BCBS) claim. (32)		
3. Generate a ledger card; post date of OV, CPT code/description, fee, copayment, and balance. (4)		
4. Note BCBS claim submission. (1)		
5. Proofread the claim for accuracy.		
Optional: May deduct points for taking more time than allowed.		

Total Points = 40

Student's Score: _____

Evaluator: _____

Comments: _____

_____

_____

_____

_____

Patient Record No. 052545

Name: Tyler Swanson   Birth Date: 01/04/2001   Sex: M

Address: 529 Parkway   City/State/Zip: Middletown, XT 12345
                                   Phone: 555-766-1100

Employer/Occupation: student

Employer Address/Phone No.: _____

Responsible Party (Spouse/Parent/Guardian): Connie Templeton (same address)

Relationship to Patient: legal guardian   DOB: 04/22/1968

Occupation/Employer: Administrative Assistant

Employer Address/Phone No.: Superior Insurance Adjustment Bureau

Primary Insurance: Blue Cross/Blue Shield** Subscriber: Connie Templeton

Policy No.: QXY654321100 Group No.: XYZ12   Effective Date: 12/31/1998

Other Insurance: _____ Subscriber: _____

Policy No.: _____ Group No.: _____ Effective Date: _____

Medicare No.: _____ Medicaid No.: 13647780 SSN: 654-00-1111

Name/NPI of Referring Provider: _____

Referring Provider's Address/Phone No.: _____

PROGRESS NOTES

2/04/20XX	Tyler is a new patient to the practice. He complains of R ear pain and sore throat of two days' duration.
PX	See health record
ASSESSMENT	Acute tonsillitis
PLAN	Bedrest and fluids. Amoxicillin, 250 mg. x 12. Rtn 1 wk PRN.
DX	Otitis media, acute (H65.01) *M. Lucero*
Charges:	99202 OV New PT $65.00

**Patient is covered under his guardian's BCBS plan. Medicaid coverage is under his name only. Connie is not a Medicaid recipient.

ICD-10 code (H65.01) indicates the right ear is affected.

Fig. 8.13 Medical record (Swanson).

Performance Objective 8.3: Medicare/Medicaid Claim

Conditions: Student will complete a Medicare/Medicaid claim and ledger card using the information in Patient Record No. 052548.

Supplies/Equipment: Patient Record No. 052548 (Fig. 8.14), CMS-1500 claim form (paper or electronic), and blank ledger card (paper or electronic)

Time Allowed: 50 minutes

Accuracy Needed to Pass: 90%

Procedural Steps	Points Earned	Comments
Evaluator: Note time began: _____		
1. Carefully read and study Patient Record No. 052548.		
2. Complete ALL blocks required for a Medicare/Medicaid claim. (30)		
3. Generate a ledger card; post date of OV, CPT code/description, fee, copayment, and balance. (14)		
4. Note insurance claim submission. (1)		
5. Proofread the claim for accuracy.		
Optional: May deduct points for taking more time than allowed.		

Total Points = 40

Student's Score: _____

Evaluator: _____

Comments: _____

_____

_____

_____

_____

Patient Record No. 052548

Name: Margaret R. Phillips   Birth Date: 03/21/1940   Sex: F

Address: 1893 Edgewood Place   City/State/Zip: Middletown, XT 12345

                                                  Phone: 555-985-2318

Employer/Occupation: retired

Employer Address/Phone No.: _____

Responsible Party (Spouse/Parent/Guardian): Frederick Phillips (son)

Relationship to Patient: son

Occupation/Employer: farmer – self-employed

Employer Address/Phone No.: _____

Primary Insurance: _____ Subscriber: _____

Policy No.: _____ Group No.: _____ Effective Date: _____

Other Insurance: _____ Subscriber: _____

Policy No.: _____ Group No.: _____ Effective Date: _____

Medicare No.: 666554444B   Medicaid No.: 123321456   SSN: 666-55-4444

Name/NPI of Referring Provider: Olin Swenson, MD   0814551100

Referring Provider's Address/Phone No.: _____

PROGRESS NOTES

4/22/20XX

CC   Margaret is here again today complaining of redness and "crusting" of the L eyelid, which began yesterday morning. She is accompanied by her son who reports that several of the residents at WondraCare Assisted Living are suffering from similar complaints.

PX   See patient's health record for PX

ASSESSMENT   Chronic follicular conjunctivitis (H10.432)

PLAN   Patient was advised not to rub her eyes. Apply cool compresses to the affected eye several times a day. Trifluridine 1%. Rtn 1 wk PRN.

                           R. L. Jones

Charges: 99212   OV Est Pt. $60.00

Fig. 8.14 Medical record (Phillips).

Performance Objective 8.4: Medicaid/Commercial Claim

Conditions: Student will complete a Medicaid/Commercial claim and ledger card using the information in Patient Record No. 052543.

Supplies/Equipment: Patient Record No. 052543 (Fig. 8.15), CMS-1500 claim form (paper or electronic), and blank ledger card (paper or electronic)

Time Allowed: 50 minutes

Accuracy Needed to Pass: 90%

Procedural Steps	Points Earned	Comments
Evaluator: Note time began: _____		
1. Carefully read and study Patient Record No. 052543.		
2. Complete ALL blocks required for a Commercial/Medicaid claim. (30)		
3. Generate a ledger card; post date of OV, CPT code/description, fee, copayment, and balance. (14)		
4. Note insurance claim submission. (1)		
5. Proofread the claim for accuracy.		
Optional: May deduct points for taking more time than allowed.		

Total Points = 45

Student's Score: _____

Evaluator: _____

Comments: _____

_____

_____

_____

_____

Patient Record No. 052543

Name: Inga M. Jones   Birth Date: 8/10/1962   Sex: F

Address: 600 Lincoln Way   City/State/Zip: Middletown, XT 12345

Employer/Occupation: Daycare aide at Babes R Us DayCare

Employer Address/Phone No.: 2551 Ridgemont, Middletown, XT 12345

Responsible Party (Spouse/Parent/Guardian): self   (NO PHONE)

Relationship to Patient: _____

Occupation/Employer: _____

Employer Address/Phone No.: _____

Primary Insurance: Allgood Life & Health   Subscriber: Inga Jones

Policy No.: 44355QWP   Group No.: 55X9L   Effective Date: 01/01/1999

Other Insurance: _____   Subscriber: _____

Policy No.: _____   Group No.: _____   Effective Date: _____

Medicare No.: _____   Medicaid No.: 44637620011   SSN: 444-44-4444

Name/NPI of Referring Provider: _____

Referring Provider's Address/Phone No.: _____

PROGRESS NOTES

11/06/20XX

CC	New pt Inga Jones is in the office today with complaints of headache, fever, and cough of 2 days' duration. Pt works at a daycare center and reports that many of the children have colds and flu.
PX	See H&P in patient health record.
ASSESSMENT	Influenza w/cold (J10.1)
PLAN	Bedrest, fluids and OTC cold remedies. No prescriptions at this time. Rtn 1 wk PRN if symptoms don't improve.
11/07/20XX	Pt returns today with worsening symptoms of a "tight feeling" in her chest, nausea, and sore throat. Reported fever of 102.3 last night. Chest x-ray was clear.
ASSESSMENT	Acute bronchitis (J20.9) *R. L. Jones*
PLAN	Penicillin 5cc IM. Rtn 1 wk PRN.
CHARGES:	99202 OV New Pt. $55.00 99214 OV Est. PT $170.00

Fig. 8.15 Medical record (Jones).

Performance Objective 8.5: Posting Payments from Medicaid Remittance Advice (RA)

Conditions: Student will post payments from a Medicaid RA on ledger cards for five patients.

Supplies/Equipment: Pen, RA No. 433900 (Fig. 8.16) from XT Department of Human Services; and five patient ledger cards (Figs. 8.17 through 8.21)

Note: For Inga Jones, Allgood Life & Health paid $0 on this claim and then "crossed it over" to Medicaid.

Time Allowed: 50 minutes

Accuracy Needed to Pass: 90%

Procedural Steps	Points Earned	Comments
Evaluator: Note time began: _____		
1. Carefully read and study RA #433900; note the Medicaid patients in this clinic must pay 10% co-payment for office visits on the day they are seen.		
2. RA and Medicaid check was received on 11/28/20XX.		
3. Correctly post payments on the ledger cards for these patients:		
I. M. Jones (8)		
C. T. Brown (8)		
J. L. Doe (8)		
E. Martin (8)		
J. Ruiz (3)		
4. Proofread each ledger card for accuracy.		
Optional: May deduct points for taking more time than allowed.		

Total Points = 35

Student's Score: _____

Evaluator: _____

Comments: _____

_____

_____

_____

_____

XT DEPARTMENT OF HUMAN SERVICES
MEDICAID MANAGEMENT INFORMATION SYSTEM

REMITTANCE ADVICE

RA No. 433900
MMIS Ck No. 0098887

TO: HARPER, DANIEL, MD   PROVIDER NO.   12345678   REPORT SEQ NUMBER: 3   DATE: 11/24/20XX
606 BRIDGE STREET   POLICY/BILLING   800-555-0987   R/S NUMBER   987654343   PAGE   1
MIDDLETOWN, XT 12345

PATIENT NAME/ID NO. SERVICE DATES FROM TO	PERF PROV NO.	DAYS QTY	PROC CODE	PROCEDURE DESCRIPTION	AMOUNT BILLED	AMOUNT ALLOWED	COPAY	PAID AMOUNT	EOB CODES
PAID OR DENIED CLAIMS									
JONES, I.M./44637620011 11/06/20XX 11/07/20XX	81234123 81234123	1 1	99202 99214	OFFICE/OP VISIT–NEW PT OFFICE/OP VISIT–ESTABL PT	55.00 170.00	49.50 152.00	5.50 17.00	44.00 135.00	12 12
BROWN, C.T./44637112001 11/09/20XX	12345678	1	99202 73600	OFFICE/OP VISIT–NEW PT XRAY ® ANKLE	65.00 40.00	50.50 38.00	6.50 4.00	44.00 34.00	12 12
DOE, J.L./44637220887 11/11/20XX	12345678	1	99218	INITIAL OBSERVATION CARE	110.00	110.00	N/A	110.00	14
MARTIN, E./4463771124 11/15/20XX 11/15/20XX 11/15/20XX	12345678 81234123 81234123	1 1 1	99205 99175 99401	OFFICE/OP VISIT–NEW PT IPECAC/SIM ADMIN FOR IND EMESIS COUNSELLING/RISK FX (15 MIN)	225.00 35.00 50.00	212.00 35.00 25.00	22.50 N/A 5.00	189.50 35.00 7.50	12 14 13
RUIZ, JUAN/446375566 11/19/20XX	81234123	1	96900	ACTINOTHERAPY (UV)	25.00	0.00	2.50	0.00	15
TOTALS					775.00	672.00	63.00	611.50	

EOB CODES:
12 Service paid at the maximum amount allowed by Medical Assistance Reimbursement policies
13 Service paid at 50% of amount allowed by Medical Assistance Reimbursement policies
14 Service paid at 100% by Medical Assistance Reimbursement policies
15 Service not allowed by Medical Assistance Reimbursement policies

Fig. 8.16 Medicaid remittance advice (RA).

STATEMENT

BROADMOOR MEDICAL CLINIC
4353 Pine Ridge Drive
Milton, XY 12345-0001
Telephone: 555-656-7890

INGA M. JONES
600 LINCOLN WAY
MIDDLETOWN, XT 12345

DATE 20XX	PROFESSIONAL SERVICE DESCRIPTION	CHARGE	CREDITS		CURRENT BALANCE
			PAYMENTS	ADJUSTMENTS	
11/06	99202 OV NP	55 00	5 50		49 50
11/07	99214 OV EST PT	170 00	17 00		202 50
11/08	Medicaid claim				

Due and payable within 10 days.   **Pay last amount in balance column** ⇧

Fig. 8.17 Ledger card (Jones).

STATEMENT

BROADMOOR MEDICAL CLINIC
4353 Pine Ridge Drive
Milton, XY 12345-0001
Telephone: 555-656-7890

MARVEL BROWN
55 NORTH WINSTON DR.
MIDDLETOWN, XT 12345

DATE 20XX	PROFESSIONAL SERVICE DESCRIPTION	CHARGE	CREDITS		CURRENT BALANCE
			PAYMENTS	ADJUSTMENTS	
11/09	99202 Charles OV NP	65 00	6 50		58 50
11/09	73600 X-ray ® ankle	40 00	4 00		94 50
11/10	Medicaid claim				

Due and payable within 10 days.   **Pay last amount in balance column** ⇧

Fig. 8.18 Ledger card (Brown).

STATEMENT

BROADMOOR MEDICAL CLINIC
4353 Pine Ridge Drive
Milton, XY 12345-0001
Telephone: 555-656-7890

JERAMIAH L. DOE
14 HILLCREST CIRCLE
MIDDLETOWN XT 12345

DATE 20XX	PROFESSIONAL SERVICE DESCRIPTION	CHARGE		CREDITS				CURRENT BALANCE	
				PAYMENTS		ADJUSTMENTS			
11/11	99218 Init Obs. Care	110	00					110	00
11/12	Medicaid claim								

Due and payable within 10 days.   **Pay last amount in balance column** ⇧

Fig. 8.19 Ledger card (Doe).

STATEMENT

BROADMOOR MEDICAL CLINIC
4353 Pine Ridge Drive
Milton, XY 12345-0001
Telephone: 555-656-7890

MRS. ELOISE C. MARTIN
543 MAPLE STREET
MIDDLETOWN, XT 12345

DATE 20XX	PROFESSIONAL SERVICE DESCRIPTION	CHARGE	CREDITS		CURRENT BALANCE
			PAYMENTS	ADJUSTMENTS	
11/15	99205 OV NP	225 00	22 50		202 50
11/15	99175 Ipecac Adm.	35 00	—		237 50
11/15	99401 Couns/Risk Fx	50 00	5 00		282 50
11/16	Medicaid claim				

Due and payable within 10 days.

Pay last amount in balance column ⇧

Fig. 8.20 Ledger card (Martin).

STATEMENT

BROADMOOR MEDICAL CLINIC
4353 Pine Ridge Drive
Milton, XY 12345-0001
Telephone: 555-656-7890

JUAN RUIZ
1500 SOUTH 9TH ST.
MIDDLETOWN, XT 12345

DATE 20XX	PROFESSIONAL SERVICE DESCRIPTION	CHARGE		CREDITS			CURRENT BALANCE	
				PAYMENTS	ADJUSTMENTS			
11/19	96900 Actinotherapy	25	00	2 50			22	50
11/20	Medicaid claim							

Due and payable within 10 days.   **Pay last amount in balance column** ⇧

Fig. 8.21 Ledger card (Ruiz).

Performance Objective 8.6: Posting Claims to Medical Insurance Record

Tracking Form Conditions: Student will post the claims generated in Performance Objectives 8.1 through 8.4 and patient payments and payments received from the third-party insurers, using the insurance tracking form begun in Case Study C (see Fig. 8.11).

Supplies/Equipment: Pen or computer and medical insurance record tracking form

Time Allowed: 50 minutes

Accuracy Needed to Pass: 90%

Procedural Steps	Points Earned	Comments
Evaluator: Note time began: _____		
1. Assemble the four claims generated in Performance Objectives 8.1 through 8.4.		
2. Post the applicable information to the insurance tracking form begun in Case Study C.		
3. Correctly post the applicable information for these claims:		
Brown (5)		
Swanson (5)		
Phillips (5)		
Jones (5)		
4. Proofread your entries for accuracy.		
Optional: May deduct points for taking more time than allowed.		

Total Points = 20

Student's Score: _____

Evaluator: _____

Comments: _____

_____

_____

_____

_____

APPLICATION EXERCISES

Health Insurance Professional's Notebook

Generate a section in your notebook for Medicaid information. You should include the following information and documents, as well as other information or forms that you find pertinent:

- Medicaid's contractor in your state
- Names and telephone numbers of Medicaid contractor
- Sample Medicaid ID cards with explanations
- List of procedures and services covered by Medicaid in your state
- Sample claim form required by the Medicaid contractor
- Guidelines for completing the required claim form
- Template showing blocks on the claim that require completion
- Sample Medicaid remittance advice with explanations and interpretations
- Sample completed claims for:
  - Medicaid simple
  - Medicaid secondary
  - Medicare/Medicaid
- Helpful websites for additional provider information

Chapter Checklist

Student Name: _____

Chapter Completion Date: _____

Evaluate your classroom performance. Complete the self-evaluation and submit it to your instructor. When your instructor returns this form to you, compare your self-evaluation with the evaluation completed by your instructor.

1.	Record	Your start time and date: _____
2.	Read	The assigned chapter in the textbook
3.	View	PowerPoint slides (if available)
4.	Complete	Exercises in workbook as assigned
5.	Compare	Your answers to the answers posted on the bulletin board, website, or handout
5.	Correct	Your answers
7.	Complete	All tests and required activities
8.	Read	Assigned readings (if any)
9.	Complete	Chapter performance objectives (competencies), if any
10.	Evaluate	Your personal performance and submit it to your instructor
11.	Record	Your ending time and date: _____
12.	Move on	Begin next chapter as assigned

Student Name: _____

Chapter Completion Date: _____

Evaluate your classroom performance. Compare this evaluation with the one provided by your instructor.

Skill	Student Self-Evaluation			Instructor Evaluation		
	Good	**Average**	**Poor**	**Good**	**Average**	**Poor**
Attendance/punctuality						
Personal appearance						
Applies effort						
Is self-motivated						
Is courteous						
Has positive attitude						
Completes assignments in timely manner						
Works well with others						

Student's Initials: _____   **Instructor's Initials:** _____

Date: _____   **Date:** _____

Points Possible: _____

Points Awarded: _____

Chapter Grade: _____

9 Conquering Medicare's Challenges

Medicare is the United States health insurance program for people age 65 or older, certain people with disabilities who are younger than age 65, and people of any age who have permanent kidney failure (end-stage renal disease [ESRD]). Medicare provides basic protection against the cost of healthcare, but it does not cover all medical expenses or the cost of most long-term care. The Medicare program is financed by a portion of the Federal Insurance Contributions Act (FICA) taxes paid by workers and their employers. It is also financed partly by monthly premiums paid by beneficiaries. The Centers for Medicare and Medicaid Services (CMS) (formerly the Health Care Financing Administration [HCFA]) is the federal agency in charge of the Medicare program. The Social Security Administration determines who is eligible for Medicare, enrolls individuals in the program, and distributes general Medicare information.

Medicare may be the most challenging of all healthcare reimbursement programs. It is composed of several different components (Parts A, B, C, and D). These parts and what is covered under each tend to change frequently. It is important that health insurance professionals understand the specifics of Medicare not only for their own benefit and the benefit of the providers with whom they are employed but also for the sake of the patients who are beneficiaries of this program.

The exercises and activities in this workbook chapter further educate and reinforce your understanding of and ability to deal with Medicare's challenges.

WORKBOOK CHAPTER OBJECTIVES

After completing the workbook activities for Chapter 9, the student should be able to:
1. Define the terms used in the chapter.
2. Answer the review questions according to the evaluation criteria set by the instructor.
3. Demonstrate the ability to think critically and draw conclusions from facts and information provided in scenarios and performance objectives.
4. Explore websites to acquire information needed to complete workbook activities successfully.
5. Abstract applicable information from healthcare documents necessary for completion of Medicare claims.
6. Complete specific forms common to the health insurance professional's role in Medicare claims and billing.
7. Compute mathematic calculations to arrive at correct patient statement balances.
8. Generate information and collect documents for inclusion in the student's personal Health Insurance Professional's Notebook.
9. Undertake self-analysis and self-evaluation in completed workbook activities.

DEFINING CHAPTER TERMS

Using the computer, students should write an accurate definition for each of the chapter terms listed. These definitions should be in the students' own words. When finished, students should compare their definitions with those listed in the glossary at the back of the textbook and correct any inaccuracies.

5-Star Plans
adjudicated
advance beneficiary notice (ABN)
allowable charges
appeals process
beneficiary
Beneficiary Complaint Response Program
benefit period
care coordination
Centers for Medicare and Medicaid Services (CMS)
claim adjustment reason code
Clinical Laboratory Improvement Amendments (CLIA)

coordination of benefits contractor (COBC)
cost sharing
credible coverage
demand bill
disproportionate share
donut hole
downcoding
dual eligible
electronic funds transfer (EFT)
electronic remittance advice (ERA)
end-stage renal disease (ESRD)
Federal Insurance Contributions Act (FICA)

163

health insurance claim number (HICN)
HMO with point-of-service (POS) option
initial claims
initial enrollment period
lifetime (one-time) release of information form
local coverage determination (LCD)
mandated Medigap transfer
medically necessary
Medicare
Medicare administrative contractor (MAC)
Medicare audits
Medicare gaps
Medicare limiting charge
Medicare managed care plan
Medicare nonparticipating provider (nonPAR)
Medicare Part A
Medicare Part B
Medicare Part C
Medicare Part D
Medicare participating provider (PAR)
Medicare secondary payer (MSP)
Medicare Summary Notice (MSN)
Medicare supplement policy
Medicare whistleblowers
Medigap crossover

Medigap insurance
national coverage determination (NCD)
network
noncovered services
observation care
peer review organization (PRO)
Physician Quality Reporting System (PQRS)
Program of All-Inclusive Care for the Elderly (PACE)
provider-sponsored organization (PSO)
quality improvement organization (QIO)
quality review study
recovery audit contractor (RAC)
relative value unit
remittance advice (RA)
remittance remark code
resource-based relative value system (RBRVS)
self-referring
Seniors' Health Insurance Information Program (SHIIP)
small provider
special enrollment period
special needs plan (SNP)
standard paper remittance (SPR)
TrOOP
value-based payment modifier

ASSESSMENT

Multiple Choice

Directions: In the questions and statements presented, choose the response that **best** answers or completes the stem and circle the letter that precedes it.

1. Medicare provides financial assistance with medical expenses to:
   a. People older than 65
   b. People with ESRD
   c. People younger than 65 with certain disabilities
   d. All of the above

2. Medicare requires its beneficiaries to pay premiums, deductibles, and coinsurance, which is referred to as:
   a. Medigap
   b. Taxation
   c. Cost sharing
   d. Allowable charges

3. Medicare Part A, the hospital insurance part of Medicare, is funded through:
   a. Taxes withheld from employees' wages
   b. Contributions paid by employers
   c. State funds
   d. Both a and b

4. Coverage requirements under Medicare state that for a service to be covered, it must be considered:
   a. Proper and timely
   b. Reasonable and customary
   c. Medically necessary
   d. Medicare has no coverage requirements

5. Part A coverage is available free of charge to Medicare beneficiaries age 65 or older who:
   a. Have no other insurance
   b. Have paid at least 20 quarters of work credits
   c. Are eligible to receive monthly Social Security benefits
   d. Medicare Part A is not free of charge to anyone

6. Private insurance companies that serve as the federal government's agents in the administration of the Medicare program, including the payment of claims, are called:
   a. Medicare Administrative Contractors
   b. Part A negotiators
   c. Beneficiaries
   d. PAR providers

7. Medicare Part B helps pay for:
   a. Medically necessary physicians' services
   b. Acute care hospitalization
   c. Custodial and long-term care
   d. All of the above

8. Medicare pays _____ % of allowable charges after the annual deductible is met.
   a. 20
   b. 50
   c. 80
   d. 100

9. The _____ is the duration of time during which a Medicare beneficiary is eligible for Part A benefits for services incurred in a hospital and/or skilled nursing facility (SNF).
   a. Donut hole
   b. Medicare gap
   c. Benefit period
   d. Open enrollment period

10. Managed healthcare plans that offer regular Part A and Part B Medicare coverage and additional coverage for certain other services are called:
    a. Medicare Part A
    b. Medicare Part B
    c. Medicare Part C
    d. Medicare Part D

11. The Medicare prescription drug coverage plan is called:
    a. Medicare Part A
    b. Medicare Part B
    c. Medicare Part C
    d. Medicare Part D

12. In Medicare Part D, individual plans (such as group health insurance plans that offer varying benefits) must offer no less than the standard Medicare benefit, referred to as:
    a. Medigap
    b. Credible coverage
    c. Basic prescription coverage
    d. Mandated benefit coverage

13. An individual qualifying for both Medicare and Medicaid benefits is referred to as a:
    a. Dual eligible
    b. MediMax
    c. Medical qualifier
    d. Categorically eligible

14. The program that provides community-based acute and long-term care services to Medicare beneficiaries is called:
    a. FICA
    b. PACE
    c. CLIA
    d. LCD

15. Beneficiaries can change their Medicare health or prescription drug coverage during the:
    a. Benefit period
    b. Donut hole
    c. Annual open enrollment period
    d. First 6 months of each year

16. A health insurance plan sold by private insurance companies to help pay for healthcare expenses not covered by Medicare is called a:
    a. Commercial policy
    b. Trading partner plan
    c. Prospective payment plan
    d. Supplemental policy

17. The term commonly used when another insurance policy is primary to Medicare is:
    a. Medigap
    b. Medicare Supplement Insurance
    c. Medicare Secondary Payer
    d. Other health insurance (OHI)

18. Some Medicare Advantage Plan enrollees are allowed to see specialists outside the "network" without going through a primary care physician. This is called:
    a. Self-referring
    b. Open enrollment
    c. Noncovered services
    d. Not medically necessary

19. A form that Medicare requires all healthcare providers use when a service is rendered that Medicare ordinarily covers but is likely to be denied on this particular occasion is the:
    a. SPR
    b. COB
    c. ABN
    d. EOB

20. _____ consist only of information pertaining to when a procedure is considered medically reasonable and necessary.
    a. CLIAs
    b. LCDs
    c. COBs
    d. QIOs

21. Medicare "initial claims" do *not* include:
    a. Mandated Medigap transfers
    b. Medi/Medi claims
    c. Appeal requests
    d. Previously rejected claims

22. Exceptions to mandatory electronic claims submission include:
    a. Small provider claims
    b. Roster billing
    c. Dental claims
    d. All of the above

166

23. The Patient Protection and Affordable Care Act included a provision that limited timely filing of Medicare claims to:
    a. 90 days from the date(s) of service
    b. October first of the year after the date(s) of service
    c. 1 year from the date of service(s)
    d. December 1 of the year in which services were rendered

24. There are _____ levels of the Medicare appeals process.
    a. 4
    b. 5
    c. 6
    d. 7

25. The acronym for the quality reporting system that provided an incentive payment for eligible professionals (EPs) who satisfactorily reported data on quality measures for covered services furnished to Medicare beneficiaries is:
    a. PQRS
    b. CLIA
    c. LMRP
    d. FICA

True/False

Directions: Place a "T" in the blank preceding the sentence if it is true; place an "F" if it is false.

_____ 1. Medicare Parts A and B are provided free of charge for all individuals older than 65.

_____ 2. Part A covers custodial and long-term care.

_____ 3. For durable medical equipment (DME) to qualify for Medicare payment, it must be ordered by a physician for use in the home, and items must be reusable.

_____ 4. Neither Medicare Part A nor Part B covers any preventive care services.

_____ 5. Most Medicare Part B beneficiaries pay for Part B coverage in the form of a premium deducted from their monthly Social Security check.

_____ 6. The private organization that determines payment of Part B-covered items and services is called a *peer review organization* (PRO).

_____ 7. Part A Medicare beneficiaries are allowed only one "benefit period" per year.

_____ 8. If individuals do not sign up for Medicare Part B when first becoming eligible and later decide to enroll, the monthly premiums may be higher due to penalties.

_____ 9. An individual must be eligible for Part A or B to enroll in a Medicare Advantage Plan.

_____ 10. If a beneficiary has a Medicare Advantage Plan, he or she still needs a supplemental policy.

_____ 11. An individual who has original Medicare Parts A and B must have a supplemental policy.

_____ 12. When an individual turns 65 and enrolls in Medicare Part B, federal law forbids insurance companies from denying eligibility for Medigap policies for 6 months.

_____ 13. Workers' compensation would likely be a primary payer to Medicare.

_____ 14. Medicare HMOs typically have no yearly cap on how much the enrollee pays for Parts A and B services during the year.

_____ 15. Under certain circumstances, a signed release of information form for Medicare beneficiaries can be valid for more than 1 year.

_____ 16. Medicare's definition of medical necessity must meet specific criteria.

_____ 17. Medicare HICNs are typically in the format of nine numeric characters followed by one alpha character.

_____ 18. The Medicare physicians' fee schedule has been changed from a fee-for-service to a resource-based relative value system (RBRVS).

167

_____ 19. Medicare nonPARs do not have to submit claims for their Medicare patients.

_____ 20. ASC X12 Version 5010 has been replaced by Version 4010/4010A1 as the standard for all HIPAA-covered transactions.

Short Answer/Fill-in-the-Blank

Directions: Read the statements; then, using the textbook for review, insert the correct word or words that complete the sentence or answer the question.

1. The second cost-sharing requirement in Medicare Part B is an annual deductible of $_____, after which Medicare pays _____ % of _____.

2. The duration of time Medicare uses for hospital and skilled nursing facility (SNF) services is called a(n) _____.

3. This duration of time begins the day an individual is _____ to a hospital or SNF and ends when the beneficiary has not received care in a hospital or SNF for _____ days in a row.

4. Medicare Part _____ is free for qualifying individuals who are eligible on the basis of wages on which *sufficient* Medicare payroll taxes were paid, which is _____ quarters of Social Security work credits.

5. The Balanced Budget Act of 1997, which went into effect in January 1999, expanded the role of private plans to include _____ _____ plans.

6. List four managed care plan choices included under Medicare Part C.

   _____

   _____

   _____

7. Medicare Part C coverage not only includes Part A and Part B coverage but may also pay for services not covered under the original Medicare plan, such as:

   _____

   _____

   _____

8. What does Medicare Part D offer to all seniors eligible for Medicare?

   _____

   _____

9. How does Medicare's Part D payment structure differ for dual eligibles compared with that of Medicare beneficiaries who do not qualify for dual eligibility?

   _____

10. Plans that are not Medicare Advantage Plans but are still part of Medicare include:

_____

_____

_____

11. The Medigap Crossover program requires that the Medigap policy information be shown in Blocks 9 through 9d on the CMS-1500 claim form and includes these two elements:

_____

_____

12. List five items contained on the MSN:

_____

_____

_____

_____

_____

Matching

Directions: Place the letter that precedes the word or words that correctly answer the question or statement. (**Note:** Not all answers will be used.)

_____ 1. The program that provides community-based long-term care services

_____ 2. A health insurance plan sold by private insurance companies to help pay for expenses not covered by Medicare

_____ 3. The time frame Medicare allows for enrolling in a Medicare supplement plan without penalty

_____ 4. The term used when Medicare is not the primary payer and the beneficiary is covered under another insurance policy

_____ 5. The entity responsible for the mandatory Medicare supplemental (Medigap) insurance crossover program

a. COB contractor
b. MSP (Medicare secondary payer)
c. PACE
d. Medigap
e. Open enrollment
f. Medi/Medi
g. PPO

CRITICAL THINKING ACTIVITIES

A. You are employed as a health insurance professional at Broadmoor Medical Clinic, where there is a standing policy that patients cannot be seen until they produce "proof of insurance." When you ask Averil Potter, a 76-year-old new patient, for his Medicare ID card, he informs you that he does not carry it with him because he is afraid of "identify theft." He informs you that he has memorized his Medicare number, which is his Social Security number with an ending alpha character. In light of the growing incidence of identity theft and the fact that some insurance companies may still use Social Security numbers as policy identifiers, would you recommend that the clinic's policy be changed? If so, how; if not, why not?

B. Members of the healthcare team of the Broadmoor Medical Center's emergency department are not allowed to ask for proof of insurance before treating a patient who has arrived for emergency treatment. What is the rationale for this difference in policy as opposed to that of the clinic?

C. Because a Medicare nonPAR can charge 15% more than the Medicare allowable charge and bill the patient for this excess amount, why do many providers become Medicare PARs?

D. Frieda Dawson is a 66-year-old Medicare-established patient. She was seen on March 16, 20XX, and had a mammogram the next day. Frieda returns on November 30 of that same year for treatment of a severe urinary tract infection, at which time she requests another mammogram. She is worried because her 73-year-old sister was recently diagnosed with breast cancer. You schedule the second mammogram as Frieda requests; however, Medicare disallows it as not being "medically necessary." You failed to get an ABN because you thought Medicare paid for mammograms. Why did Medicare disallow this procedure? How should you handle this situation?

PROBLEM-SOLVING/COLLABORATIVE (GROUP) ACTIVITIES

Study Table 9.1. Then solve these problems. (**Note:** The deductible and beneficiary copay amounts are subject to change every year.)

Table 9.1 2016 Medicare Benefits Table—Part A	
	Beneficiary Pays
Inpatient Hospital	
Days 1–60	Deductible of $1228 per benefit period*
Days 61–90	$322 per day
Days 91–150 (*lifetime reserve days*)	$644 per day
After 150 days	All charges
Skilled Nursing Facility	
Days 1–20	Nothing
Days 21–100	$161.00 per day
Beyond 100 days	All charges
Home Health	
Part-time care	Nothing (if approved)
Hospice	Nothing if doctor certifies care except limited costs for drug and respite care
Blood	First 3 pints

*A benefit period begins when a person is admitted to a hospital and ends 60 days after discharge from a hospital or a skilled nursing facility.
Note: For more detailed information on preventive and other benefits, see http://www.Medicare.gov.

170

A. Alfred Winters was admitted to Broadmoor Medical Center on November 11, 20XX, which began a new inpatient benefit period for him. Alfred's hospital stay was 98 days.
   1. How much of the cost for Alfred's hospital stay is his responsibility?

      Days 1 to 60: _____

      Days 61 to 90: _____

      Days 91 to 98: _____

      Total due from Alfred: _____

   2. How many lifetime reserve days would be left if Alfred were to be admitted again as an inpatient? (Note: the days he is out of the hospital do not count toward his lifetime reserve days.)

      1 month later: _____

      6 months later: _____

B. Sylvia Thompson is a Medicare beneficiary with Medicare Parts A and B. Follow her through a series of hospitalizations and subsequent care and write the Medicare inpatient hospital deductible amount that Sylvia was responsible for at each point, using Table 9.1 for calculating Part A benefits and Table 9.2 for Part B benefits. Write the Medicare inpatient hospital deductible amount that Sylvia was responsible for at each point in the blanks in Table 9.3. (Assume this is her first hospitalization.)

Table 9.2 2016 Medicare Benefits Table—Part B

Benefits	Individual Pays
Premium	$104.90 per month plus 20% of Medicare approved amount
Deductible	$166.00 a year
Physician and other medical services	
MD accepts assignment	20% coinsurance
MD does not accept assignment	20% coinsurance plus up to 15% over Medicare-approved fee[a]
Outpatient hospital care	20% coinsurance
Ambulatory surgical services	20% coinsurance
X-rays	20% coinsurance
Durable medical equipment	20% coinsurance
Physical, occupational, and speech therapy	20% coinsurance[b]
Clinical diagnostic laboratory services	No coinsurance
Home healthcare	No coinsurance
Outpatient mental health services	50% coinsurance
Preventive services	
Flu shots, pneumococcal vaccines, colorectal and prostate cancer screenings, Pap smears, mammograms	Part B deductible and 20% coinsurance are waived for certain preventive services
Bone mass measurement, diabetes monitoring, glaucoma screening	20% coinsurance

[a]Referred to as the Medicare Limiting Charge Law, the limit on the percentage higher than the Medicare-approved amount that a physician can charge is less than 15% in some states.
[b]There is an annual coverage limit on Medicare outpatient therapy services, which are subject to change every year. These limits can be found in the *Medicare & You* handbook published yearly.
Note: For more detailed information on preventive and other benefits, see http://www.Medicare.gov.

Table 9.3 Inpatient Hospital Benefits Exercise (Using 2013 Figures)

	Day of Admission
February 27: Sylvia is admitted to the hospital as an inpatient for removal of her gallbladder. She remains in the hospital for 5 days before being discharged.	February 27 (5 days) _____
March 11: Sylvia returns to the hospital with a severe infection. This time, her hospital stay is 10 days.	March 11 (10 days) _____
April 20: Sylvia returns to the hospital for chest pains. Her stay for this problem is 3 days.	April 20 (3 days) _____
August 22: Sylvia is admitted to the hospital for bladder cancer surgery. She remains for 7 days.	August 22 (7 days) _____
November 17: Sylvia is hospitalized with complications from the cancer surgery. She remains in the hospital for 60 days before being transferred to a skilled nursing facility.	November 17 (60 days) _____

C. Louise Mayfair visits Broadmoor Medical Clinic on January 2, 20XX, and sees two different participating (PAR) providers. Dr. Aldrich charges $85; Dr. Bennett charges $78. Medicare approves $55 for Dr. Aldrich and $45 for Dr. Bennett.

1. If these were Mrs. Mayfair's first medical expenses of the year, and she has no other insurance, calculate how much Mrs. Mayfair owes each provider. **Note:** Use the information in Table 9.2 for this exercise.

   Dr. Aldrich: $_____

   Dr. Bennett: $_____

2. If Mrs. Mayfair's visits were to PAR providers, and Medicare pays 80% of the "approved" charges, why must she pay these fees?
3. If Drs. Aldrich and Bennett had been nonPARs, how much more could they have charged Mrs. Mayfair?
4. On May 23, 20XX, Mrs. Mayfair visits Dr. Carbolla (a PAR provider) at Broadmoor Medical Clinic. Dr. Carbolla's charge for services was $130, and the Medicare-approved amount was $100. Calculate the amount Mrs. Mayfair owes for this encounter. (Assume she has now met her deductible.)

Amount charged by Dr. Carbolla	$ _____
Medicare-approved amount	$ _____
Medicare will pay	$ _____
Mrs. Mayfair owes	$ _____

5. Is Mrs. Mayfair responsible for the difference between the amount Dr. Carbolla charged ($130) and the Medicare-approved amount ($100)? Why or why not?
6. Do you as the health insurance professional need to address this $30 difference on Mrs. Mayfair's account? If so, how do you handle it?
7. Mrs. Mayfair was referred to Dr. Dykstrom on April 14, 20XX, a nonPAR provider (does not accept assignment). Dr. Dykstrom's charge was $115, of which Medicare approves $100. How much does Mrs. Mayfair owe in this scenario?

Dr. Dykstrom's charge (limiting)	$115
Medicare-approved amount	$100
Medicare pays	$ _____
Mrs. Mayfair's coinsurance amount	$ _____
Allowed excess charge	$ _____
Total owed by Mrs. Mayfair	$ _____

D. Alicia Freemont, a 66-year-old patient with Medicare Part B, comes to see Dr. Beverly Carson, a dermatologist at Broadmoor Medical Clinic, and asks for dermabrasion treatments to reduce an unsightly scar on her face. You advise Ms. Freemont that this procedure may not be covered by Medicare; however, she insists that she wants it anyway.

1. What do you do?
2. Ms. Freemont remarks, "Well, if Medicare won't pay for it, my Medigap supplement policy will." Is she correct? Why or why not?

E. What is the deadline for submitting a Medicare claims for services rendered October 14, 2016?

PROJECTS/DISCUSSION TOPICS

A. The Medicare Fee Schedule is published yearly by the Centers for Medicare and Medicaid Services (CMS). According to the fee schedule, a medical practice will be reimbursed a prespecified rate for each service identified on the fee schedule. Discuss the pros and cons of such a method of determining Medicare's payment for healthcare services.

B. Debate the advantages and disadvantages of a PAR versus a nonPAR Medicare provider.

C. Generate a chart comparing traditional fee-for-service Medicare with Medicare managed care options (Medicare Advantage).

D. Search the Internet and find a good website for information on how to appeal a denied Medicare claim. Create a page for the Office Procedures Manual detailing a step-by-step procedure for appealing a denied Medicare claim.

CASE STUDIES

A. **Medicare Part B benefits:** When Phyllis Trent, age 72, was in the hospital, she received services from several providers in addition to the hospital. Some providers were PAR; some were nonPAR. Use the information provided in Table 9.2.
   1. The first provider to visit Phyllis was Dr. Frank McDonald, her internist (a PAR provider) and her regular physician. Dr. McDonald examined Phyllis and referred her to a surgeon, Dr. Maxwell Leonard. (**Note:** Phyllis has not met her deductible for the year.) Dr. McDonald's charges to Medicare were processed as follows:

      Charged for professional services: $500

      Medicare-approved charges: $400

      Phyllis owes deductible of: _____

      Medicare paid _____ % × $ _____ = $ _____

      Phyllis owes coinsurance of _____ % × $ _____ = $ _____

   2. Dr. Leonard, the surgeon, is a Medicare PAR provider. He bills Medicare as follows:

      Charges for professional services: $1800

      Medicare-approved charges: $1200

      Medicare paid _____ % × $ _____ = $ _____

      Phyllis owes deductible of _____

      Phyllis owes coinsurance of _____ % × $ _____ = $ _____

   3. Phyllis received a statement from the anesthesiologist, who is nonPAR with Medicare and does not accept assignment. The anesthesiologist billed Medicare as follows:

      Charges for professional services: $920

      Medicare-approved charges: $800

      Medicare paid _____ % × $ _____ = $ _____

      Phyllis owes deductible of _____

      Phyllis owes coinsurance of _____ % × $ _____ = $ _____

      Plus excess charges of _____ % × $ _____ = $ _____

174

Chapter **9 Conquering Medicare's Challenges**

4. Phyllis was transported to the hospital by ambulance. Medicare determined it was medically necessary because it was an emergency. The ambulance claim was processed as follows:

Charges for ambulance transport: $720

Medicare-approved charge: $300

Medicare paid _____ % × $ _____ = $ _____

Phyllis owes deductible of _____

Phyllis owes coinsurance of _____ % × $ _____ = $ _____

Plus excess charges of _____ % × $ _____ = $ _____

Note: Ambulance transport for Medicare-approved emergency carries a mandatory assignment.

5. Phyllis had a series of clinical diagnostic laboratory tests when in the hospital. This claim was processed as follows:

Blood series charge: $280

Medicare-approved charge: $220

Phyllis owes coinsurance of _____ % × $ _____ = $ _____

Plus excess charges of _____ % × $ _____ = $ _____

6. How would Phyllis's responsibility for the laboratory tests change if she had not yet satisfied her Part B deductible?

7. Medicare denied one laboratory test as "not medically necessary." What was Phyllis's responsibility for this charge?

B. **Interpreting a Medicare Summary Notice (MSN):** Study the MSN in Fig. 9.1 and then answer these questions.
   1. What does the "A" indicate after this patient's Medicare ID number?
   2. If the alpha character had been a "D," what would that indicate?

   3. This claim was for a _____-day _____.
   4. Has the patient met the deductible for this benefit period?
   5. What is the total amount the patient may have to pay out of pocket?

Medicare Summary Notice

Jane Beneficiary
123 Any Street
Anytown, Iowa 50000

Customer Service Information

Your Medicare Number: 123-45-6789A

If you have questions, write or call:
Medicare
555 Medicare Blvd.
Suite 200
Medicare Building
Medicare, US XXXXX-XXXX

Local: (XXX)XXX-XXXX
Toll-free: 1-800-XXX-XXXX
TTY for Hearing Impaired: 1-800-XXX-XXXX

HELP STOP FRAUD: Beware of door-to-door solicitors offering free or discounted Medicare items or services.

This is a summary of claims processed from 09/15/20XX through 10/15/20XX.

PART A HOSPITAL INSURANCE – INPATIENT CLAIMS

Dates of Service	Benefit Days Used	Amount Charged	Non-Covered Charges	Deductible and Coinsurance	You May Be Billed	See Notes Section
Claim number 0000-0000-0000 Broadmoor Medical Clinic Milton, XY 12345 R. L. Jones, MD						a
09/06/XX-09/08/XX	2 days	$2,399.55	$34.00	$776.00	$810.00	b,c,d

Notes Section:

a. This information is being sent to your private insurer(s). Send any questions regarding benefits to them.
b. $776.00 was applied to your inpatient deductible.
c. Days used are being subtracted from your total inpatient benefits for this benefit period.
d. $34.00 for noncovered charges for which you are liable.

Deductible Information:

You have now met the Part A deductible for this benefit period.

General Information:

If you were offered free items or services but Medicare was billed, please call your local Customer Service at (XXX)XXX-XXXX or toll-free 1-800-XXX-XXXX.

Appeals Information – Part A

If you disagree with any claims decision on this notice, you can request an appeal by **December 15, 20XX.** Follow the instructions below:

1) Circle the item(s) you disagree with and explain why you disagree.

2) Send this notice, or a copy, to the address in the "Customer Service Information" box on Page 1.

3) Sign here _____ Phone number (___)_____

THIS IS NOT A BILL – Keep this notice for your records.

Fig. 9.1 Medicare Summary Notice (MSN).

C. Elizabeth Franklin has a Medicare supplement policy with Blue Cross and Blue Shield of Iowa. Study the EOB in Fig. 9.2 and answer these questions.

1. What was the date of service? _____

2. Gastroenterologists PC charged _____.

3. Medicare-approved charge is _____.

4. How much did Medicare pay? _____

5. How much did BCBS pay? _____

6. How much does Ms. Franklin owe on this claim? _____

BlueCross BlueShield of Iowa

Explanation of Health Benefits
Medicare Supplement

Page   1

Identification Number:

Claim Number: 43900190CLJX

Provider Number: 4486942

Provider Name: MILTON GASTROENTEROLOGY CLINIC

This is not a bill. It is a statement showing how we applied your Blue Cross and Blue Shield of Iowa coverage to claims submitted to us. If you have a question, please detach the top of this form and send it to us with a letter or call: Customer Service is available to answer calls Mon.–Fri. 8:00 a.m.–4:00 p.m.

Date of Service From	Date of Service Through	SER-VICE CODE	Charge	Medicare Approved	Medicare Benefit Amount	BC/BS Benefit Amount	Notes	Claim Summary
11-01	11-01-20XX	3G	50 00	26 99	21 59	5 40		Total Charges Submitted
								50.00
								Medicare Approved
								26.99
								Medicare Benefit Amount
								21.59
								Noncovered Services
								.00
								Amount You Owe*
								.00
								Blue Cross Blue Shield Benefit Amount For This Claim

This is not a bill and you should not send us money. However, if you have not paid for the service shown here, you may owe the provider. You may want to keep this statement for your records.	5.40

Notes

*This is the amount you owe the provider indicated above. If you have already paid this provider, please disregard this amount.

Identification Number	Group Number	Claim Number	Account Number
Claim Received 12-22-20XX	Claim Processed 01-13-20XX	Provider Name MILTON GASTROENTEROLOGY CLINIC	Patient Name

Fig. 9.2 Blue Cross and Blue Shield Explanation of Benefits (EOB).

D. Study the EOB from the Medicare Supplemental Policy in Fig. 9.3.

Page 1 of 1

Medicare Summary Notice

Customer Service Information

Your Medicare Number: 123-45-6789A

If you have questions, write or call:
Medicare
555 Medicare Blvd.
Suite 200
Medicare Building
Medicare, US XXXXX-XXXX

Local: (XXX)XXX-XXXX
Toll-free: 1-800-XXX-XXXX
TTY for Hearing Impaired: 1-800-XXX-XXXX

Harold Shalladay
1552 Airline Drive
Milton, XY 12345

HELP STOP FRAUD: Beware of door-to-door solicitors offering free or discounted Medicare items or services.

This is a summary of claims processed from 02/15/20XX through 03/15/20XX.

PART B MEDICAL INSURANCE – ASSIGNED CLAIMS

Dates of Service	Services Provided	Amount Charged	Medicare Approved	Medicare Paid Provider	You May Be Billed	See Notes Section
Claim number 0000-0000-0000 Broadmoor Medical Clinic Milton, XY 12345 R. L. Jones, MD						a
01/31/XX	1 Office/Outpatient visit, Est. (99212)	$32.00	$17.17	$0.00	$17.17	b

Notes Section:
a. This information is being sent to your private insurer(s). Send any questions regarding benefits to them.
b. $17.17 of this approved amount has been applied toward your deductible

Deductible Information:

You have now met $38.73 of your Part B deductible.

General Information:

If you were offered free items or services but Medicare was billed, please call your local Customer Service at (XXX)XXX-XXXX or toll-free 1-800-XXX-XXXX.

Appeals Information – Part B

If you disagree with any claims decision on this notice, you can request an appeal by **September 15, 20XX.** Follow the instructions below:

1) Circle the item(s) you disagree with and explain why you disagree.

2) Send this notice, or a copy, to the address in the "Customer Service Information" box on Page 1.

3) Sign here _____ Phone number ( )_____

THIS IS NOT A BILL – Keep this notice for your records.

Fig. 9.3 Medicare Summary Notice (Shalladay).

1. Dr. Jones charged Harold Shalladay $32 for an office visit on 01/03/20XX, and Medicare approved $17.17. Did Medicare pay anything on this claim? If so, why? If not, why not?
2. Medicare sent Mr. Shalladay's claim to his Medicare supplemental carrier, Mutual of Omaha Companies. How much, if anything, did Mutual of Omaha pay toward this claim?
3. What amount can you bill Mr. Shalladay after Medicare and Mutual of Omaha have paid their share of the claim?
4. Can you determine from the EOB if Dr. Jones is Medicare PAR or nonPAR?
5. If Mr. Shalladay were eligible for the QMB Program, how much would he have to pay out of pocket for this claim?

INTERNET EXPLORATION

A. Visit http://www.medicare.gov and research the wealth of information available on this site. Choose a topic of interest to you—for example, "Medicare basics." You might also want to study the relevant information about Medicare Part D or Medigap plans in your state. Compare this information with that of neighboring states.

B. You can find an overview and general information regarding the coordination of benefits contractor (COBC) on the http://www.cms.gov website. There are also other CMS links on this page that might be of interest to you.

C. Medicare's general claim processing manual can be found at http://www.cms.gov/Regulations-and-Guidance/Guidance/Manuals/downloads/clm104c26.pdf. This is an excellent information source for health insurance professionals. Keep this web link in your "favorites" for frequent reference.

D. Visit http://www.cms.gov/MLNMattersArticles/ for current and past articles of interest to you. Your instructor may assign a particular topic for a discussion or oral report.

PERFORMANCE OBJECTIVES

For Performance Objectives 1 through 4, use the blank CMS-1500 forms and ledger cards (back of workbook) or the practice management software (if available).

Special Notes:

1. The providers at Broadmoor Medical Clinic are PARs.
2. All patients have a current release of information on file.
3. All claims are assigned.
4. Names and addresses of FIs or carriers are listed in Fig. 9.4.
5. Use the guidelines provided in Appendix B of the textbook that follow the Medicare Claims Processing Manual at http://www.cms.gov/Regulations-and-Guidance/Guidance/Manuals/downloads/clm104c26.pdf

Names and Addresses of FIs and/or Insurance Carriers	
Medicare FI/Carrier	TRISTATE MEDICARE CARRIER PO BOX 8885A ZENOBIA, ZT 5555-8885
Blue Cross/Blue Shield XY	BLUE CROSS AND BLUE SHIELD OF XTRA PO BOX 1212 DUBUQUE, XT 44444-1212
Medicaid FI	MEDICAID FISCAL INTERMEDIARY PO BOX 4692J PORT HURON, XY 51111-0002

Fig. 9.4 Names and addresses of fiscal intermediaries and carriers. Note: Address on CMS-1500 form must be four lines. If the address is not four lines, leave the third line blank.

Provider Block	
Broadmoor Medical Clinic 4353 Pine Ridge Drive Milton, XY 12345-0001 Telephone: 555-656-7890 Clinic EIN No. 42-1898989	Clinic NPI X100XX1000 Dr. Robert L. Jones NPI 1234567890 Dr. Marilou Lucero NPI 2907511822 Date claims 1 day after encounter Referring provider = DN Ordering provider = DK Supervising provider = DQ

Performance Objective 9.1: Medicare-Only Claim

Conditions: Student will complete a Medicare-only claim using the information in Patient Record No. 052547.
Supplies/Equipment: Patient Record No. 052547, CMS-1500 claim form or practice management software, if available
Time Allowed: 50 minutes
Accuracy Needed to Pass: 90%

Procedural Steps	Points Earned	Comments
Evaluator: Note time began: _____		
1. Carefully read and study Patient Record No. 052547.		
2. Complete all blocks required for a Medicare claim. (35)		
3. Proofread the claim for accuracy.		
Optional: May deduct points for taking more time than allowed.		

Total Points = 35

Student's Score: _____

Evaluator: _____

Comments: _____

_____

_____

_____

_____

Patient/Insurance Information	Billing Information
Vivian R. Ross	Record No. 052547
DOB: 04/15/1952; widow	02/03/20XX; 99203—$81
688 Plum Street	02/03/20XX; 73560—$98
Middletown, XT 12345	Diagnosis: Knee Pain ICD-10 code: M25.569
555-455-6009	Ordering Provider (DK): Marilou Lucero, M.D.
Med. No. 200-00-2222D	
No secondary insurance	

Performance Objective 9.2: Medicare Secondary Claim

Conditions: Student will complete a Medicare secondary claim using the information in Patient Record No. 052548.
Supplies/Equipment: Patient Record No. 052548, CMS-1500 claim form or practice management software, if available
Time Allowed: 50 minutes
Accuracy Needed to Pass: 90%

Procedural Steps	Points Earned	Comments
Evaluator: Note time began: _____		
1. Carefully read and study Patient Record No. 052548.		
2. Complete all blocks required for a Medicare Secondary claim. (45)		
3. Proofread for accuracy.		
Optional: May deduct points for taking more time than allowed.		

Total Points = 45

Student's Score: _____

Evaluator: _____

Comments: _____

_____

_____

_____

_____

Patient/Insurance Information	Billing Information
Paul C. Robertson	Record No. 052548
DOB: 06/22/1948	02/03/20XX; 99213—$75
1555 Westlawn	02/03/20XX; 11730—$40
Middletown, XT 12345	02/03/20XX; 85025—$25
555-455-2333	Diagnosis: Ingrowing Nail ICD-10 Code: L60.0
Med. No. 122-00-4444A	Anemia NOS (ICD-10 Code: D64.9)
Group insurance through spouse's employer	Supervising Provider (DQ): Robert L. Jones, M.D.
Employer: R & T Bottling Company	
Nelda S. Robertson (wife); DOB: 10/04/1950	
Blue Cross Blue Shield XQZ8463112	

Performance Objective 9.3: Medicare/Medicaid Claim

Conditions: Student will complete a Medicare/Medicaid claim using the information in Patient Record No. 052549.

Supplies/Equipment: Patient Record No. 052549, CMS-1500 claim form (or practice management software, if available)

Time Allowed: 50 minutes

Accuracy Needed to Pass: 90%

Procedural Steps	Points Earned	Comments
Evaluator: Note time began: _____		
1. Carefully read and study Patient Record No. 052549.		
2. Complete all blocks required for a Medicare/Medicaid claim. (50)		
3. Proofread the claim for accuracy.		
Optional: May deduct points for taking more time than allowed.		

Total Points = 50

Student's Score: _____

Evaluator: _____

Comments: _____

_____

_____

_____

_____

Patient/Insurance Information	Billing Information
Dorothy R. Stevens (single)	Record No. 052549
DOB: 02/26/1939	02/03/20XX; 99213—$75
2934 Valley View	02/03/20XX; 82270—$25
Middletown, XT 12345	02/03/20XX; 81000—$15
555-478-9011	02/04/20XX; 90732—$10
Medicare No. 134-55-6666D	Diagnosis: Hypertension, benign (ICD-10 Code: I10)
Medicaid No. 22334567HIJ	Palpitations (ICD-10 Code: R00.2)
	Heartburn (ICD-10 Code: R12)
	Supervising Provider (DQ): Robert L. Jones, M.D.

Performance Objective 9.4: Medicare/Medigap Claim

Conditions: Student will complete a Medicare/Medigap claim using the information in Patient Record No. 052550.

Supplies/Equipment: Patient Record No. 052550, CMS-1500 claim form or practice management software, if available

Time Allowed: 50 minutes

Accuracy Needed to Pass: 90%

Procedural Steps	Points Earned	Comments
Evaluator: Note time began: _____		
1. Carefully read and study Patient Record No. 052550.		
2. Complete ALL blocks required for a Medicare/Medigap claim. (35)		
3. Proofread the claim for accuracy.		
Optional: May deduct points for taking more time than allowed.		

Total Points = 35

Student's Score: _____

Evaluator: _____

Comments: _____

_____

_____

_____

_____

_____

Patient/Insurance Information	Billing Information
Lewis A. Barnes (married)	Record No. 052550
DOB: 10/22/1950	02/03/20XX; 99221—$150
92 Hwy 34 West	Diagnosis: Chest pain (ICD-10 Code R07.9)
Middletown, XT 12345	Dyspnea/Resp Abn (ICD-10 Code: R06.9)
555-452-8888	Ordering Provider (DK): Marilou Lucero, M.D.
Med. No. 211-11-2222A	
Medigap based COBA ID: BAN55000	
Medigap Policy No. 8299466J	

Performance Objective 9.5: Interpreting a Medicare Remittance Advice (RA)

Conditions: Student will correctly answer questions using the information found on the Medicare remittance advice (RA) #09876 shown in Fig. 9.5.

Supplies/Equipment: Pen or computer and printer and Medicare RA #09876

Time Allowed: 30 minutes

Accuracy Needed to Pass: 90%

Procedural Steps	Points Earned	Comments
Evaluator: Note time began: _____		
1. Carefully read and study Medicare RA No. 09876.		
2. Correctly answer the following:		
Question No. 1 (2)		
Question No. 2 (2)		
Question No. 3 (2)		
Question No. 4 (2)		
Question No. 5 (2)		
Question No. 6 (2)		
3. Proofread/recheck your answers. (2)		
Optional: May deduct points for taking more time than allowed.		

Total Points = 14

Student's Score: _____

Evaluator: _____

Comments: _____

_____

_____

_____

_____

GREAT PLAINS HEALTH CARE ALLIANCE
REMITTANCE ADVICE

Broadmoor Medical Clinic
4353 Pine Ridge Drive
Milton, XY 12345-0001

PO Box 89774
Omaha, NE 66677

RA # 09876
Check No./Date: 23445 09/01/20XX
Page 1 of 1
EIN # 42-1898989

Recipient Name/ID	Service Dates	Days/ Units	Paid Claims – Medical	Total Billed	Total Allowed	Paid Amount	Reason Codes
Ross, Vivian R. 200002222D		1	Claim Number: 10202020999CLIXX MEDREC 052547				
	02/03/20XX	1	99203	112.00	108.00	00.00	100
	02/03/20XX		73560	98.00	98.00	32.00	101
Robertson, Paul C. 122004444A			Claim Number: 102020201000CLIXX MEDREC 052548				
	02/03/20XX	1	99213	75.00	72.50	58.00	
	02/03/20XX	1	11730	40.00	30.00	24.00	
	02/03/20XX	1	85025	25.00	25.00	25.00	101
Stevens, Dorothy R. 134556666D CrOv Medicaid22334567HIJ			Claim Number: 102020201001CLIXX MEDREC 052549				
	02/03/20XX	1	99213	75.00	72.50	58.00	
	02/03/20XX	1	82270	25.00	22.50	18.00	
	02/03/20XX	1	81000	15.00	15.00	15.00	101
	02/04/20XX	1	90732	10.00	10.00	10.00	102
			Suspended Claims - Medical				
Barnes, Lewis A. 211112222A CrOv Medigap 8299466J	02/03/20XX	1	Claim Number: 102020201002LIXX MEDREC 052550 99221	150.00	00.00	00.00	103
			Denied Claims - Medical				
Goodman, Julia B. 143880909B	01/15/20XX		Claim Number: 10202020925XX MEDREC 052533				
		1	99223	200.00	00.00	00.00	104
		1	99261	150.00	00.00	00.00	104
TOTALS				**944.00**	**422.50**	**240.00**	

RA Reason/Remark Codes:
100 = applied to patient deductible
101 = Medicare allows 100% of charge
102 = Beneficiary copay doesn't apply
103 = Claim under review
104 = Claim denied (second provider filed claim on same service date)

Fig. 9.5 Remittance Advice No. 09876.

1. Medicare allowed $77 for Mrs. Ross's office visit on 02/03/20XX; however, it paid nothing toward this charge. Explain why Medicare did not pay 80% of this service.

   _____

2. Show your calculations to prove that the amount Medicare paid on Mrs. Ross's second charge (73560) was correct.

   _____

3. Has Mr. Robertson met his deductible for 20XX? If so, how do you know?

   _____

4. Explain why Medicare allowed 100% of Mr. Robertson's procedure No. 85025.

   _____

5. What rationale can you give for the RA to include Ms. Stevens' Medicaid number and her Medicare number?

   _____

6. The RA shows that Mr. Barnes' claim was "suspended." What does that tell you?

   _____

Performance Objective 9.6: Posting Claims to Medical Insurance Record Tracking Form

Conditions: Student will post the claims generated in Performance Objectives 9.1 through 9.4 and patient payments and payments received from third-party insurers, using the medical insurance record tracking form shown in Fig. 9.6.

Supplies/Equipment: Pen or typewriter and medical insurance record tracking form

Time Allowed: 50 minutes

Accuracy Needed to Pass: 90%

Procedural Steps	Points Earned	Comments
Evaluator: Note time began: _____		
1. Post the four claims created in Performance Objectives 9.1 through 9.4 to the insurance tracking form.		
Vivian R. Ross (8)		
Paul C. Robertson (13)		
Dorothy R. Stevens (16)		
Lewis A. Barnes (6)		
2. RA and Medicare check was received on 11/28/20XX. Correctly post payments on the insurance tracking form for these patients:		
Vivian R. Ross (6)		
Paul C. Robertson (6)		
Dorothy R. Stevens (8)		
Lewis A. Barnes (2)		
3. Proofread each entry for accuracy.		
Optional: May deduct points for taking more time than allowed.		

Total Points = 65

Student's Score: _____

Evaluator: _____

Comments: _____

_____

_____

_____

_____

Name: <u>Broadmoor Med. Clinic</u>

Year: <u>20XX</u>   Page: <u>122</u>

**Medical Insurance
Record Tracking Form**

Service Provided			Medicare/Medicaid						Private Insurance			Patient Responsibility	
Date of Service	Patient Name & ID Number	CPT Service Codes	Assigned Y or N	Amount Billed	Amount Approved	Applied To Deductible	Amount Paid Provider	Amount Paid Patient	Date Sent	Amount Paid Provider	Amount Paid Patient	Amount Patient Paid	Date Paid Check #

Fig. 9.6 Medical insurance record tracking form.

APPLICATION EXERCISES

Health Insurance Professional's Notebook

A. Because this chapter covers Medicare, students should have accumulated information that will be helpful for filing Medicare claims when they become employed. These documents are some suggestions for inclusion in the Health Insurance Professional's Notebook:

- Sample Medicare ID cards
- Charts and tables noting what Medicare Parts A and B cover
- Sample "lifetime" release of information forms
- Name, address, and telephone numbers along with specific personnel to contact for local and state:
  - Medicare Part A fiscal intermediary
  - Medicare Part B carrier
  - Medicare Advantage carrier(s)
- Templates and completed examples of:
  - Medicare-only claims
  - Medicare secondary payer (LGHI)
  - Medicare/Medicaid claims
  - Medicare/Medigap claims
  - A sample of a current Medicare fee schedule along with an explanation of how PAR and nonPAR charges are calculated.
  - A Medicare Summary Notice (Beneficiary) along with explanation for interpretation
  - A Medicare Remittance Advice (with explanations)
  - Samples of miscellaneous forms
  - Samples of miscellaneous correspondence

SELF-EVALUATION

Chapter Checklist

Student Name: _____

Chapter Completion Date: _____

Evaluate your classroom performance. Complete the self-evaluation and submit it to your instructor. When your instructor returns this form to you, compare your self-evaluation with the evaluation completed by your instructor.

1.	Record	Your start time and date: _____
2.	Read	The assigned chapter in the text
3.	View	PowerPoint slides (if available)
4.	Complete	Exercises in the workbook as assigned
5.	Compare	Your answers to the answers posted on the bulletin board, website, or handout
6.	Correct	Your answers
7.	Complete	All tests and required activities
8.	Read	Assigned readings (if any)
9.	Complete	Chapter performance objectives (competencies), if any
10.	Evaluate	Chapter performance and submit to your instructor
11.	Record	Your ending time and date: _____
12.	Move on	Begin next chapter as assigned

Student Name: _____

Chapter Completion Date: _____

Evaluate your classroom performance. Compare this evaluation with the one provided by your instructor.

Skill	Student Self-Evaluation			Instructor Evaluation		
	Good	Average	Poor	Good	Average	Poor
Attendance/punctuality						
Personal appearance						
Applies effort						
Is self-motivated						
Is courteous						
Has positive attitude						
Completes assignments in timely manner						
Works well with others						

Student's Initials: _____   **Instructor's Initials:** _____

Date: _____   **Date:** _____

Points Possible: _____

Points Awarded: _____

Chapter Grade: _____

10 Military Carriers

TRICARE (formerly CHAMPUS) provides coverage to the families of active duty service members, families of service members who died when on active duty, and retirees and their families, whether or not the veteran is disabled. TRICARE is administered by the Department of Defense (DoD).

CHAMPVA is a health benefits program in which the Department of Veterans Affairs (VA) shares the cost of certain healthcare services and supplies with eligible beneficiaries—qualified disabled veterans and certain dependents of deceased veterans. CHAMPVA is managed by the VA's Health Administration Center (HAC) in Denver, Colorado. TRICARE and CHAMPVA are federal programs; however, an individual who is eligible for TRICARE is not eligible for CHAMPVA.

Some medical practices see few patients eligible for either the TRICARE or the CHAMPVA program; however, the health insurance professional still should be familiar with these two programs, what they cover, the rules and regulations for submitting claims, and how to interpret the explanation of benefits (EOB). The activities and exercises contained in this workbook chapter are designed to help prepare the health insurance professional for these tasks.

WORKBOOK CHAPTER OBJECTIVES

After completing the workbook activities for Chapter 10, the student should be able to:
1. Define the terms used in the chapter.
2. Answer the review questions according to the evaluation criteria set by the instructor.
3. Demonstrate the ability to process information to find thoughtful solutions to problems, to make judgments or decisions, or to reason.
4. Explore websites to acquire information needed to complete workbook activities.
5. Complete specific forms common to the health insurance professional's role in military claims.
6. Generate information and collect documents applicable to military claims for inclusion in the student's personal Health Insurance Professional's Notebook.
7. Undertake self-analysis and evaluation in completed workbook activities.

DEFINING CHAPTER TERMS

Using the computer, students should write an accurate definition for each of the chapter terms listed. These definitions should be in the students' own words. When finished, students should compare their definitions with those listed in the glossary at the back of the textbook and correct any inaccuracies.

accepting assignment
balance billing
beneficiary
catastrophic cap (cat cap)
CHAMPVA for Life (CFL)
Civilian Health and Medical Program of the Department of Veterans Affairs (CHAMPVA)
Civilian Health and Medical Program of the Uniformed Services (CHAMPUS)
claims processor
copayment
cost share
covered charges
custodial care
Defense Enrollment Eligibility Reporting System (DEERS)
Defense Health Agency (DHA)

eZ TRICARE
Military Health System (MHS)
military treatment facilities (MTFs)
minimum essential coverage
network providers
nonavailability statement (NAS)
nonnetwork providers
other health insurance (OHI)
regional contractor
sponsor
TRICARE Extra
TRICARE for Life (TFL)
TRICARE's Maximum Allowable Charge (TMAC)
TRICARE Prime
TRICARE Prime Remote
TRICARE provider

193

TRICARE Regional Office (TRO)   TRICARE Supplemental Insurance
TRICARE Standard   XPressClaim

ASSESSMENT

Multiple Choice

Directions: In the questions and statements presented, choose the response that **best** answers or completes the stem by circling the letter that precedes it.

1. TRICARE is organized into geographical regions in the United States and "areas" overseas. How many total regions and areas are there?
   a. 3
   b. 4
   c. 5
   d. 6

2. The name for the global, comprehensive, integrated system that includes combat medical services, health readiness futures, a healthcare delivery system, public health activities, medical education and training, and medical research and development is:
   a. Military Health System
   b. Military treatment facility
   c. Department of Defense
   d. Department of Health and Human Services

3. Each TRICARE region is headed by a(n) _____ who works with the DoD to administer the TRICARE benefits in that region.
   a. Claims review officer
   b. Regional contractor
   c. Fiscal intermediary
   d. Area commander

4. A clinic or hospital operated by the DoD, located on a military base, that provides care to military personnel, retirees, and dependents is called a:
   a. VA hospital
   b. Military treatment facility (MTF)
   c. Civilian healthcare center
   d. Regional management base

5. The responsibilities of a TRICARE regional contractor include all *except:*
   a. Establishing provider networks
   b. Operating TRICARE service centers
   c. Overseeing conduct on military bases
   d. Providing healthcare services and support

6. On October 1, 2013, the Department of Defense (DoD) established (the) _____ to take over management of the Military Health System (MHS) activities, replacing the former Tricare Management Activity (TMA), which ceased operations on that same date.
   a. Defense Enrollment Eligibility Reporting System (DEERS)
   b. TRICARE Regional Offices
   c. Defense Health Agency (DHA)
   d. CHAMPVA

7. The computerized data bank that lists all active and retired military service members is called:
   a. TMA
   b. FEMA
   c. DEERS
   d. COBRA

8. Similar to Medicaid and Medicare, TRICARE-eligible individuals are commonly referred to as:
   a. Enrollees
   b. Plan members
   c. Beneficiaries
   d. Covered personnel

9. Which of these categories of people are *not* covered under TRICARE?
   a. Medal of Honor recipients
   b. Active duty service members (ADSMs)
   c. Spouses and unmarried children of ADSMs
   d. Parents and parents-in-law of ASDMs

10. The Affordable Care Act (ACA) requires that individuals maintain health insurance or other coverage that meets the definition of minimum essential coverage that include all *except:*
    a. Employer-sponsored coverage and retiree coverage
    b. Coverage purchased in the individual market, including a qualified health plan offered by the Health Insurance Marketplace (also known as an Affordable Insurance Exchange)
    c. Workers' compensation coverage
    d. Medicare Part A coverage and Medicare Advantage (MA) plans

11. Which of these is *not* one of the three main program options available under TRICARE?
    a. Extra
    b. Prime
    c. Complete
    d. Standard

12. _____ provides health benefits to beneficiaries living and traveling overseas when they are eligible for TRICARE.
    a. TRICARE Worldwide
    b. TRICARE Overseas Program
    c. TRICARE Abroad
    d. TRICARE Eurasia

13. TRICARE pays for only *allowed* services, supplies, and procedures, which are referred to as TRICARE:
    a. Covered charges
    b. Authorized charges
    c. Certified charges
    d. Recommended charges

14. If needed treatment is unavailable at an MTF and it becomes necessary for the individual to seek inpatient treatment in a civilian hospital, he or she sometimes must obtain a:
    a. Letter of intent
    b. Certificate of credible coverage
    c. Release of information
    d. Nonavailability statement

15. If a TRICARE-eligible beneficiary has additional healthcare coverage through an employer or a private insurer, TRICARE considers this:
    a. Credible coverage
    b. Other health insurance
    c. Incidental coverage
    d. Both a and c

16. TRICARE's Medicare-wraparound coverage available to Medicare-eligible TRICARE beneficiaries is called:
    a. TRICARE Extended
    b. TRICARE Gap Insurance
    c. TRICARE for Life
    d. TRICARE Forever

195

17. A hospital or institutional provider, physician, or other provider of services or supplies specifically authorized to provide benefits under TRICARE is commonly referred to as a:
   a. TRICARE authorized provider
   b. TRICARE contractual provider
   c. TRICARE participating provider
   d. TRICARE approved provider

18. By law, TRICARE nonPARs cannot charge more than _____% higher than the TRICARE maximum allowable charge.
   a. 10
   b. 15
   c. 20
   d. 25

19. Providers submitting paper claims should use the:
   a. UB-04
   b. NAS form
   c. Form 2642
   d. CMS-1500

20. Which of these is *not* an authorized method for submitting claims to TRICARE electronically?
   a. EFT
   b. eZ TRICARE
   c. EDI Gateway
   d. Claims clearinghouse

21. CHAMPVA is a federal health benefits program administered by the:
   a. Social Security Administration
   b. CMS
   c. VA
   d. Individual state governments

22. CHAMPVA eligibility can be lost if certain demographic changes occur, such as:
   a. A widow remarrying
   b. Divorcing the sponsor
   c. Becoming eligible for Medicaid
   d. Both a and b

23. CHAMPVA is managed by the VA's Health Administration Center located in:
   a. Denver, Colorado
   b. Los Angeles, California
   c. Boston, Massachusetts
   d. Chicago, Illinois

24. In general, CHAMPVA covers _____% of most healthcare services and supplies that are medically and psychologically necessary.
   a. 25
   b. 50
   c. 75
   d. 100

25. To provide financial protection against a potential financial crisis of a long-term illness or serious injury, CHAMPVA has established a(n):
   a. Stop-loss clause
   b. Annual catastrophic (cat) cap
   c. Premium limit
   d. Deductible

26. CHAMPVA pays for covered services and supplies when they are received from an authorized provider and:
    a. Approved by the regional claims processor
    b. Within the scope of a Medicare contractor
    c. Medically necessary
    d. Performed at an MTF

27. CHAMPVA is the last payer after all other third-party payers have met their obligations except for:
    a. Medicaid
    b. CHAMPVA supplemental insurance
    c. OHI
    d. Both a and b

28. The deadline for filing military claims is:
    a. 60 days
    b. 90 days
    c. 1 year
    d. 2 years

29. The annual cat cap for CHAMPVA is:
    a. $1000
    b. $3000
    c. $5000
    d. $10,000

30. When completing a claim, the health insurance professional should remember that the active-duty service member is the:
    a. Patient
    b. Sponsor
    c. Custodian
    d. Beneficiary

True/False
Directions: Place a "T" in the blank preceding the sentence if it is true; place an "F" if it is false.

_____ 1. The sponsor's relationship to the beneficiary creates eligibility under TRICARE.

_____ 2. Military retirees and their family members are not eligible for TRICARE.

_____ 3. TRICARE pays for "allowed" services, supplies, and procedures only.

_____ 4. There is no "cost sharing" under TRICARE regulations.

_____ 5. Active duty, guard, and reserve members are automatically enrolled in TRICARE Standard.

_____ 6. TRICARE coverage is lost when a sponsor separates from active duty.

_____ 7. Although TRICARE healthcare benefits are broad, there is no dental coverage available.

_____ 8. OHI does not include TRICARE supplemental insurance or Medicaid.

_____ 9. Under TRICARE for Life, TRICARE pays Medicare deductibles and coinsurance or copayment amounts up to 115% of Medicare-allowable charges.

_____ 10. Eligibility for patients claiming TRICARE and CHAMPVA coverage should be verified immediately.

_____ 11. Every TRICARE-eligible ADSM, family member older than age 10, and retiree must have a Common Access Card (CAC), uniformed services identification (ID) card, or eligibility authorization letter.

_____ 12. TRICARE participating providers (PARs) must accept the TRICARE allowable charge as payment in full for the healthcare services provided and cannot balance bill.

_____ 13. Patients using TRICARE Standard may be responsible for submitting their own claims.

_____ 14. In the case of nonparticipating providers (nonPARs), TRICARE Standard patients must file their own claims; however, the reimbursement check is sent to the provider.

_____ 15. TRICARE claims must be submitted electronically without exception.

_____ 16. The deadline for submitting military claims varies from region to region.

_____ 17. When an individual becomes eligible for CHAMPVA, he or she is guaranteed coverage for life.

_____ 18. There is no cost to CHAMPVA beneficiaries when they receive healthcare treatment at a VA facility.

_____ 19. CHAMPVA eligibles may see any provider they choose as long as the provider is appropriately licensed.

_____ 20. CHAMPVA beneficiaries have no cost-sharing requirements.

_____ 21. CHAMPVA is always the payer of last resort.

_____ 22. When a beneficiary is eligible for healthcare benefits under both Medicare and CHAMPVA, Medicare is the primary payer.

_____ 23. Both PAR and nonPAR providers must accept CHAMPVA's allowable rate and cannot balance bill.

_____ 24. Both PAR and nonPAR providers are required to submit claims on behalf of CHAMPVA beneficiaries.

_____ 25. All CHAMPVA appeals should be in writing.

Short Answer/Fill-in-the-Blank

(Note: May have to research the CHAMPVA website or handbook for complete answers to some of these questions.)

1. List the three basic plan options available under the TRICARE program.

_____

_____

_____

2. The service member, whether in active duty, retired, or deceased, is called the _____.

3. List the various categories of TRICARE-eligible individuals.

_____

_____

_____

4. Name TRICARE'S six geographical regions and areas.

_____

_____

_____

5. List the responsibilities of the TRICARE regional contractor.

_____

_____

_____

6. To be eligible for TRICARE, an individual must be registered in the _____.

7. Explain the purpose of a nonavailability statement.

_____

_____

8. TFL is available for all TRICARE-Medicare-eligible uniformed services retirees including:

_____

_____

_____

9. How might the health insurance professional verify eligibility for benefits under one of the military's healthcare programs?

_____

_____

_____

10. List the categories of individuals who are eligible for CHAMPVA benefits.

_____

_____

_____

11. Under CHAMPVA, preauthorization is required for certain types of medical services, such as:

_____

_____

_____

_____

12. How is a TRICARE provider defined?

_____

_____

_____

13. List the advantages of submitting electronic claims.

_____

_____

_____

14. Identify the categories of people who are eligible for CHAMPVA for Life.

_____

_____

_____

15. The two cost-sharing responsibilities of CHAMPVA beneficiaries for outpatient services are:

_____

_____

CRITICAL THINKING ACTIVITIES

A. Patient Betsy Froman, who is enrolled in TRICARE Standard, has been referred to you, the health insurance professional at Broadmoor Clinic, with this question: "I am scheduled for an outpatient echocardiogram at Broadmoor Medical Center next week. What, if anything, needs to be done before I have this procedure?" What should you tell Ms. Froman? Will she need an NAS?

B. Assume that the Broadmoor providers are nonPARs for military claims and require patients to file their own claims. Patient Arnold Chessworth, a CHAMPVA-eligible patient, asks you for help in getting claims filing information. Generate an instruction sheet for military patients on where to find this information; include online sources and toll-free telephone numbers.

CASE STUDIES

Refer to Tables 10.1 and 10.2 for help with these case studies.

Table 10.1 TRICARE Cost Comparison Chart: Active Duty Family Members			
	TRICARE Prime	**TRICARE Extra**	**TRICARE Standard**
Annual Deductible	None	$150/individual or $300/ family for E-5 and higher; $50/$100 for E-4 and lower	$150/individual or $300/ family for E-5 and higher; $50/$100 for E-4 and lower
Annual Enrollment Fee	None	None	None
Civilian Outpatient Visit	No cost	15% of negotiated fee	20% of negotiated fee
Civilian Inpatient Admission	No cost	Greater of $25 or $15.65/ day	Greater of $25 or $15.65/ day
Civilian Inpatient Mental Health	No cost	$20/day	$20/day
Civilian Inpatient Skilled Nursing Facility Care	$0 per diem charge per admission; no separate co-payments/cost share for separately billed professional charges	$15.65/day (multiday stay) or $25 per admission, whichever is greater	$15.65/day rate (multiday stay) or $25 charge per admission, whichever is greater

200

Table 10.2 TRICARE Cost Comparison Chart: Retirees, Their Families, and Others

	TRICARE Prime	TRICARE Extra	TRICARE Standard
Annual Deductible	None	$150/individual or $300/family	$150/individual or $300/family
Annual Enrollment Fee	$230/individual or $460/family	None	None
Civilian Copayments	$12	20% of negotiated fee	25% of allowed charges for covered service
Emergency Care	$30		
Mental Health Visit	$25; $17 for group visit		
Civilian Inpatient Cost Share	Greater of $11/day or $25 per admission; no separate copayment for separately billed professional fees	Lesser of $250/day or 25% of negotiated charges plus 20% of negotiated fees	Lesser of $535/day or 25% of billed charges plus 25% of allowed professional fees
Civilian Inpatient Skilled Nursing Facility Care	Greater of $11/day or $25 per admission; no separate copayment for separately billed professional fees	$250 per diem cost share or 20% cost share of total charges, whichever is less; institutional services, plus 20% cost share of separately billed professional charges	25% cost share of allowed charges for institutional services, plus 25% cost share of allowable for separately billed professional charges
Civilian Inpatient Behavioral Health	$40/day; no charge for separately billed professional charges	20% of total charge, plus 20% of the allowable charge for separately billed professional services	**High-volume hospitals:** 25% hospital specific per diem, plus 25% of the allowable charge for separately billed professional services **Low-volume hospitals:** $193 per day or 25% of the billed charges, whichever is lower, plus 25% of the allowable charge for separately billed services

A. Christine Moss comes to Broadmoor Medical Clinic complaining of upper gastrointestinal pain. She is subsequently admitted to Broadmoor Medical Center on an outpatient basis for endoscopy. These are the procedures performed on Mrs. Moss along with the charges:

Date of Service	CPT Code	Procedure/Service	TRICARE-Approved Charge
11/29/20XX	99244	Office consultation	$166
11/30/20XX	43239	Upper GI endoscopy with biopsy*	$625
11/30/20XX	43453-78	Dilate esophagus*	$670

*Outpatient procedure

Aaron Moss, her husband, is currently on active duty in Afghanistan with an E-4 ranking. They have no children, so Mrs. Moss has "individual" coverage.

1. If Mrs. Moss is covered under TRICARE Prime, what is her annual deductible? _____

2. If she had TRICARE Extra, what would her annual (individual) deductible be? _____
3. Would Mrs. Moss's deductible be greater if she had enrolled in TRICARE Standard? If so, how much greater? _____

4. Assuming that Mrs. Moss has TRICARE Standard and she has met her deductible for the year, what would her copayment be for (a) the office consultation and (b) the outpatient procedures? Assume that the charges listed are the same as TRICARE's "allowable charges." _____

5. If Mrs. Moss was enrolled in TRICARE Extra, what would be the total amount she would have to pay out of pocket for all procedures and services rendered on 11/29/20XX and 11/30/20XX (a) if she had not yet met her annual deductible and (b) if she had met her annual deductible? _____

B. Patrick Olson is a retired colonel of the US Army. He is admitted as an inpatient to Broadmoor Medical Center for a knee replacement. The colonel only has to pay the individual deductible of $150. Other family members pay the balance. The orthopedic surgeon's bill for Col. Olson's hospitalization for $8825 is broken down as follows:

Date of Service	Procedure/Service	TRICARE-Approved Charge
11/29/20XX	Initial hospital visit	$150
11/30/20XX	Nonchemo IV infusion (Vancomycin) for MRSA	$8000
12/01/20XX through 12/05/20XX	Subsequent hospital visits × 5	$550
12/06/20XX	Discharge visit	$125

1. Assuming this patient has a family policy and has met any required annual deductibles, what would be the total out-of-pocket amount Col. Olson would have to pay for just the professional service listed (not including the enrollment fee) if he was enrolled in (a) TRICARE Prime, (b) TRICARE Extra, or (c) TRICARE Standard? Assume that the fees charged are the same as the "allowed fees." _____

2. Assuming this patient had not met his annual deductible, what would be the total out-of-pocket amount Col. Olson would have to pay if he was enrolled in (a) TRICARE Prime, (b) TRICARE Extra, or (c) TRICARE Standard? _____

3. In this scenario, after Col. Olson was discharged from Broadmoor Medical Center, he was transferred to a civilian inpatient skilled nursing facility (SNF) for a 10-day stay. If the SNF charges $180/day, how much did this stage of his rehabilitative care cost him if he was enrolled in (a) TRICARE Prime, (b) TRICARE Extra, or (c) TRICARE Standard?

INTERNET EXPLORATION

A. The health insurance professional should have ready access to the latest handbooks available for guidance in submitting claims. Visit these websites and peruse the electronic versions of the provider handbooks. (**Note:** Because websites change frequently, these links may change. If this happens, use "TRICARE provider handbook [year]" or "CHAMPVA provider handbook [year]" as search words. Note that each region's contractor has its own separate provider handbook, so students may wish to select which one is applicable in their area.)
   1. Example: TRICARE website for the north region: https://www.hnfs.com/content/hnfs/home/tn/prov/res/prov_manuals.html
   2. CHAMPVA website: https://www.va.gov/purchasedcare/pubs/champva_policy.asp

B. Create a list of addresses where the various military claims (TRICARE and CHAMPVA) should be sent and a list of telephone numbers to call for questions and claims processing assistance.

C. The website "http://www.tricare.mil/FAQs" provides extensive information and answers to frequently asked questions regarding TRICARE. Visit this website and search for information that may be helpful to a health insurance professional.

D. The health insurance specialist should keep up to date with all major carriers. Visit these websites to find out what's new with TRICARE and CHAMPVA.
   http://www.tricare.mil/tma/tai/new.aspx
   https://www.va.gov/homeless/Whats_New_Archives.asp

PERFORMANCE OBJECTIVES

For Performance Objectives 1 through 4, use the blank CMS-1500 forms and ledger cards (back of workbook) or the practice management software (if available). Use the claims completion instructions provided in Appendix B in the back of the textbook or those provided by the regional contractor or claims coordinator in your service area.

Performance Objective 10.1: Claim for TRICARE Patient with Standard Coverage Only

Conditions: Student will complete a claim for a patient with TRICARE Standard (only) using the information in Patient Record No. 052555.

Supplies/Equipment: Patient Record No. 052555, CMS-1500 claim form or practice management software

Time Allowed: 50 minutes

Accuracy Needed to Pass: 90%

Procedural Steps	Points Earned	Comments
Evaluator: Note time began: _____		
1. Carefully read and study Patient Record No. 052555.		
2. Complete *all* blocks required for a TRICARE claim.		
3. Proofread claim for accuracy.		
Optional: May deduct points for taking more time than allowed.		

Total Points = _____

Student's Score: _____

Evaluator: _____

Comments: _____

_____

_____

_____

Note: Use the information in this provider block for all CMS-1500 claims in this chapter.

Provider Block	
Broadmoor Medical Clinic	Clinic EIN # 421898989
4353 Pine Ridge Drive	Dr. Robert L. Jones NPI 1234567890
Milton, XY 12345-0001	Dr. Marilou Lucero NPI # 2907511822
Clinic NPI X100XX1000	Date claims 1 day after examination
Telephone: 555-466-3422	Supervising Provider: DQ Ordering Provider: DK Referring Provider: DN

Patient/Insurance Information	Billing Information
Marie I. Carson	Record No. 052555
DOB: 08/29/1975	11/16/20XX; 99395—$150
2334 Apple Tree Cove	11/16/20XX; 85025—$40
Middletown, XT 12345	11/16/20XX; 36415—$15
555-466-3422	11/16/20XX; 88142—$35
ID # 111-22-3333	Diagnosis: Annual physical examination ICD-10 Code: Z00.00
Relationship to sponsor: Spouse	Supervising (DQ) Physician: Marilou Lucero, M.D.
Employer: Unemployed	
Sponsor Name: Alan V. Carson; USMC/AD	
Sponsor's Address: APO 47349A, NY, NY 22222	
Sponsor's DOB: 03/18/1972	
Sponsor's ID # 111010122	

Performance Objective 10.2: Claim for TRICARE Prime with Other Health Insurance (OHI)

Conditions: Student will complete a claim for a patient with TRICARE Prime and group health insurance (OHI) using the information in Patient Record No. 052556.

Supplies/Equipment: Patient Record No. 052556, CMS-1500 claim form or practice management software

Time Allowed: 50 minutes

Accuracy Needed to Pass: 90%

Procedural Steps	Points Earned	Comments
Evaluator: Note time began: _____		
1. Carefully read and study Patient Record No. 052556.		
2. Complete *all* blocks required for a TRICARE claim.		
3. Proofread claim for accuracy.		
Optional: May deduct points for taking more time than allowed.		

Total Points = _____

Student's Score: _____

Evaluator: _____

Comments: _____

_____

_____

_____

_____

_____

206

Patient/Insurance Information	Billing Information
Wyatt D. Peters	Record No. 052556
DOB: 12/13/2012	11/15/20XX; 99383—$125
811 Linden Circle	11/20/20XX; 92506—$110
Middletown, XT 12345	11/21/20XX; 99241—$65
555-321-5050	Diagnosis: Autism (ICD-10 Code: F84.01) F84.0
	Supervising (DQ) Physician: Robert L. Jones, M.D.
Relationship to sponsor: Child	
Sponsor name: David R. Peters	
Sponsor DOB: 04/28/1977	
Sponsor DBN: 43435559881	
Sponsor service status: USN	
Relationship to sponsor: Child	
Other insurance: Metropolitan Group Health	
Policy holder: Helen Peters; DOB: 01/01/1980	
Employer: Clinton County School District	
Policy # 655778111	

Performance Objective 10.3: Claim for CHAMPVA Coverage Only

Conditions: Student will complete a claim for a patient with CHAMPVA (only) coverage using the information in Patient Record No. 052557.

Supplies/Equipment: Patient Record No. 052557, CMS-1500 claim form or practice management software

Time Allowed: 50 minutes

Accuracy Needed to Pass: 90%

Procedural Steps	Points Earned	Comments
Evaluator: Note time began: _____		
1. Carefully read and study Patient Record No. 052557.		
2. Complete CHAMPVA claim.		
3. Proofread claim for accuracy.		
Optional: May deduct points for taking more time than allowed.		

Total Points = _____

Student's Score: _____

Evaluator: _____

Comments: _____

_____

_____

_____

_____

Patient/Insurance Information	Billing Information
Edward (Eddie) T. Houston	Record No. 052557
DOB: 01/10/1965	11/21/20XX; 80053—$37
14 Baluster Road	11/21/20XX; 80061—$48
Middletown, XT 12345	11/21/20XX; 85025—$35
555-366-1222	11/21/20XX; 84153—$63
DBN 00966098765	11/21/20XX; 36415—$14
Employer: Unemployed	Diagnosis: Hypertension, benign ICD-10 Code: I10
Sponsor name: Self (single)	Diagnosis: Long-term drug use ICD-10 Code Z79.899
Sponsor service status: USAF Ret.	Supervising (DQ) Physician: Robert L. Jones, M.D.
No secondary insurance	Patient paid the 25% copayment

Performance Objective 10.4: Claim for Medicare and CHAMPVA

Conditions: Student will complete a claim for a patient with Medicare and CHAMPVA coverage using the information in Patient Record No. 052558.

Supplies/Equipment: Patient Record No. 052558, CMS-1500 claim form or practice management software

Time Allowed: 50 minutes

Accuracy Needed to Pass: 90%

Procedural Steps	Points Earned	Comments
Evaluator: Note time began: _____		
1. Carefully read and study Patient Record No. 052558.		
2. Complete *all* blocks required for a Medicare/CHAMPVA claim.		
3. Proofread claim for accuracy		
Optional: May deduct points for taking more time than allowed.		

Total Points = _____

Student's Score: _____

Evaluator: _____

Comments: _____

_____

_____

_____

_____

_____

Patient/Insurance Information	Billing Information
Dora L. Michaels	Record No. 052558
DOB: 10/23/1941	11/21/20XX; 74400-26—$140
29 Orchard Meadows	11/21/20XX; 71020-26—$55
Middletown, XT 12345	11/21/20XX; 76770-26—$108
555-444-6666	Diagnosis: Bladder neck obstruction ICD-10 Code: N32.0
ID # 222-11-4567	Diagnosis: Respiratory distress ICD-10 Code: R06.00
Medicare ID # 222-11-4567B	Supervising (DQ) Physician: Robert L. Jones, M.D.
Sponsor name: Alvin Michaels; DOB: 02/18/1937	POS: 22
Sponsor SSN: 220-00-0001	
Sponsor service status: USMC	
Relationship to sponsor: Spouse	
Employer: Unemployed	

Performance Objective 10.5: Posting to the Insurance Record Tracking Form

Post the four military claims completed in Performance Objectives 10.1 through 10.4 to the insurance record tracking form (Fig. 10.1).

Conditions: Student will post the claims generated in Performance Objectives 10.1 through 10.4 to the insurance tracking form (see Fig. 10.1).

Supplies/Equipment: Pen or computer and medical insurance record tracking form

Time Allowed: 50 minutes

Accuracy Needed to Pass: 90%

Procedural Steps	Points Earned	Comments
Evaluator: Note time began: _____		
1. Assemble the claims generated in Performance Objectives 10.1 through 10.4.		
M. Carson (8)		
W. Peters (8)		
E. Houston (8)		
D. Michaels (8)		
2. Insert correct page heading. (3)		
3. Proofread each entry for accuracy.		
Optional: May deduct points for taking more time than allowed.		

Total Points = 35

Student's Score: _____

Evaluator: _____

Comments: _____

_____

_____

_____

_____

Name: _____

Year: _____ **Page:** _____

Medical Insurance
Record Tracking Form

Service Provided			Medicare/Medicaid						Private Insurance			Patient Responsibility	
Date of Service	Patient Name & ID Number	CPT Service Codes	Assigned Y or N	Amount Billed	Amount Approved	Applied To Deductible	Amount Paid Provider	Amount Paid Patient	Date Sent	Amount Paid Provider	Amount Paid Patient	Amount Patient Paid	Date Paid Check #

Fig. 10.1 Medical Insurance Record tracking form.

APPLICATION EXERCISES

Health Insurance Professional's Notebook

Because this chapter covers TRICARE and CHAMPVA claims, students should have accumulated information that would be helpful for filing military-associated claims when they become employed. Some suggestions for inclusion in the Health Insurance Professional's Notebook are:

- Sample TRICARE and CHAMPVA ID cards
- Current charts and tables noting what various military plans cover
- Name, address, and telephone number(s) along with specific personnel to contact for:
  - TRICARE claims
  - Current CHAMPVA claims
  - Local military healthcare facilities (if any)
- Templates and completed examples of:
  - TRICARE-only claims
  - TRICARE with OHI
  - CHAMPVA-only claims
  - MEDICARE/CHAMPVA claims
- Representative examples of TRICARE and CHAMPVA EOBs (with explanations)
- Samples of miscellaneous forms affiliated with military claims processing
- Other documents as applicable

"JUST FOR FUN!"

A. Develop a crossword puzzle of chapter terms.

B. Generate a matching exercise using the chapter terms.

Chapter Checklist

Student Name: _____

Chapter Completion Date: _____

Evaluate your classroom performance. Complete the self-evaluation and submit it to your instructor. When your instructor returns this form to you, compare your self-evaluation with the evaluation completed by your instructor.

1.	Record	Your start time and date: _____
2.	Read	The assigned chapter in the textbook
3.	View	PowerPoint slides (if available)
4.	Complete	Exercises in the workbook as assigned
5.	Compare	Your answers to the answers posted on the bulletin board, website, or handout
6.	Correct	Your answers
7.	Complete	All tests and required activities
8.	Read	Assigned readings (if any)
9.	Complete	Chapter performance objectives (competencies), if any
10.	Evaluate	Chapter performance and submit to your instructor
11.	Record	Your ending time and date: _____
12.	Move on	Begin next chapter as assigned

PERFORMANCE EVALUATION

Student Name: _____

Chapter Completion Date: _____

Evaluate your classroom performance. Compare this evaluation with the one provided by your instructor.

Skill	Student Self-Evaluation			Instructor Evaluation		
	Good	Average	Poor	Good	Average	Poor
Attendance/punctuality						
Personal appearance						
Applies effort						
Is self-motivated						
Is courteous						
Has positive attitude						
Completes assignments in timely manner						
Works well with others						

Student's Initials: _____

Date: _____

Points Possible: _____

Points Awarded: _____

Chapter Grade: _____

Instructor's Initials: _____

Date: _____

Miscellaneous Carriers: Workers' Compensation and Disability Insurance

Up to now, the textbook has been presenting information regarding healthcare insurance for individuals with illness or injuries that are not related to employment. Workers' compensation is different from all the other types of insurance because to be eligible for benefits, the individual's injury or illness must be work related. As we learned from the text, most workers in the United States are covered by the workers' compensation laws, and the employer, not the employee, pays the premiums.

Disability insurance, another type of insurance discussed in Chapter 11, differs from regular health insurance and workers' compensation. Disability insurance replaces a portion of an individual's earned income in the event he or she is unable to work because of accident or sickness. An individual might have disability insurance through his or her employer or a private policy unrelated to work. Two well-known federal disability insurance programs are Social Security Disability Insurance (SSDI) and Supplemental Security Income (SSI).

This workbook chapter presents activities and exercises that reinforce the information presented in Chapter 11 of the text and helps prepare the health insurance professional for on-the-job tasks associated with workers' compensation and disability claims.

WORKBOOK CHAPTER OBJECTIVES

After completing the workbook activities for Chapter 11, the student should be able to:
1. Define the terms used in the chapter.
2. Answer the review questions according to the evaluation criteria set by the instructor.
3. Demonstrate the ability to process information to find thoughtful solutions to problems, to make judgments or decisions, or to reason.
4. Participate in classroom discussions on workers' compensation and disability insurance topics at an informed level.
5. Find and explore websites to obtain information needed for successful completion of workbook activities.
6. Complete specific forms common to the health insurance professional's role in workers' compensation and disability insurance claims and reports.
7. Generate information and collect documents applicable to workers' compensation and disability insurance for inclusion in the student's personal Health Insurance Professional's Notebook.
8. Undertake self-analysis and evaluation in completed workbook activities.

DEFINING CHAPTER TERMS

Using the computer, students should write an accurate definition for each of the chapter terms listed. These definitions should be in the students' own words. When finished, students should compare their definitions with those listed in the glossary at the back of the textbook and correct any inaccuracies.

activities of daily living (ADLs)
Americans with Disabilities Act (ADA)
benefit cap
coming and going rule
disability income insurance
earned income
egregious
employment network
Energy Employees Occupational Illness Compensation
   Program Act (EEOICP)
exemptions
Federal Black Lungs Benefits Program
Federal Employment Compensation Act (FECA)

Federal Employment Liability Act (FELA)
financial means test
instrumental activities of daily living (IADLs)
job deconditioning
Longshore and Harbor Workers' Compensation Act
long-term disability
Merchant Marine Act (Jones Act)
modified own-occupation policy
no-fault insurance
occupational therapy
ombudsman
own-occupation policy
permanent and stationary

215

permanent disability
permanent partial disability
permanent total disability
progress or supplemental report
protected health information (PHI)
short-term disability
Social Security Disability Insurance (SSDI)
supplemental security income (SSI)

temporarily disabled
temporary disability
temporary partial disability
temporary total disability
Ticket to Work program
vocational rehabilitation
workers' compensation

ASSESSMENT

Multiple Choice

Directions: In the questions and statements presented, choose the response that **best** answers or completes the stem and circle the letter that precedes it.

1. Workers' compensation got its start in the 1800s in:
   a. The United States
   b. England
   c. Germany
   d. Japan

2. In workers' compensation insurance, the premiums are paid by:
   a. The employee
   b. The employer
   c. Split equally between employer and employee
   d. There are no premiums with workers' compensation

3. The federal program that establishes workers' compensation for federal and postal workers is known by the acronym:
   a. OSHA
   b. FEMA
   c. FECA
   d. FELA

4. The federal program that establishes workers' compensation for railroad workers engaged in interstate commerce is known by the acronym:
   a. OSHA
   b. FEMA
   c. FECA
   d. FELA

5. An individual responsible for investigating and resolving workers' complaints against the employer or insurance company that is denying the benefits is called a(n):
   a. Ombudsman
   b. Lead agent
   c. Fiscal intermediary
   d. Claims investigator

6. The time limit for filing a workers' compensation claim is established by the:
   a. Employer
   b. Federal government
   c. Individual state statutes
   d. Insurance company that issues the policy

7. An injury or illness that is job related typically must be reported to the employer:
   a. Within 24 hours
   b. Within 2 days
   c. There are no time limits
   d. Time limits vary from state to state

216

8. A patient's inability to perform normal job duties at the previous level of expertise as a result of being absent from work is called:
   a. Acquiescing
   b. Noncompliance
   c. Job deconditioning
   d. Job reclassification

9. After the initial attending physician report has been filed, periodic updates must be provided to the employer and insurer; these updates are called:
   a. Progress reports
   b. Supplemental reports
   c. Period update reports
   d. Both a and b

10. The type of insurance that replaces a portion of earned income when an individual is unable to perform the requirements of his or her job because of non–job-related injury or illness is called:
    a. SSDI
    b. Workers' compensation
    c. Indemnity insurance
    d. Disability insurance

11. When determining SSDI eligibility, the government looks at _____ that are accumulated as the individual works and pays into Social Security through FICA payroll taxes.
    a. Work credits
    b. Dollars
    c. Hours
    d. Days

12. The income limit for the SSI program is based on:
    a. Earned income
    b. Exemptions
    c. Federal benefit rate
    d. Activities of daily living

13. The maximum amount of benefits that can be received in a specific period is called:
    a. A benefit cap
    b. Liability limit
    c. Payment closure
    d. A catastrophic cap

14. After eliminating all items not considered income and applying all appropriate exclusions to the items that are income, what's left is referred to as:
    a. Net income
    b. Countable income
    c. Gross income
    d. Taxable income

15. The federal act established in 1990 that protects the civil rights of individuals with disabilities is called the:
    a. Consolidated Omnibus Budget Reconciliation Act (COBRA)
    b. Occupational Safety and Health Administration (OSHA) Act
    c. Social Security Disability Insurance (SSDI)
    d. Americans with Disabilities Act (ADA)

16. The examining body that determines whether an applicant qualifies for SSDI is the:
    a. State Disability Determination unit
    b. Social Security Administration
    c. Centers for Medicare and Medicaid Services (CMS)
    d. Department of Health and Human Services

17. The method of determining whether an individual is eligible for SSI benefits is through a(n):
    a. Activities of daily living evaluation
    b. Financial means test
    c. Spend-down process
    d. Patient–provider interview

18. Social Security disability benefits do not cover the first _____ of the disability.
    a. 2 weeks
    b. Month
    c. 3 months
    d. 6 months

19. The program whose goal is to increase opportunities and choices for Social Security disability beneficiaries to obtain employment and other support services is:
    a. ADA
    b. FELA
    c. Ticket to Work Program
    d. Temporary Work Program

20. The _____ initiates an SSI or SSDI claim by going to the nearest Social Security office in person or by telephoning and arranging for a telephone interview to file the claim.
    a. Patient
    b. Physician
    c. Employer
    d. Health insurance professional

True/False

Directions: Place a "T" in the blank preceding the numbered statement if it is true; place an "F" if it is false.

_____ 1. All employers must purchase workers' compensation policies from the state in which their business operates.

_____ 2. In the United States, any employee who is injured on the job or develops an employment-related illness that prevents the individual from working is likely to be eligible to collect workers' compensation benefits.

_____ 3. If an employee is injured on the job, the employer can be penalized if the cause of injury or illness was conspicuous negligence on the part of the employer.

_____ 4. Most state workers' compensation laws include coverage for injuries sustained when an employee is commuting to and from work.

_____ 5. If a workers' compensation claim is denied, the worker may file a claim with his or her health insurance carrier only after all workers' compensation appeals have been exhausted.

_____ 6. The first thing an injured employee must do is call his or her family physician.

_____ 7. Workers' compensation claims must be submitted on the universal CMS-1500 claim form.

_____ 8. As long as a workers' compensation claim is pending, the provider cannot bill the patient.

_____ 9. Workers' compensation patients are not required to sign a release of information form for a claim form to be filed.

_____ 10. An individual may receive benefits from only one federal disability program even if he or she meets all the eligibility requirements for several.

_____ 11. The SSI program provides monthly cash payments to low-income aged, blind, and disabled individuals.

_____ 12. The health insurance professional typically does not get involved in the SSDI or SSI claim process.

_____ 13. The SSDI and SSI programs share various concepts and terms; however, there are many important differences in the rules affecting eligibility and benefit payments.

_____ 14. The HIPAA privacy rule does not permit covered entities to disclose PHI to workers' compensation insurers without patients signing a release of information.

_____ 15. The premium costs of a managed care option cannot be less than a fee-for-service (FFS) option that states offer for workers' compensation insurance.

Short Answer

Note: If space provided is not adequate, use a separate piece of blank paper.

1. List four work-related incidents in which injury occurs that would be exceptions to the employee drawing workers' compensation benefits.

_____

_____

_____

_____

2. List five classifications of businesses that do not have to provide workers' compensation for their employees.

_____

_____

_____

_____

_____

3. Workers' compensation insurance is no-fault insurance. Explain what this means.

_____

4. List the four major benefit components to workers' compensation.

_____

_____

_____

_____

5. List the physician's two distinct roles in workers' compensation claims.

_____

_____

6. List and explain the various classifications of workers' compensation disability cases as mandated by federal law.

_____

_____

_____

Chapter **11** **Miscellaneous Carriers: Workers' Compensation and Disability Insurance**

7. List and explain the two major classifications of disability coverage.

_____

_____

8. List five pertinent items the attending physician's statement must include when filing a disability claim.

_____

_____

_____

_____

_____

9. List the nine federal disability programs.

_____

_____

_____

_____

_____

_____

_____

_____

_____

10. Define *disability*.

_____

_____

_____

_____

11. Name at least four of the commonly used factors federal programs look at in assessing disability.

_____

_____

_____

_____

12. Name the two criteria an individual must meet to become eligible for SSDI.

_____

_____

13. List the three ways disabled individuals can receive SSDI.

_____

_____

_____

14. Discuss the health insurance professional's role in the disability claims process.

_____

_____

_____

15. List at least three differences between SSDI and SSI.

_____

_____

_____

_____

CRITICAL THINKING ACTIVITIES

A. Casey Belmont, a 33-year-old established patient, comes to Broadmoor Medical Clinic for treatment of a back injury. Casey, who is employed by National Parcel Delivery Service, claims he was injured at work when lifting a heavy box onto a conveyor. When Casey's chart arrives in your office for claims processing, you notice that the clinical notes from this visit are added to his ongoing health record. Is this appropriate? Why or why not?

B. You also note from Casey's chart that his employer has not notified Broadmoor Medical Clinic of this alleged work-related injury. How does this affect the case? Can you telephone Casey's employer to confirm or disaffirm this injury without jeopardizing patient confidentiality?

C. On the Patient Information form, Casey has listed his primary health insurance carrier as Fortune Health through National Parcel. There is no completed "First Report of Injury" form; is it okay to go ahead and file a claim with Fortune Health?

D. During a telephone conversation with the Human Resources Department at National Parcel, you are informed that the department does not consider Casey Belmont's claim valid because he did not attend the mandatory safety meetings the company provides periodically, and he did not follow the instructions in the company's safety manual for proper procedure in lifting heavy containers. How does this affect the case?

Chapter **11** **Miscellaneous Carriers: Workers' Compensation and Disability Insurance**

PROBLEM-SOLVING/COLLABORATIVE (GROUP) ACTIVITIES

Along with the members of your group, study this scenario. Prepare a short, 3-minute presentation responding to the questions.

You are employed by Broadmoor Medical Clinic as a health insurance professional. Your vacation is coming up, and you are training temporary employee Tessy Banks to take your place when you are gone. Tessy informs you that she was previously employed at Halcyon Health Care Center in Kenobi, Michigan, for 5 years as a health insurance professional, and she is familiar with the workers' compensation claim filing process from her previous job.

A. Should you be comfortable in assuming that Tessy can handle your job without further training because of her experience in claims processing? Why or why not?
B. What problems might Tessy experience if she has no further instruction?
C. Generate an outline for a suitable training schedule for Tessy.

PROJECTS/DISCUSSION TOPICS

Be prepared to discuss (1) what you, the health insurance professional, should do when you suspect workers' compensation fraud and (2) how the Health Insurance Portability and Accountability Act's (HIPAA) confidentiality regulations apply to patients being treated for workers' compensation illnesses and injuries.

CASE STUDIES

Determine the amount each workers' compensation patient can be billed in these scenarios and briefly explain your answer.

1. Brett Swanson, a constructor worker, was treated in your office for a fractured leg sustained in a fall into a footing excavation. Total charges were $1875, and workers' compensation paid $1400.

   Patient can be billed: _____

2. Part-time worker Effie Brockett was treated for a cut above her right eye sustained during an altercation with a fellow worker. Total charges were $256.50. Workers' compensation denied the claim. She has no healthcare coverage.

   Patient can be billed: _____

3. John Stevens underwent surgery for carpal tunnel syndrome caused by repetitive motion from assembly line work. Total charges were $7345. Workers' compensation paid $3500, and his group health insurance paid $2500.

   Patient can be billed: _____

4. Antonio Estabon was treated for a dislocated shoulder sustained when performing his duties as a county roads engineer. Total charges were $3900. Workers' compensation case is pending.

   Patient can be billed: _____

5. Salid Mufazi was treated for an acute case of bronchitis, which he claims was caused by breathing dust when cleaning a grain elevator at his jobsite. Charges totaled $730. Workers' compensation denied the claim, and Mr. Mufazi informs you that he is appealing the decision.

   Patient can be billed: _____

6. Sally Forsythe was treated in the office for injuries sustained in an automobile accident when delivering flowers for Elegant Arrangements. Total charges were $1600. Workers' compensation charges allowed in your state for the services and procedures provided to Sally are $1195; however, the claim was denied.

   Patient can be billed: _____

INTERNET EXPLORATION

A. Explore websites on workers' compensation. Determine the:
1. Specific rules and regulations for filing claims in your state
2. Your state's approved claim form

B. Explore the Ticket to Work program's website at https://yourtickettowork.com/.

C. Using search words such as *state disability programs,* use the Internet to determine what programs, if any, your state provides to disabled workers and what the eligibility requirements are.

D. Explore the Internet using search words such as *disability* and *HIPAA.* Determine how HIPAA affects workers' compensation and disability claims.

Performance Objective 11.1: Workers' Compensation Claim

Referring to the information in the patient record (#052560), complete a workers' compensation claim using the universal CMS-1500 form or the practice management software, if available. Follow the guidelines provided in Appendix B for workers' compensation claims. (A blank CMS-1500 form can be found at the back of this workbook.)

Note: Student should add all claims in the workbook chapter to the ongoing insurance tracking form.

Conditions: Student will complete a workers' compensation claim using the information in Patient Record No. 052560.

Supplies/Equipment: Patient Record No. 052560 (on next page) and CMS-1500 claim form (or practice management software)

Time Allowed: 50 minutes

Accuracy Needed to Pass: 90%

Procedural Steps	Points Earned	Comments
Evaluator: Note time began: _____		
1. Carefully read and study Patient Record No. 052560.		
2. Complete *all* blocks required for a workers' compensation claim (30).		
3. Proofread claim for accuracy.		
Optional: May deduct points for taking more time than allowed.		

Total Points = 30

Student's Score: _____

Evaluator: _____

Comments: _____

_____

_____

_____

_____

Note: Use the information in the provider block for all CMS-1500 claims in this chapter.

Provider Block	
Broadmoor Medical Clinic	Clinic EIN # 42-1898989
4353 Pine Ridge Drive	Dr. Robert L. Jones NPI 1234567890
Milton, XY 12345-0001	Dr. Marilou Lucero NPI #2907511822
Clinic NPI X100XX1000	Date claims 1 day after examination
Telephone: 555-656-7890	Referring provider = DN
Clinic EIN # 42-1898989	Ordering provider = DK
Dr. Robert L. Jones NPI 1234567890	Supervising provider = DQ

Patient/Insurance Information	Billing Information
Julia Elenstein	Record No. 052560
DOB: 04/11/1984	Claim # 83104900HJX
1800 Aspen Circle	"First Report of Injury" Date: 11/23/20XX
Milton, XY 12345	11/23/20XX; 99203—$130
555-551-1115	11/24/20XX; 73030—$55
SSN: 333-33-0000	Diagnosis: ICD-10 Code: S43.006A
Employer: Milton Basket Works	Unable to work from 11/23/20XX through 12/21/20XX
Address: 2799 Industrial Complex, Milton, XY 12345	NUCC does not provide a two-character code for "attending physician;" therefore, we will use "Supervising (DQ)" in all exercises. Physician: Robert L. Jones, M.D.
555-566-9988	
Occupation: Sorter/Packer	
Primary Insurance: BCBS XYZ333330000; Group # 1414XL	

Performance Objective 11.2: Completing an Attending Physician's Statement for a Workers' Compensation Claim

Using the information in the Patient Record No. 052561 and the patient's clinical notes in Fig. 11.1, complete the attending physician's statement for a workers' compensation case in Fig. 11.2.

Conditions: Student will complete an attending physician's statement using the information in Patient Record No. 052561 and chart notes in Fig. 11.1.

Supplies/Equipment: Pen or computer, Patient Record No. 052561, chart notes, and attending physician's statement form

Time Allowed: 50 minutes

Accuracy Needed to Pass: 90%

Procedural Steps	Points Earned	Comments
Evaluator: Note time began: _____		
1. Carefully read and study Patient Record No. 052561.		
2. Complete *all* applicable blanks on the attending physician's form. (30)		
3. Proofread claim for accuracy.		
Optional: May deduct points for taking more time than allowed.		

Total Points = 30

Student's Score: _____

Evaluator: _____

Comments: _____

_____

_____

_____

_____

Patient/Insurance Information	Billing Information
Frank E. Messmer	Record No. 052561
DOB: 01/16/1953	11/23/20XX; 99202—$140
601 Butternut Lane	DX: ICD-10 Code: S39.82XA
Milton, XY 12345	Supervising (DQ) physician: Robert L. Jones, M.D.
555-521-2226	
SSN: 321-00-5555	
Employer: Milton Creamery	
555-521-2226	
Occupation: Bottler	

```
CHART NOTES                          Record # 052561

11/23/20XX        Frank E. Messmer        DOB: 01/16/1953

HX    This 53-year-old white male presents to the clinic today for
      chief complaint of a sharp pain in the left groin after loading
      a truck at his place of work yesterday. His work is
      repetitious, and patient recalls lifting something "the wrong
      way" after which he felt "sort of a dull pain." Patient states
      this has never occurred before. He denies bulging in the
      area of the lower abdomen, scrotal swelling, or scrotal pain.
      Patient denies urgency, frequency, or dysuria.
      PAIN ASSESSMENT:  Scale 0-10, 3-4 involving the left
      groin area.
      ALLERGIES: NKA
      CURRENT MEDS: None

PE    NAD. Ambulatory. Appears well
      VS:   BP: 116/80   P: 82   R: 18   WT: 193#
      ENT: TMs:  Clear bilaterally without inflammation,
                 bulging, or retraction
      NOSE:      Clear
      SINUS:     Nontender to palpation and percussion
      THROAT:    Clear without tonsillar enlargement,
                 inflammation, or exudates
      NECK:      Supple, not rigid, without adenopathy or
                 thyropathy
      LUNGS:     CTA all fields with good breath sounds heard
      throughout. No wheezes or rales. Normal vocal fremitus
      without egophony change. Respiratory excursion is
      symmetric and equal.
      ABDOMEN: Soft with active bowel sounds in all
      quadrants. No hepatosplenomegaly or palpable masses.
      No involuntary guarding or rebound tenderness. Patient
      has a mild palpable pain on the left side of the groin along
      the inguinal ligament. There is no obvious bulging.
      GU EXAM:  Testes are descended bilaterally, normal
      size, shape, and consistency without nodularity. Cord
      structure is normal, nontender. There is no swelling.
      Patient was checked for hernia, and none was noted,
      though there is some mild laxity in the left inguinal ring.
      Penis is without urethral discharge, circumcised, no
      lesions.
IMP.  Left inguinal groin strain with no evidence of hernia
      at this time.
PLAN  Recommended no work for one week. When he returns to
      work, he should decrease his activity to lifting no greater
      than 10-15 pounds. This decreased activity should
      continue until his return visit in two weeks. I also
      counseled patient on signs/symptoms of hernias, and if he
      notes any changes, he should return for follow up at that
      time.
      Routine follow up 2 wk.


      R. L. Jones
      R. L. Jones, MD/xxx
```

Fig. 11.1 Chart notes for Messmer.

OFFICE OF STATE EMPLOYER
ATTENTING PHYSICIAN'S STATEMENT

Patient Information

Name: _Frank E. Messmer_ Social Security #: _321-00-SSSS_ Medical Record # _OS261_
First Name   Middle Name   Last Name

Address: _601 Butternut Lane, Milton   XY   12345_
Street #   Street   City   State   Zip

Current Department: _Bottling_   Agency: _N/A_

I hereby authorize any agency of the State of Michigan insurance company, prepayment organization, employer, hospital, or physician, to release all information with respect to myself or any of my dependents which may have a bearing on the benefits payable under this or any other plan providing benefits or services.
I certify that the information furnished by me in support of this claim is true and correct.

Date _11/23/20XX_   Employee's Signature _Frank E Messmer_

History

When did symptoms first appear or accident happen?   Mo. _____ Day _____ Year _____
Date doctor authorized patient to cease work because of disability?   Mo. _____ Day _____ Year _____
Has patient ever had same or similar condition?   ❑ Yes ❑ No
If yes, state when and describe

Present Condition

Subjective symptoms _____

Is the condition due to injury or sickness arising out of the patient's employment? ❑ Yes ❑ No If "yes" please explain. _____

Objective findings. (Include results of current X-rays, EKGs or any other special tests). _____

Is patient...Ambulatory?❑ Bed Confined?❑ House Confined?❑ Hospital Confined?❑ Contagious?❑ On Narcotic Medication?❑

Restrictions/limitations

Diagnosis

Diagnosis _____   ICD Code _____
Name Of Hospital _____   Anticipated Length of Hospitalization _____
Surgical Procedure _____   Date of Surgery _____
If Pregnancy, date of LMC _____   EDC Date _____   Delivery Date _____

Treatment

Date of first visit for this period of disability   Month _____ Day _____ Year _____
Frequency of visits   ❑ Weekly   ❑ Monthly   ❑ Other _____
When did you last examine/treat the patient?   Month _____ Day _____ Year _____
Date of next scheduled visit   Month _____ Day _____ Year _____
Progress ....Recovered ❑   Improved ❑   Unimproved ❑   Retrogressed ❑

Extent Of Disability

	FOR ANY OCCUPATION	FOR USUAL OCCUPATION
Is patient now totally disabled?	❑ Yes ❑ No	❑ Yes ❑ No
If no, when was patient able to go to work?	Month ___ Day ___ Year ___	Month ___ Day ___ Year ___
If yes, when do you think patient will be able to resume any work?	Month ___ Day ___ Year ___	Month ___ Day ___ Year ___
	Never ❑	Never ❑

If yes, is patient a suitable candidate for a return to work program? ❑ Yes ❑ No If yes, please complete the appropriate return to work assessment form.
Is the patient competent to endorse the checks and direct the proceeds thereof? ❑ Yes   ❑ No

Print Name _____ Street Address _____ City or Town _____ State _____ Zip Code _____

Signature (Attending Physician/Mental/Health Provider) _____ Date _____ Degree _____ Telephone Number _____

Fig. 11.2 Attending physician's statement for Messmer.

Performance Objective 11.3: Employer-Sponsored Disability Claim

Using the information in Patient Record No. 052572, complete the attending physician's form shown in Fig. 11.3.
Conditions: Student will complete an attending physician's statement using the information in Patient Record No. 052572.
Supplies/Equipment: Pen or computer, Patient Record No. 052572, and attending physician's statement form
Time Allowed: 50 minutes
Accuracy Needed to Pass: 90%

Procedural Steps	Points Earned	Comments
Evaluator: Note time began: _____		
1. Carefully read and study Patient Record No. 052572.		
2. Complete *all* applicable blanks on the attending physician's form. (30)		
3. Proofread claim for accuracy.		
Optional: May deduct points for taking more time than allowed.		

Total Points = 30

Student's Score: _____

Evaluator: _____

Comments: _____

_____

_____

_____

_____

Patient/Insurance Information	Billing Information
Benjamin R. Shalimar	Record No. 052572 (New Patient)
DOB: 10/06/1950	Date of accident: 11/23/20XX
82 Sylvan Annex	TRF # 00233389XYZ
Milton, XY 12345	S: Pt was knocked unconscious as a result of a fall from a grain bin this AM. He fell about 8 ft, landing on his R side. He was "out for a spell." Complains of a severe left frontal headache. Cannot walk w/o assistance; R arm/hand numbness; blurred vision.
555-533-6665	O: See emergency department report in patient record.
SSN: 766-55-7777	A: Diagnosis: ICD-10 Code: S09.90XA
Employer: Farm Ag Resources	P: Referred to the Neurology Clinic for CT scan and/or MRI. See chart for meds. Scheduled follow-up OV 11/25/20XX at 8 a.m. Return to work: unknown
555-511-0087	11/23/20XX; 99283 ER visit—$180
Occupation: Livestock Inspector	Supervising (DQ) physician: Marilyn. Lucero, M.D.
Policy #8 692G	

Chapter **11** **Miscellaneous Carriers: Workers' Compensation and Disability Insurance**

ATTENDING PHYSICIAN'S STATEMENT	REFERENCE NUMBER

THE INSURED IS RESPONSIBLE FOR COMPLETION OF THIS FORM
WITHOUT EXPENSE TO THE COMPANY

POLICY NUMBER (with Prefix)

SEX: M OR F   D.O.B.:

PATIENT'S NAME AND ADDRESS ....
....
WHAT IS DISABLING PATIENT? ....
Please give a complete diagnosis of this condition ....
....
....
....

HISTORY:

1.   When did patient first receive medical treatment?..
2.   (a) Was there a previous history of this or a similar condition? Yes/No ....
     (b) If Yes, please state condition and advise when previous treatment was given.................................
....
....

3.   (a) How long have you known the patient?..
     (b) Are you the regular general practitioner? Yes/No .... If not, please advise who is......................
....

IF INJURY:

1.   When did patient suffer the injury?..
2.   What were the circumstances surrounding the injury?..

IF SICKNESS:

1.   When was sickness first contracted?..
2.   When did symptoms become evident?..

DEGREE OF DISABILITY:

1.   Patient's occupation?..
2.   When was patient obliged to cease work?..
3.   If patient is still disabled, when approximately will the patient be able to resume:

                                                      (a)   Some Duties? ....
                                                      (b)   Full Duties?...

OR

4.   If patient has recovered, when was patient able to resume:

                                                      (a)   Some Duties? ....
                                                      (b)   Full Duties?...

Fig. 11.3 Attending physician's statement for Shalimar.

Performance Objective 11.4: Private Disability Claim with Attending Physician's Report

Using the information in Patient Record No. 052573 and the chart notes in Fig. 11.4, complete the employer-sponsored disability claim form shown in Fig. 11.5. For questions that you do not know the answer to, indicate "unknown." When asked for facts and information, indicate that a copy of the patient's medical record is attached. Dr. Jones has been in practice for 22 years and received his education at the University of Xanthia.

Conditions: Student will complete an attending physician's statement using the information in Patient Record No. 052573 and the chart notes in Fig. 11.4.

Supplies/Equipment: Pen or computer, Patient Record No. 052573, and attending physician's statement form

Time Allowed: 50 minutes

Accuracy Needed to Pass: 90%

Procedural Steps	Points Earned	Comments
Evaluator: Note time began: _____		
1. Carefully read and study Patient Record No. 052573.		
2. Complete *all* applicable blanks on the attending physician's form. (35)		
3. Proofread claim for accuracy.		
Optional: May deduct points for taking more time than allowed.		

Total Points = 35

Student's Score: _____

Evaluator: _____

Comments: _____

_____

_____

_____

_____

Patient/Insurance Information	Billing Information
Shaley Sue Graham	Record No. 052573
DOB: 07/24/1970	TRF # 00087878IJ
1846 Creamery Row	11/23/20XX; 99202-25—$180
Milton, XY 12345	11/24/20XX; 20610—$45
555-526-6622	11/24/20XX; J3301 × 4—$100
SSN: 123-32-2222	Diagnosis: ICD-10 Codes: M75.42; M75.02; S49.92A
Employer: Milton Community College	Supervising DQ physician: Robert L. Jones, M.D.
555-566-3222	
Occupation: Instructor	

CHART NOTES

PATIENT NAME: Shaley Sue Graham   RECORD NO.   052573

DATE OF VISIT: 11/23/20XX   DATE OF BIRTH   7/24/1970

S: Shaley is a new pt to me. She is here with complaints of shoulder pain. On Nov. 23 she was working at home in the storage area of the garage. When she went to lift down a box of books from a high shelf, she felt a catching sensation in her L shoulder along with pain and pulling sensation in her shoulder. She reports limited ROM from the very beginning. There is severe pain with overhead activity.

ROS: Denies any numbness or tingling in the upper extremity.
PFSH: See Form 811A (in chart)
ALLERGIES: Penicillin and aspirin
PMH: Usual childhood diseases and occasional headaches

O: Vitals are stable. She is alert and oriented x 3 and does not appear to be in acute distress. On exam of the L shoulder, she has no deltoid or parascapular atrophy. No evidence of winging with wall pushup. She has no warmth or erythema of the shoulder. Good grip strength bilaterally and positive radial pulses. She does have positive impingement. No signs of instability. There is pain with empty-can supraspinatus testing, and there is posterior capsular tightness. Pt does have weakness with external rotation with arm at her side secondary to pain. No weakness with internal rotation with the arm at the side. Lift off sign is negative. She does have an intact Napoleon's sign. Spurling's sign for cervical radiculopathy is negative. ROM is 85 degrees abduction, active assist to 120-130 degrees before pain. Active ROM is 105 degrees with pain.

A: Rotator cuff tendonitis/impingement syndrome

P: I went over the MRI with the patient, which we had ordered this morning, and it shows rotator cuff tendonitis and impingement syndrome. I have recommended an intra-articular injection in the L shoulder. Pt consents for injection. I advised no work for the next 2 weeks. She is not to do any overhead activity and is not to lift more than 15 pounds. F/U in two weeks. I recommend PT and Celebrex. Papers for disability were filled out today and given to pt.

PROCEDURE: L shoulder Injection: The pt is in the sitting position on the examining table. The shoulder joint is palpated. Plan is to inject from a posterior portal into the joint itself. The area is sterilely prepped followed by inserting the needle into the shoulder joint itself.   1 cc of Kenalog, 40 mg, and 5 cc of Xylocaine was injected in L joint. Needle is removed and pressure applied. The shoulder is placed through an ROM to disseminate the fluid.

R. L. Jones

R. L. Jones, MD/xxx

CPT: 20610*, 99202-25 & J3301 x 4
DX: M75.102; W11.XXXD

Fig. 11.4 Chart notes for Graham.

ATTENDING PHYSICIAN'S STATEMENT

PRIVACY NOTICE		
Patient Name (Last, First, Middle)	Social Security Number	TRF Number
Date of Birth (MM/DD/YY)	Marital Status Single	Sex (circle one) Male Female	Phone Number ( ) -

PATIENT HISTORY	
How long have you personally known patient?	Date of your first visit with patient for illness claimed to have brought about present condition?
Number of visits?	Date of last visit?

What organ, system, or parts of the body have been affected?

Describe fully the course of the disease—its initial symptoms—history of its progress.

Has patient suffered from any ailments other than those above mentioned? If so, describe each case, and state how long it lasted and if recovery was complete?

Has patient been attended to or prescribed for by any other physician or surgeon within three years? If so, what was the reason? Give name and addresses of all such physicians and surgeons:

Is patient wholly and continuously unable to perform any work, or follow any occupation for compensation or profit?

If so, how long has patient been totally disabled?

Fig. 11.5 Attending physician's statement for Graham.

Continued

Chapter **11   Miscellaneous Carriers: Workers' Compensation and Disability Insurance**

If not so disabled, is patient wholly and continuously unable to perform the work of a community college instructor?		
Is the disability, in your opinion, likely to be temporary; permanent and total; or permanent and partial?		
Please give any other facts or information, which in your judgment will aid in the correct solution of the claims presented.		
How long have you practiced as a physician and where did you receive your medical education?		
Signature of Physician	Printed Name of Physician	Date
Signature of Patient for the release of this information *Shaley Sue Graham*	Printed Name of Patient Shaley Sue Graham	Date 11/23/20XX
Address of Physician	City	
State	ZIP	Phone Number ( ) -

Fig. 11.5 cont'd

Performance Objective 11.5: Supplemental Security Income Claim

Using the information in the patient record (#052530) and the chart notes in Fig. 11.6, complete the application for SSI disability form in Fig. 11.7. Under items 8 and 10 on the form, indicate that a copy of the patient's recent health record is attached.

Conditions: Student will complete an SSI disability application (see Fig. 11.7) using the information in Patient Record No. 052530 and chart notes in Fig. 11.6.

Supplies/Equipment: Pen or computer, Patient Record No. 052530, and attending physician's statement form

Time Allowed: 50 minutes

Accuracy Needed to Pass: 90%

Procedural Steps	Points Earned	Comments
Evaluator: Note time began: _____		
1. Carefully read and study Patient Record No. 052530.		
2. Complete *all* applicable blanks on the attending physician's form. (35)		
3. Proofread claim for accuracy.		
Optional: May deduct points for taking more time than allowed.		

Total Points = 35

Student's Score: _____

Evaluator: _____

Comments: _____

_____

_____

_____

_____

Patient/Insurance Information	Billing Information
Lynette Kay Burns	Record No. 052530
DOB: 05/06/1961	11/26/20XX; 99455-32—$225
156 Castle Courts	Diagnosis: ICD-10 Codes: E66.01, I10, B37.89, F32.9
Milton, XY 12345	Supervising DQ physician: Marilyn Lucero, M.D.
No telephone	
SSN 456-65-4321	
Employer: Unemployed	
Primary insurance: None	

CHART NOTES

PATIENT NAME: Lynette K. Burns   DOB: 05/06/1961

DATE OF EXAM: 11/26/20XX   RECORD NO.   052530

S: Lynette presents today at the request of the Social Security Administration. She
has applied for disability based on her morbid obesity. I have been asked by the
SSA to do a physical exam. Lynette is a longtime pt of mine. I have been
managing her chronic diseases since 4/6/1995.

    FH: Non-contributory
    SH: Single, does not smoke; drinks 1 or 2 beers a wk
    PMH: HTN, arthritis, morbid obesity, depression
    MEDS: Prozac/HCTZ

O: BP 142/105, P 90, R 19, W 355, H 5'2". Patient appears to not be in distress. On
asking her questions she does not show good eye contact; her affect is flat. She
seems more depressed today than usual. Abd is obese but soft. Heart RRR,
Lungs CTA. Skin: there is a candidiasis infection under her breast. She has a
Grade I-II stasis ulcer on her R ankle. Pt has bilateral varicose veins due to poor
circulation. Pt becomes SOB when she walks less than 100 yards and she
becomes tachycardic. She has chronic complaint of knee, ankle, and back pain.
Legs show mild edema. She has arthritis of the knees, and today on exam they
show crepitus bilaterally. Patient is unable to bend or stoop. She cannot stand for
prolonged periods of time and needs rest in between.

A: Physical exam, requested by State of XY.

    1. Morbid obesity
    2. HTN, elevated
    3. Candidiasis, skin of breast
    4. Depression

P: I have been educating and working with Lynette since 1995, trying to get her
motivated for weight loss and exercise program consisting of walking. She has
tried a walking program of walking less than 100 yards the first week, then
increasing her distance as tolerated week by week. She is encouraged to walk to
help increase her tolerance. She has been on an 1800-cal. diet and low salt diet
with no success. She is instructed to continue with her Prozac 20mg d, and
HCTZ 25mg d for her leg edema and HTN. Rtn 1 mo.

Marilou Lucero
_____
M. Lucero, MD/xx

CPT: 99455-32
DX: ICD-10 Codes: E66.01; I10; B37.89; F32.9;

Fig. 11.6 Chart notes for Burns.

APPLICATION FOR SSI DISABILITY

MEDICAL PROVIDER'S STATEMENT

1. PATIENT'S NAME: _____ DATE OF BIRTH: ____ / ____ / ____
             (First)   *(Middle)*   *(Last)*   *MM*   *DD* *YYYY*

2. CURRENT MEDICAL CONDITION(s):

   PRIMARY DIAGNOSIS: _____ ICD CODE: _____

   SECONDARY DIAGNOSIS: _____ ICD CODE: _____

3. DATE THAT SYMPTOMS FIRST APPEARED OR ACCIDENT HAPPENED: ____ / ____ / ____
                                                            (Month) *(Day)* *(Year)*

4. DATE THAT PATIENT FIRST CONSULTED YOU FOR THIS CONDITION: ____ / ____ / ____
                                                             (Month) *(Day)* *(Year)*

5. DATE YOU LAST TREATED THE PATIENT: ____ / ____ / ____
                                                             (Month) *(Day)* *(Year)*

6. IS THIS CONDITION RELATED TO PATIENT'S EMPLOYMENT?   YES ☐   NO ☐

7. WAS PATIENT REFERRED TO YOU BY ANOTHER PRACTITIONER? YES ☐   NO ☐
   (If "yes," please provide the name and address of that practitioner): _____

   _____

8. OBJECTIVE FINDINGS *(Include x-rays, lab results and clinical findings. If pregnancy, also give LMP and EDC):* _____

   _____

   _____

9. HAS PATIENT BEEN HOSPITALIZED? YES ☐   NO ☐ *(if "yes," provide reason, hospital name and*
   dates of confinement): _____

10. NATURE OF TREATMENT CURRENTLY BEING PROVIDED OR PLANNED: *(Include surgery and medications*
    prescribed if applicable):

    _____

    _____

11. HAVE YOU REFERRED THE PATIENT TO ANOTHER PRACTITIONER? YES ☐ NO ☐ *(If "yes," please provide the*
    name and address of all applicable physicians or practitioners): _____

    _____

12. IN YOUR OPINION IS THE PATIENT ABLE TO WORK AT THIS TIME?   YES ☐   NO ☐
    IF "NO," WHEN DO YOU EXPECT THAT THE
    PATIENT WILL BE ABLE TO PERFORM SOME WORK?   ____ / ____ / ____
                                                              (Month) *(Day)* *(Year)*

13. IS THERE ANY TYPE OF JOB MODIFICATION OR ACCOMMODATION THAT WOULD
    ENABLE THE PATIENT TO WORK AT THIS TIME? YES ☐ NO ☐ *(If "yes," please describe):* _____

    _____

Fig. 11.7 Application for Supplemental Security Income benefits for Burns.   *Continued*

14. BASED ON OBJECTIVE FINDINGS AND YOUR MEDICAL OPINION:

a) THE PATIENT WAS TOTALLY DISABLED FROM: ___/___/___ THROUGH: ___/___/___
   (Mo.) (Day) (Year)   (Mo.) (Day) (Year)

b) THE PATIENT WAS PARTIALLY DISABLED FROM: ___/___/___ THROUGH: ___/___/___
   (Mo.) (Day) (Year)   (Mo.) (Day) (Year)

15. LIST ALL CURRENT RESTRICTIONS AND LIMITATIONS YOU HAVE PLACED ON THE
    PATIENT'S WORK AND PERSONAL ACTIVITIES DUE TO HIS OR HER MEDICAL
    CONDITION *(If none, indicate "NONE")*: _____

    _____

    _____

16. HAS THE PATIENT BEEN RELEASED FROM YOUR CARE? YES ☐ NO ☐

    IF "YES," DATE RELEASED   IF "NO," DATE OF NEXT SCHEDULED
    FROM YOUR CARE: TREATMENT OR EVALUATION:

    ___/___/___   ___/___/___
    (MO) (DAY) (YEAR)   (MO) (DAY) (YEAR)

ANY PERSON WHO KNOWINGLY AND WITH THE INTENT TO DEFRAUD ANY INSURANCE COMPANY OR OTHER PERSON FILES AN APPLICATION FOR INSURANCE OR STATEMENT OF CLAIM CONTAINING ANY MATERIALLY FALSE INFORMATION, OR CONCEALS FOR THE PURPOSE OF MISLEADING, INFORMATION CONCERNING ANY FACT MATERIAL THERETO, COMMITS A FRAUDULENT INSURANCE ACT, WHICH IS A CRIME AND SUBJECTS SUCH PERSON TO CRIMINAL AND CIVIL PENALTIES.

MEDICAL PROVIDER'S DECLARATION AND SIGNATURE

I declare that the answers on this statement are complete and true to the best of my knowledge and belief. I understand that periodic updates (including providing copies of medical records when requested) will be required in the event of a continuing claim.

_____   _____   ( ) _____
PROVIDER'S NAME/SPECIALTY   TAX ID/SOCIAL SECURITY #   TELEPHONE NUMBER
    (PLEASE PRINT)

_____   _____
STREET ADDRESS   CITY   STATE   ZIP CODE

_____   _____
PROVIDER'S SIGNATURE   DATE SIGNED

Please return completed forms to:

State of XY Services
Attn: Disability Department
PO Box 22333
Crescent City, XY 21112

Fig. 11.7 cont'd

Performance Objective 11.6: Employer-Sponsored Expanded Disability Certification

Patient Benjamin Shalimar returns to the clinic for follow-up. Because his disability continues, students must complete a "Disabled Expanded Certification Verification" form using the information in the patient record (#052572) and the form in Fig. 11.8. (Mother's maiden name is Lutz.)

Conditions: Student will complete an "expanded" disability form using the information in Patient Record No. 052572.

Supplies/Equipment: Pen or computer, Patient Record No. 052572, and disabled expanded certification verification form (see Fig. 11.8)

Time Allowed: 50 minutes

Accuracy Needed to Pass: 90%

Procedural Steps	Points Earned	Comments
Evaluator: Note time began: _____		
1. Carefully read and study Patient Record No. 052572.		
2. Complete *all* applicable blanks on the attending physician's form. (30)		
3. Proofread claim for accuracy.		
Optional: May deduct points for taking more time than allowed.		

Total Points = 30

Student's Score: _____

Evaluator: _____

Comments: _____

_____

_____

_____

_____

Patient/Insurance Information	Billing Information
Benjamin R. Shalimar	Record No. 052572
DOB: 10/06/1950	Progress report: 12/07/20XX
82 Sylvan Annex	Patient returns to the office today. He continues to have blurred vision and tremors from this farm accident on 11/23/XX. There is still weakness in R hand and leg. He is able to walk with a cane.
Milton, XY 12345	It is my opinion that this patient's head injury significantly restricts his ability to perform his usual job and any related occupation and is likely permanent.
555-533-6665	Continue PT; return 2 wk
SSN: 766-55-7777	Supervising DQ physician: Marilyn Lucero, M.D.
Employer: Farm Ag Resources	
555-511-0087	
Occupation: Livestock Inspector	
Policy #8 692G	

239

DISABLED EXPANDED CERTIFICATION VERIFICATION

<u>APPLICANT, SEND COMPLETED FORM TO</u>:

Disabled Certification Department
4526 Central Avenue
Springfield, XY 12345

APPLICANT'S SOCIAL SECURITY
NUMBER (or assigned 9-digit number)

MOTHER'S MAIDEN NAME (enter your mother's maiden name or another
name or word that will serve as an additional identifier to make your applicant record unique)

NAME (please print Last Name, First Name)

ADDRESS (please print mailing address, city, state, and zip code)

TELEPHONE NO.

RELEASE OF INFORMATION AUTHORIZATION

I authorize you to release the information requested on this form to the Division of Merit Recruitment and Selection. I understand that this information will be used only to determine my eligibility for the Disabled Expanded Certification Program.

Benjamin R Shalimar   12/01/20XX

APPLICANT'S SIGNATURE   DATE

* *

DOES THE PERSON NAMED ABOVE HAVE A PERMANENT PHYSICAL OR MENTAL DISABILITY THAT SUBSTANTIALLY LIMITS THE MAJOR LIFE ACTIVITY OF WORKING? This means that the disability significantly restricts the person's ability to perform a class of jobs or broad range of jobs in different classes when compared to the average person who has comparable training, skills and abilities. **(CHECK ONE)**

YES _____   NO _____

If yes, please identify the disability and describe how it affects the person's ability to work:

NAME (PRINT): _____ DATE: _____

SIGNATURE: _____

TITLE: _____ TELEPHONE NO.: _____

ADDRESS: _____
STREET   CITY   STATE   ZIP CODE

Fig. 11.8 Expanded benefits form for Shalimar.

Performance Objective 11.7: Progress Notes—Continued Disability Form

James Morrison has returned to the clinic for a follow-up visit. He is being referred to a neurosurgeon for surgical treatment. Student must complete progress form for this patient's continued disability.

Conditions: Student will complete physician's progress notes for continued disability using the information in Patient Record No. 052576.

Supplies/Equipment: Pen or computer, Patient Record No. 052576, and progress notes form (Fig. 11.9)

Time Allowed: 50 minutes

Accuracy Needed to Pass: 90%

Procedural Steps	Points Earned	Comments
Evaluator: Note time began: _____		
1. Carefully read and study Patient Record No. 052576.		
2. Complete *all* applicable blanks on the attending physician's form. (20)		
3. Proofread claim for accuracy.		
Optional: May deduct points for taking more time than allowed.		

Total Points = 20

Student's Score: _____

Evaluator: _____

Comments: _____

_____

_____

_____

_____

_____

Patient/Insurance Information	Billing Information
James T. Morrison	Record No. 052576
DOB: 03/18/1951	Progress notes: 11/25/20XX
916 Brown Street	Professor Morrison is in my office again for a follow-up and test results of his acute back injury sustained after a fall from a ladder when cleaning the gutters on his house 2 days ago. He continues his daily PT at Milton Rehab Center.
Milton, XY 12345	MRI shows vertebral dislocation (L4-5). He is referred to Dr. Jonas Palmer, neurosurgeon at this same clinic, for lumbar laminotomy and decompression on 11/30/20XX.
555-566-2047	It is estimated that patient will be unable to work for 6–8 wks after his surgery.
SSN: 110-01-0101	Recommendations: No work until further notice; walking on level ground; PT.
Employer: Harvest College	Diagnosis ICD-10 Codes: S39.82XA, S33.101A
Occupation: Director, Human Resources	Supervising DQ physician: Marilyn Lucero, M.D.
Primary Insurance: BCBS XWQ110010101	

HARVEST COLLEGE CERTIFICATION FORM
Progress Report

Section I:	**To Be Completed by EMPLOYEE**

Employee Name: **JAMES T. MORRISON**   Harvard I.D. **110-01-0101PHR**

Home Address: **916 Brown St.**   Office Address:
Milton, XY 12345

Home Telephone: **SSS-S66-2047**   Office Telephone: **SSS-780-1000 EX 8112**

Job Title: **Dir. H.R.**   Work Schedule: **N/A** days/week **N/A** hours/day

Employment Date: **08-31-1993**   Last Day Worked: **Salaried 11-22-20XX**

Employee Signature: **James T. Morrison**   Date: **11/25/20XX**

In some cases, it may be necessary to request medical information and records. I agree to release medical information and records related to my current disability, if requested, by the Disability Claims Unit (DCU) of Harvest College within 10 days of the request by the DCU. I understand that I may not receive benefits until the necessary medical information is received and reviewed. I understand that such information will be used solely to determine my eligibility for STD benefits.

Section II:	**To Be Completed by HEALTH CARE PROVIDER**

Date of examination leading to disability determination ___/___/___   Date of onset of disability ___/___/___

Please indicate ICD Diagnosis Code: _____

Is surgery expected? If yes, give date: _____   Is illness/injury acute? _____

Is illness chronic? _____ If so, what has led to disability at this time? _____

Is disability related to work activities? _____

Is employee treating with any other physician(s)? _____ If so, please provide name, address and specialty:

Is employee compliant with treatment recommendations? _____

Expected duration of incapacity (Please note that re-certification is required every 60 days):

Is a return to work on a reduced work schedule or modified work duties appropriate at this time?   Yes _____ No _____

Will one of those options become appropriate within the next 60 days?   Yes _____ No _____

Expected date of return to work ___/___/___

Name of Health Care Provider: Telephone Number:

Name and Address of Practice:

Signature of Health Care Provider: Date

Revised: 7/03

Fig. 11.9 Progress notes for Morrison.

Chapter **11** **Miscellaneous Carriers: Workers' Compensation and Disability Insurance**

Performance Objective 11.8: Release to Return to Work

Patient Shaley Graham has been released to return to work. Student must complete a Release to Return to Work form.
Conditions: Student will complete a Release to Return to Work form using the information in Patient Record
   No. 052573 and chart notes in Fig. 11.10.
Supplies/Equipment: Pen or computer, Patient Record No. 052573, and Release to Return to Work form (Fig. 11.11)
Time Allowed: 50 minutes
Accuracy Needed to Pass: 90%

Procedural Steps	Points Earned	Comments
Evaluator: Note time began: _____		
1. Carefully read and study Patient Record No. 052573.		
2. Complete *all* applicable blanks on the attending physician's form. (25)		
3. Proofread claim for accuracy.		
Optional: May deduct points for taking more time than allowed.		

Total Points = 25

Student's Score: _____

Evaluator: _____

Comments: _____

_____

_____

_____

_____

Patient/Insurance Information	Billing Information
Shaley Sue Graham	Record No. 052573
DOB: 07/24/1970	TRF# 00087878IJ
1846 Creamery Row	12/14/20XX; 99213—$55
Milton, XY 12345	Diagnosis: ICD-10 Codes: M75.42; M75.02; S49.92D
555-526-6622	Follow-up appt: 2 mo
SSN: 123-32-2222	Supervising DQ physician: R. L. Jones, M.D.
Employer: Milton Community College	
555-566-3222	
Occupation: Instructor	

```
CHART NOTES

PATIENT NAME:   Shaley Sue Graham        DOB:  07/24/1970

DATE:              12/14/20XX            RECORD NO.  052573

S.    I saw Shaley today in the office for follow up.  Her shoulder pain has diminished
      considerably since I last saw her.  She believes she is well enough to return to
      work.

O.    On examination, abduction,130 degrees w/o pain; forward flexion, 180 degrees;
      extension, 45 degrees; external rotation, 90 degrees; elbow at 90 degrees with
      arm comfortable at side and with arm at 90 degrees abduction.  Internal rotation,
      90 degrees.

A:    Rotator cuff tendonitis/impingement syndrome, resolved.

P.    It is my opinion that Shaley's rotator cuff injury is resolved, and she has been
      released to return to her job without limitations.  I cautioned the patient, however,
      of certain repetitive arm/shoulder motions that could aggravate the rotator cuff
      again, such as lifting weights and certain active sports, such as tennis, golf, and
      archery—all of which she previously engaged in.  Rtn PRN.


R. L. Jones

R. L. Jones, MD/xxx
```

Fig. 11.10 Chart notes for Graham (return visit).

RELEASE TO RETURN TO WORK

Name of worker	Claim number

Please fill out this form and return it to us at the address indicated above.

1. Is the worker medically stationary? ☐ Yes ☐ No

   Date: _____ (Provide closing information and complete Form 827.)

   Next scheduled appointment date: _____

2. Worker is released to:

   ☐ full duty without limitations Date: _____ (Do not complete lines 3 through 11. Sign below.)

   ☐ modified duty from (date) _____ through (date) _____ (specify limitations below)

   ☐ modified hours — specify _____ from (date) _____ through (date) _____

	Hours:	No limitations	1	2	3	4	5	6	7	8
3. In an eight-hour workday, worker can stand/walk a total of	-----	☐	☐	☐	☐	☐	☐	☐	☐	☐
4. At one time, worker can stand/walk	-----	☐	☐	☐	☐	☐	☐	☐	☐	☐
5. In an eight-hour workday, worker can sit a total of	-----	☐	☐	☐	☐	☐	☐	☐	☐	☐
6. At one time, worker can sit	-----	☐	☐	☐	☐	☐	☐	☐	☐	☐

7. The worker is released to return to work in the following range for lifting, carrying, pushing/pulling:

Pounds	<10	10	15	20	25	30	35	40	45	50	55	60	65	70	75	80	85	90	95	100	>100
Occasionally	☐	☐	☐	☐	☐	☐	☐	☐	☐	☐	☐	☐	☐	☐	☐	☐	☐	☐	☐	☐	☐
Frequently	☐	☐	☐	☐	☐	☐	☐	☐	☐	☐	☐	☐	☐	☐	☐	☐	☐	☐	☐	☐	☐

8. Worker can use hands for repetitive:

	Right	Left	
a. Fine manipulation	☐ Yes ☐ No	☐ Yes ☐ No	
b. Pushing and pulling	☐ Yes ☐ No	☐ Yes ☐ No	Dominant hand
c. Simple grasping	☐ Yes ☐ No	☐ Yes ☐ No	☐ Right ☐ Left
d. Keyboarding	☐ Yes ☐ No	☐ Yes ☐ No	

9. Worker can use feet for repetitive raising and pushing (as in operating foot controls): ☐ Yes ☐ No

10. Worker is able to:

	Continuous 67-100% of the day	Frequently 34-66% of the day	Occasionally 6-33% of the day	Intermittently 1-5% of the day	Not at all
a. Stoop/bend	☐	☐	☐	☐	☐
b. Crouch	☐	☐	☐	☐	☐
c. Crawl	☐	☐	☐	☐	☐
d. Kneel	☐	☐	☐	☐	☐
e. Twist	☐	☐	☐	☐	☐
f. Climb	☐	☐	☐	☐	☐
g. Balance	☐	☐	☐	☐	☐
h. Reach	☐	☐	☐	☐	☐
i. Push/pull	☐	☐	☐	☐	☐

11. Other functional limitations or modifications necessary in worker's employment:

Additional comments may be written on back of form.

Signature of medical service provider*	Printed name	Date

Fig. 11.11 Return to work form for Graham.

APPLICATION EXERCISES

Health Insurance Professional's Notebook

A. Examples of forms and completion instructions for:
1. Workers' compensation claims
2. Employer/private disability claims
3. SSDI and SSI claims
4. Attending physician's statement of disability forms
5. Continued disability forms
6. Release to Return to Work forms

B. Names of agencies and telephone numbers for workers' compensation and disability claims in your state

Chapter Checklist

Student Name: _____

Chapter Completion Date: _____

Evaluate your classroom performance. Complete the self-evaluation and submit it to your instructor. When your instructor returns this form to you, compare your self-evaluation with the evaluation completed by your instructor.

1.	Record	Your start time and date: _____
2.	Read	The assigned chapter in the textbook
3.	View	PowerPoint slides (if available)
4.	Complete	Exercises in the workbook as assigned
5.	Compare	Your answers to the answers posted on the bulletin board, website, or handout
6.	Correct	Your answers
7.	Complete	All tests and required activities
8.	Read	Assigned readings (if any)
9.	Complete	Chapter performance objectives (competencies), if any
10.	Evaluate	Chapter performance and submit to your instructor
11.	Record	Your ending time and date: _____
12.	Move on	Begin next chapter as assigned

PERFORMANCE EVALUATION

Student Name: _____

Chapter Completion Date: _____

Evaluate your classroom performance. Compare this evaluation with the one provided by your instructor.

Skill	Student Self-Evaluation			Instructor Evaluation		
	Good	Average	Poor	Good	Average	Poor
Attendance/punctuality						
Personal appearance						
Applies effort						
Is self-motivated						
Is courteous						
Has positive attitude						
Completes assignments in timely manner						
Works well with others						

Student's Initials: _____

Date: _____

Points Possible: _____

Points Awarded: _____

Chapter Grade: _____

Instructor's Initials: _____

Date: _____

Chapter **11** **Miscellaneous Carriers: Workers' Compensation and Disability Insurance**

12 Diagnostic Coding

Diagnosis codes started out as a way to track morbidity and mortality. As their use evolved, changes were made to add information, resulting in a coding structure that precisely describes the clinical picture of a patient. ICD-9-CM has been used for coding diagnoses in the United States for nearly 30 years; however, ICD-9 has several drawbacks. Most important, it was running out of room. Because the classification is organized scientifically, each three-digit (or three-character) category in ICD-9-CM could have only 10 subcategories. Most numbers in the majority of categories have been assigned diagnoses. Medical science keeps making new discoveries, and there are only a limited number of categories available in ICD-9 to assign to these new diagnoses.

The structure of the ICD-10-CM coding system allows for unlimited expansion of codes. Besides allowing for unlimited expansion, other improvements have been made to coding in ICD-10-CM. For example, a single code can report a disease and its current manifestation (i.e., type 2 diabetes with diabetic retinopathy). In fracture care, the code differentiates an encounter for an initial fracture, follow-up of fracture healing normally, follow-up with fracture in malunion or nonunion, or follow-up for late effects of a fracture. ICD-10-CM codes are composed of three to seven characters with the first character being alphabetic; it is not case sensitive. As of the publication of this edition, the compliance date for conversion to the ICD-10 coding system was October 1, 2015.

Completing the exercises in this workbook chapter provides valuable practice in applying diagnostic coding conventions, interpreting coding guidelines, and assigning appropriate diagnostic codes to the highest level of specificity. It is not, however, intended to prepare students for coding certification.

WORKBOOK CHAPTER OBJECTIVES

After completing the workbook activities for Chapter 12, the student should be able to:
1. Define the terms used in the chapter.
2. Answer the review questions according to the evaluation criteria set by the instructor.
3. Use problem-solving skills (individually or in a group setting) to determine correct responses and outcomes in case studies and application exercises.
4. Identify coding conventions and their meaning.
5. Recognize the main terms in a medical diagnosis.
6. Apply the correct steps for accurate coding.
7. Assign the correct codes to clinical diagnoses to the greatest level of specificity.
8. Complete performance objectives to the criteria set by the instructor.
9. Compile a section in the Health Insurance Professional's Notebook on diagnostic coding.

DEFINING CHAPTER TERMS

Using the computer, students should type an accurate definition in their own words for each of the chapter terms listed. When finished, students should compare their definitions with those listed in the glossary at the back of the textbook and correct any inaccuracies.

adverse effects
category
code set
combination code
contraindication
conventions
covered entities
default code
diagnosis
eponym

essential modifiers
etiology
first-listed diagnosis
General Equivalence Mappings (GEMs)
histology
in situ
instructional notes
International Classification of Diseases, 10th revision (ICD-10-CM)
laterality

251

main term
manifestation
morphology
NEC (not elsewhere classifiable)
neoplasm
nonessential modifiers
NOS (not otherwise specified)

placeholder character
principal diagnosis
puerperium
sequela (*pl.* sequelae)
seventh (7th) character
subcategory
underdosing

ASSESSMENT

Multiple Choice

Directions: In the questions and statements presented, choose the response that **best** answers or completes the stem and circle the letter that precedes it.

1. A recognized process of transforming descriptions of a patient's disease process, disorder, or injury into universal numerical or alphanumerical formats is referred to as:
   a. Assignation
   b. Coding
   c. Diagnosis
   d. Insurance

2. The reason (sore throat or chest pain) that brings a patient to the healthcare facility is commonly referred to as a(n):
   a. Adverse effect
   b. Manifestation
   c. Diagnosis
   d. Condition

3. The first ICD system (ICD-1) was put into use in:
   a. 1890
   b. 1900
   c. 1950
   d. 1999

4. Diagnosis codes in the outdated ICD-9-CM system consisted of _____ digits or characters.
   a. 2 to 4
   b. 3 to 5
   c. 4 to 6
   d. 5 to 7

5. Diagnosis codes in the ICD-10-CM system consist of _____ digits or characters.
   a. 2 to 4
   b. 3 to 5
   c. 4 to 6
   d. 3 to 7

6. The Alphabetic Index in ICD-10 lists all diagnostic terms:
   a. In numerical order
   b. In alphabetic order
   c. By level of severity
   d. By anatomical site

7. Which of these *is not* a covered entity as defined by HIPAA rules?
   a. Healthcare publishers
   b. Health plans
   c. Healthcare clearinghouses
   d. Healthcare providers

8. Part III (Tabular List of Diseases and Injuries) of the ICD-10-CM coding manual is composed of _____ chapters.
   a. 10
   b. 17
   c. 21
   d. 30

9. Common uses of coding include all of these *except:*
   a. Setting health policy
   b. Establishing physician fees
   c. Monitoring resource utilization
   d. Preventing healthcare fraud and abuse

10. Valid reasons for converting to the ICD-10-CM system include all *except:*
    a. Lack of specificity in ICD-9 codes
    b. The AMA mandated the change
    c. Lack of available code numbers in ICD-9
    d. ICD-10-CM uses full code titles, reflecting advances in medical technology

11. In the current diagnostic coding system, the manual used for coding inpatient procedures is:
    a. ICD-10-CM
    b. HCPCS Volume 2
    c. ICD-10-PCS
    d. ICD-9-Volume 4

12. Diagnosis codes in ICD-10-CM are used in:
    a. All physicians' offices
    b. Outpatient clinics
    c. Inpatient hospital settings
    d. Both a and b

13. In fracture care, a seventh character A indicates:
    a. An initial encounter
    b. A subsequent encounter
    c. A sequela (follow-up) for late effects
    d. Fracture care does not require a seventh character.

14. After the diagnosis has been determined, the _____ in the diagnosis should be identified.
    a. Main term
    b. Etiology
    c. Lead term
    d. Either a or c

15. When diseases, procedures, or syndromes are named after the individual who discovered or first used them, they are commonly referred to as:
    a. Modifiers
    b. Eponyms
    c. Manifestations
    d. Subcategories

16. Identify the main term in the diagnosis of premature atrial contraction (PAC):
    a. Premature
    b. Atrial
    c. Contraction
    d. Heart

17. Some categories, mainly those subject to notes linking them with other categories, require multiple indexing steps. To avoid repeating multiple steps for each of the additional terms involved, a _____ is used.
    a. Modifier
    b. Seventh character
    c. Cross-reference
    d. Place-holder character

18. After the provisional code is located in the _____, the coder should verify the code by locating it in the _____ to ensure that the diagnosis has been coded to the optimal specificity.
    a. Alphabetic Index/Tabular List
    b. ICD-10-CM/ICD10-PCS
    c. Tabular List/Alphabetic Index
    d. Both a or c

19. Codes are arranged in the Tabular and divided into chapters based on _____.
    a. Anatomical site
    b. Body system
    c. Etiology
    d. All of the above

20. In ICD-10 diagnostic coding, the letter "x":
    a. Allows for future expansion of the code
    b. Is used to fill out empty characters when a code contains fewer than six characters and a seventh character applies
    c. Indicates that the code is new in this coding edition
    d. Both a and b

21. The Index to Diseases in the ICD-10-CM coding manual is organized:
    a. By anatomical sites
    b. Alphabetically by main terms
    c. Numerically
    d. By body systems

22. Diseases, procedures, or syndromes named for individuals who discovered or first used them are called:
    a. Eponyms
    b. Main terms
    c. Modifiers
    d. Diagnoses

23. Essential modifiers describe:
    a. Various anatomical sites
    b. The cause or origin of a disease or condition
    c. Clinical types
    d. All of the above

24. Terms enclosed in parentheses after main terms are called:
    a. Subterms
    b. Essential modifiers
    c. Nonessential modifiers
    d. Eponyms

25. If a patient's condition has not been specifically diagnosed, the health insurance professional must code the:
    a. "Suspected" disease(s)
    b. Disease(s) to be "ruled out"
    c. Probable disease(s)
    d. Signs or symptoms

26. Which of these is considered a "main term"?
    a. Heart
    b. Fracture
    c. Shoulder
    d. Groin

27. The _____ code represents the condition that is most commonly associated with the main term or is the unspecified code for the condition.
    a. First-listed
    b. Default
    c. Combination
    d. Subcategory

28. The main term for *acute depressive reaction* is:
    a. Acute
    b. Depressive
    c. Reaction
    d. Either a or c

29. In the ICD-10-CM system, all letters of the alphabet are used ***except***:
    a. The letter U
    b. The letter X
    c. The letters X, Y and Z
    d. The letter O

30. When a term has many modifiers that might be listed beneath more than one term; what cross-reference is used?
    a. *See*
    b. *See also*
    c. NOS
    d. NEC

31. In most ICD-10-CM manuals, main terms in the index appear in:
    a. Italics
    b. Bold type
    c. Upper case (capital) letters
    d. Parentheses

32. The "placeholder character" in ICD-10-CM utilizes:
    a. The letter "x"
    b. Either the letters "X," "Y," or "Z"
    c. The numeral zero (0)
    d. The point dash (.-)

33. In ICD, rules and guidelines used in coding are commonly referred to as:
    a. Standards
    b. Directives
    c. Conventions
    d. Parameters

34. Identify the symbol that typically is used in the Tabular List when an addition digit (or digits) is needed to code a diagnosis to its greatest specificity:
    a. Asterisk
    b. Bullet
    c. Triangle
    d. Right-facing arrow

35. Which of these *are not* used in ICD-10-CM?
    a. Symbols
    b. Punctuation marks
    c. Abbreviations
    d. Quotation marks

36. NEC in the ICD-10-CM system represents:
    a. Other specified
    b. New etiology code
    c. Not elsewhere classified
    d. Both a and c

37. In ICD-10, when a code appears with a Type 1 Excludes note, it means:
    a. Do not use a seventh character
    b. Exclude any manifestations
    c. Not coded here
    d. Laterality

38. In medicine, _____ is a sign or symptom of a disease.
    a. A manifestation
    b. Etiology
    c. Laterality
    d. A diagnosis

39. A _____ code is a single code used to classify two diagnoses or a diagnosis with an associated secondary process (manifestation).
    a. Default
    b. Combination
    c. Laterality
    d. Etiology

40. In medicine, the study of the form and structure of organisms and their specific structural features is:
    a. Etiology
    b. Utility
    c. Morphology
    d. Laterality

41. A code listed next to a main term in the ICD-10-CM Index is referred to as a:
    a. Combination code
    b. Prerequisite code
    c. Condition code
    d. Default code

42. Sequelae are the _____ of injury or illness.
    a. Anatomical sites
    b. Late effects
    c. Manifestations
    d. Signs and symptoms

43. Which character in an ICD-10-CM code indicates laterality for bilateral sites?
    a. The first character in a five-character code
    b. The seventh character
    c. The character preceding the decimal point
    d. The last character in a six-character code

44. The coder should always begin the search for the correct code assignment in the:
    a. Alphabetic Index
    b. The ICD manual guidelines
    c. The Tabular List
    d. The appendices

45. Examples of adverse effects include all of these *except:*
    a. Vomiting
    b. Tachycardia
    c. Fracture
    d. Respiratory failure

46. Under HIPAA, a _____ is any set of codes used for encoding data elements, such as tables of terms, medical concepts, or medical diagnosis codes.
    a. Crosswalk
    b. Code set
    c. National coverage determination
    d. Supplementary set

47. What must be coded if a patient's condition has not been specifically diagnosed?
    a. Signs or symptoms
    b. Manifestations
    c. Suspected condition
    d. Adverse effect

48. Identify what must be coded first if the patient's diagnosis is *diabetic ulcer of the heel:*
    a. Heel
    b. Ulcer
    c. Diabetes
    d. Signs and symptoms

49. If a patient has both scarlet fever and strep throat:
    a. Code only the scarlet fever
    b. Code only the strep throat
    c. Use a combination code that represents both disorders
    d. Two separate codes must be used

50. Which of these *is not* considered a code set by HIPAA rules?
    a. ICD-10
    b. CPT-4
    c. HCPCS
    d. GEMs

True/False
Directions: Place a "T" in the blank preceding each of these statements if it is true; place an "F" if it is false.

_____ 1. A diagnosis should never be coded from the alphabetic list alone.

_____ 2. A diagnosis must be determined by the healthcare professional providing the medical care.

_____ 3. When the healthcare insurance professional generates an insurance claim for payment of the provider's services, the written diagnosis must appear on the claim.

_____ 4. The U.S. healthcare system currently uses six major coding structures.

_____ 5. A covered entity under the HIPAA Privacy Rule refers to health plans, healthcare clearinghouses, and healthcare providers that transmit health information electronically.

_____ 6. One of the primary concerns with the former ICD-9 system was the lack of specificity expressed in the codes.

_____ 7. All publishers must format and arrange the ICD-10 codes identically.

_____ 8. The Tabular List lists all diagnostic codes in alphanumerical order.

_____ 9. Anatomical sites are often listed as main terms in ICD-10-CM.

_____ 10. Essential modifiers must be a part of the diagnosis documented in the health record.

_____ 11. Nonessential modifiers frequently are not a part of the diagnostic statement but are provided to assist the coder in locating the correct code.

_____ 12. Main terms cannot be anatomical sites.

_____ 13. If a patient has a diagnosis of deviated nasal septum, the main term is _nasal._

_____ 14. _See_ or _see also_ tells the coder to continue the search under another main term.

_____ 15. The Alphabetic Index to Diseases contains a Hypertension table and a Neoplasm table.

_____ 16. In the Tabular List, a bullet symbol preceding the code indicates the code is no longer in use.

_____ 17. The Table of Drugs and Chemicals contains a classification of drugs and other chemical substances to identify poisoning states and external causes of adverse effects.

_____ 18. In ICD-10, an unspecified side code should be used if laterality is not identified in the diagnostic statement.

_____ 19. In ICD-10-CM, any poisoning that was intentional is classified as "poisoning, intentional, self-harm."

_____ 20. Bold type is used in ICD-10 for all exclusion notes and to identify codes that should not be used for describing the first-listed diagnosis.

_____ 21. When the notation "code first underlying disease" is seen, the etiology is coded before the manifestation.

_____ 22. Colons are used in the Tabular List after an incomplete term that needs one or more of the modifiers after the colon to make it assignable to a given category.

_____ 23. ICD-10-CM codes may consist of up to seven characters, with the seventh character extensions representing visit encounter or sequela for injuries and external causes.

_____ 24. The first character of an ICD-10-CM code is always an alphabetic letter.

_____ 25. All alpha characters in the ICD-10-CM coding system are case sensitive.

_____ 26. In ICD-10-CM, codes longer than three characters always have a decimal point after the first three characters.

_____ 27. Categories of injuries are arranged alphabetically under the main term "Injury" rather than by type of injury, such as dislocation.

_____ 28. Indented subterms are never used in combination with the main term.

_____ 29. In ICD-10-CM, if a code has only three characters (e.g., B03 Smallpox), the coder can generally assume that the category has not been further subdivided.

_____ 30. If a code that requires a seventh character is not six characters long, the placeholder "x" must be used to fill in the empty character(s).

Short Answer/Fill-in-the-Blank

Note: If space provided is not adequate, use a separate piece of blank paper.

1. Define _diagnosis_ in your own words.

_____

2. ICD-10-CM stands for _____.

3. Provide a brief explanation of the diagnostic coding process.

_____

_____

_____

4. Explain where the diagnosis can be found in a patient's record.

_____

_____

_____

5. The text states that coding of healthcare data allows access to health records according to diagnoses and procedures for use in clinical care, research, and education. List other common uses of coding data.

_____

_____

_____

6. List the seven essential steps to ICD-10 diagnostic coding.

_____

_____

_____

7. Why is it important for the health insurance professional to use the most recent diagnostic coding manual?

_____

_____

8. List the four ways main terms appear in the Alphabetic Index to Diseases and give an example of each.

_____

_____

_____

_____

_____

9. The first character in an ICD-10-CM diagnosis code is always a(n) _____, and all letters of the alphabet are used

except the letter _____.

10. The second section of the ICD-10-CM manual is the Tabular List. Explain what this section contains and how the information is arranged.

_____

_____

259

11. In ICD-10-CM, if no bilateral code is provided and the condition is bilateral, what should the coder do?

_____

_____

12. Explain the two uses of the "placeholder" character in ICD-10 coding.

_____

_____

_____

_____

13. Explain the difference between etiology and manifestation.

_____

_____

_____

_____

14. Explain what the point dash (.-) indicates in the Tabular List section of ICD-10-CM.

_____

_____

15. Explain the function of the General Equivalence Mappings (GEMs).

_____

_____

_____

_____

CRITICAL THINKING ACTIVITIES

A. Create a one-page essay on the history, development, and use of the ICD system.

B. Underline the main term in each of these:
   1. Breast mass
   2. Deviated nasal septum
   3. Heel spurs
   4. Excessive eye strain
   5. Tension headache
   6. Bronchial croup
   7. Senile cataract
   8. Paranoid delusions
   9. Acute hemorrhagic otitis media with effusion
   10. Coronary insufficiency

260

C. Underline the main terms in these diseases and conditions and assign the correct ICD-10-CM code according to your instructor's directions.

1. Angina pectoris, unspecified: _____

2. Asthma, unspecified (uncomplicated): _____

3. Excessive and frequent menstruation w/ irregular cycle: _____

4. Parkinson disease: _____

5. Urethral abscess: _____

D. Explain each of these conventions and symbols used in ICD-10-CM:

NOS: _____

NEC: _____

- (dash): _____

- (point dash): _____

E. A diagnostic statement from the physician may contain many medical terms, but only one main term describes the patient's illness or injury. All accompanying words that describe the main term further are called *modifiers*. These are found in the Alphabetic Index after (or indented under) the main terms in ICD-10-CM.
1. Name the two types of modifiers.

_____

_____

2. Explain how these two types of modifiers are differentiated, how they are used, and their effect on assigning a correct diagnostic code.

_____

_____

_____

_____

F. Cross-references in the index of both coding manuals assist the coder in locating the appropriate code. Name two types of cross-references (e.g., *see* and *see also*) and explain what each means.

_____

_____

_____

G. These instructional notes appear in the ICD-10 coding manual. Explain what each means in your own words.
■ And

_____

■ With

_____

- Other and other specified

_____

- Unspecified

_____

- Code first

_____

- Code also

_____

H. These instructional notes appear only in the Tabular List of Diseases and Injuries. Explain what each means in your own words.
- Includes

_____

- Excludes

_____

- Use additional code

_____

- Code first underlying disease

_____

I. Frequently, a bullet precedes a code in the Tabular List of Diseases and Injuries. What does this indicate?

_____

_____

PROBLEM-SOLVING/COLLABORATIVE (GROUP) ACTIVITIES

A. Code these accidents using ICD-10-CM codes. (Hint: Accident codes can be located in Chapter 20 [V01–Y99].)
- Exposure to flames in controlled building fire, initial encounter: _____
- Injury to car driver in collision with pedestrian in nontraffic accident, subsequent encounter: _____
- Injury to occupant of train in collision with rolling stock, sequela: _____

B. Using ICD-10-CM, code these diagnoses, which were documented in the health records of various patients. (Keep in mind that you must code the symptoms only.)
- Chest pain (suspected myocardial infarction): _____
- Abdominal discomfort: _____
- Fatigue (suspected iron deficiency anemia):   _____
- Head trauma (possible cerebral concussion):   _____

C. In the front part of the coding manual is a list of symbols and conventions that indicate revisions and additions to the Tabular List. Study these and prepare a group activity to familiarize yourself and those in your group with these items to enhance your coding proficiency.

D. There are 21 chapters in the ICD-10-CM Tabular List of Diseases and Injuries. Generate a five-column table, identifying each chapter number with its corresponding alpha character, the category or body system the chapter contains, code range, and the beginning page number. For example:

Chapter No.	Alpha Prefix	Content	Code Range	Page
1	A & B	Certain Infectious and Parasitical Diseases	A00–B99	479*

*Page numbers will differ depending which coding manual is used.

E. The Centers for Medicare and Medicaid (CMS) has a PowerPoint presentation providing an overview of ICD-10 at https://www.cms.gov/Medicare/Medicare-Contracting/ContractorLearningResources/downloads/ICD-10_Overview_Presentation.pdf. View and review this PowerPoint presentation and then prepare a short oral presentation on key points.

F. Using your ICD-10-CM manual, code these diagnoses:

a. Stress fracture, unspecified ankle, initial encounter

_____

b. Spotting complicating pregnancy, first trimester

_____

c. Cellulitis of right axilla

_____

d. Stuttering

_____

e. Rubella w/complications

_____

PROJECTS/DISCUSSION TOPICS

A. Make a table of coding conventions and symbols used in ICD-10-CM with examples for quick reference to use when coding diagnoses.

B. Participate in a class discussion on HIPAA's effect on ICD coding.

A. Aileen Fortune visited Broadmoor Medical Clinic on 12/29/20XX. On examining her health record, you find these diagnoses. Underline the main terms and assign the correct ICD-10-CM codes to each:

Hypertension, essential, benign: _____   _____

Urinary incontinence: _____   _____

Vesicovaginal fistula of bladder: _____   _____

B. Patient Marcus Aberle's chief complaint and diagnoses are documented as follows:
CC: shortness of breath, chest discomfort, nausea, and profuse sweating
DX: (1) probable myocardial infarction; (2) rule out gastroesophageal reflux disease
What is the correct ICD-10-CM code(s) for this patient?

C. A 51-year-old man is seen at Broadmoor Medical Clinic for an annual health maintenance examination. In addition to the examination, three diagnoses are listed in his health record as follows. Underline the main terms for this patient's diagnoses or conditions and assign the proper ICD-10 code to each:

1. Health maintenance examination, 51-year-old male: _____   _____

2. Tobacco dependence: _____   _____

3. Gastroesophageal reflux disease: _____   _____

4. Arthritis of spine (degenerative): _____   _____

D. Archie Simpson, a 14-year-old boy, presents to the clinic with an insect bite to the right hand, etiology unknown. What is the correct ICD-10-CM code?

E. Katie Olivier, a 6-year-old girl, comes to the clinic with complaints of fever of 101.5°F, chills, sweats, mild earache, stuffy nose, sinus pain and pressure, an episodic cough that is worse in the evening, wheezing, and dyspnea that started approximately 5 days ago. The diagnosis documented in Katie's health record is *acute upper respiratory infection with mild sinusitis, possibly allergy related.* How many diagnostic codes would you list on the claim form? Assign the correct code(s) for ICD-10-CM.

F. Provide the correct answer in these scenarios:
1. David Scott presented to the clinic as a new patient on 08/05/20XX. The documentation in his health record states a diagnosis of ulcer of the left midfoot on this first visit.
2. Over the next 2 years, Mr. Scott continues to come to the clinic on follow-up visits for treatment of his foot ulcer, which tends to heal and then recur. Would the ICD-10-CM code be the same for this patient's follow-up visit 2 years later?
3. If not, what is the correct ICD-10 code for this follow-up visit?

G. Marcie Emerson, a 22-year-old female, presents to the clinic with a chief complaint of sore throat, mild discomfort with swallowing, hoarseness in her voice, nasal congestion with a greenish nasal discharge, and slight postnasal drainage. She denies sinus pain and pressure. She has had a minimal cough with no wheezing, shortness of breath, or dyspnea. The patient is afebrile. Impression: Acute pharyngitis.
1. How many diagnosis codes are needed for this patient's claim form?
2. State the diagnosis(es).
3. Using the steps learned from the text, assign the correct ICD-10 code(s).

A. This website contains helpful information and ICD-10-CM coding resources: https://www.cms.gov/ICD10/. Explore this expansive website for additional information on diagnostic coding. Be prepared for exercises and/or class activities.

B. Using the URL listed in "A," locate and download these topics:
- ICD-10-CM Quick Reference Guide
- 2010 ICD-10-CM Indexes to Diseases and Injuries, Neoplasm, External Cause, and Drug
- 2010 ICD-10-CM Tabular List of Diseases and Injuries
- 2010 ICD-10-CM Official Coding Guidelines

C. The Medicare Learning Network (MLN) publishes periodic articles of interest to health insurance professionals. Visit https://www.cms.gov/MLNMattersArticles/, locate the current year's index, and search for pertinent articles on ICD-10-CM coding.

Performance Objective 12.1: Identifying Format Components of the ICD-10-CM Manual

Conditions: Student will identify the various format components of the ICD-10-CM Manual.
Supplies/Equipment: Pen, current ICD-10-CM manual, and instruction sheet (Fig. 12.1)
Time Allowed: 30 minutes
Accuracy Needed to Pass: 90%

Procedural Steps	Points Earned	Comments
Evaluator: Note time began: _____		
1. Carefully read and study the instruction sheet in Fig. 12.1.		
2. Correctly label the format components by writing or typing the correct term that identifies the component in its corresponding numbered blank.		
Item A—5 points		
Item B—4 points		
Item C—3 points		
3. Proofread your answers for accuracy.		
Optional: May deduct points for taking more time than allowed.		

Total Points = 12

Student's Score: _____

Evaluator: _____

Comments: _____

_____

_____

_____

_____

Identifying Format Components in the ICD-10-CM Manual

The following are sections taken from the ICD-10-CM manual. Identify each component by labeling the corresponding number with the correct name/term of that portion of the disease/condition:

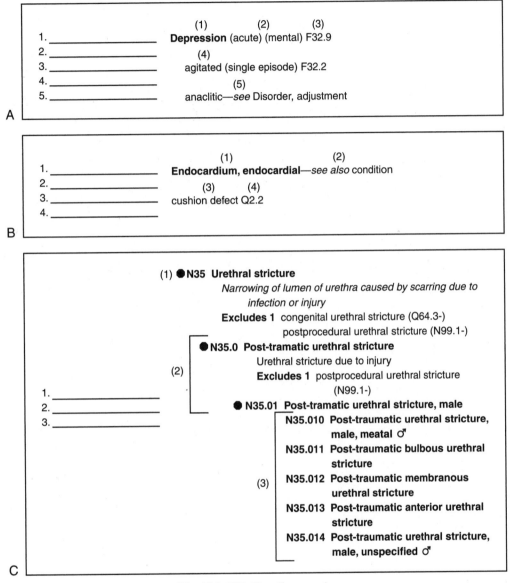

         (1)   (2)   (3)

1. _____   **Depression** (acute) (mental) F32.9
2. _____   (4)
3. _____   agitated (single episode) F32.2
4. _____   (5)
5. _____   anaclitic—*see* Disorder, adjustment

A

                 (1)   (2)

1. _____   **Endocardium, endocardial**—*see also* condition
2. _____   (3)   (4)
3. _____   cushion defect Q2.2
4. _____

B

    (1) ● **N35 Urethral stricture**
           Narrowing of lumen of urethra caused by scarring due to infection or injury
           Excludes 1 congenital urethral stricture (Q64.3-)
                     postprocedural urethral stricture (N99.1-)
    (2) ● **N35.0 Post-tramatic urethral stricture**
           Urethral stricture due to injury
           Excludes 1 postprocedural urethral stricture (N99.1-)
1. _____
2. _____   ● **N35.01 Post-tramatic urethral stricture, male**
3. _____   **N35.010 Post-traumatic urethral stricture, male, meatal** ♂
                     N35.011 Post-traumatic bulbous urethral stricture
    (3)   **N35.012 Post-traumatic membranous urethral stricture**
                     N35.013 Post-traumatic anterior urethral stricture
                     N35.014 Post-traumatic urethral stricture, male, unspecified ♂

C

Fig. 12.1 ICD-10 coding exercise.

Performance Objective 12.2: Assigning ICD-10-CM Diagnosis Codes

Conditions: Student will study the 10 health status and injuries listed on the instruction sheet in Fig. 12.2, after which he or she will assign the correct code to each.

Supplies/Equipment: Pen, current ICD-10-CM manual, and instruction sheet (see Fig. 12.2)

Time Allowed: 30 minutes

Accuracy Needed to Pass: 90%

Procedural Steps	Points Earned	Comments
Evaluator: Note time began: _____		
1. Carefully read and study the instruction sheet in Fig. 12.2.		
2. Review the instructions given for coding health status and injuries.		
3. Using the most current ICD-10-CM manual, identify the underline each main term, then code each of the 10 diagnoses to it greatest specificity. (30)		
4. Proofread your answers for accuracy.		
Optional: May deduct points for taking more time than allowed.		

Total Points = 30

Student's Score: _____

Evaluator: _____

Comments: _____

_____

_____

_____

_____

Instructions: (1) Determine the main term in each of the following diagnoses and underline it. (2) Using the "steps to accurate diagnostic coding" outlined in the book, code each disease/condition to its greatest specificity.

(*Important Note:* Some of the following diagnoses/conditions cannot be used as *first-listed* diagnoses. Also, ICD-10 Codes can have up to 7 digits.)

Diagnostic statement	ICD-10 Code
1. Allergy to eggs	_____
2. Family history of asthma	_____
3. Supervision of high-risk pregnancy w/ history of infertility	_____
4. Routine health checkup (18 y/o male)	_____
5. Dietary counseling and surveillance	_____
6. HIV screening	_____
7. Injury sustained by a pedestrian hit by a car (initial encounter)	_____
8. Patient injury due to fall from a snowmobile (driver) (subsequent encounter)	_____
9. Injury sustained due to (rider) being thrown from a horse (sequelae)	_____
10. Diabetes mellitus screening in asymptomatic patient	_____

Score 1 point for correct selection of main term; 2 points for accurate code assignment.

Fig. 12.2 Coding exercise.

Performance Objective 12.3: Assigning ICD-10-CM Diagnostic Codes

Conditions: Student will study the 10 diseases and conditions listed on the instruction sheet in Fig. 12.3; then he or she will underline the main term and apply the applicable steps for diagnostic coding to locate the correct ICD-10-CM code (to the greatest level of specificity).

Supplies/Equipment: Pen, current ICD-10-CM manual, and instruction sheet (see Fig. 12.3)

Time Allowed: 30 minutes

Accuracy Needed to Pass: 90%

Procedural Steps	Points Earned	Comments
Evaluator: Note time began: _____		
1. Carefully read and study the instruction sheet in Fig. 12.3.		
2. Determine and underline the main term for each of the 10 diseases or conditions listed. (10)		
3. Apply the steps to accurate diagnostic coding, and assign the correct code (to the greatest specificity) to each of the 10 diagnoses. (20)		
4. Proofread your answers for accuracy.		
Optional: May deduct points for taking more time than allowed.		

Total Points = 30

Student's Score: _____

Evaluator: _____

Comments: _____

_____

_____

_____

_____

Instructions: (1) Determine the main term in each of the following diagnoses.
(2) Using the steps to accurate diagnostic coding, code each disease/condition to its greatest specificity.

(*Note:* Never code from the Index alone. Find the main term in the Index to Diseases, and then turn to the Tabular Section and code to the greatest specificity. Remember: ICD-10 Codes can have up to 7 characters.)

Diagnostic statement	ICD-10 Code
1. Urinary incontinence	_____
2. Vesicovaginal fistula	_____
3. Carcinoma *in situ* of prostate	_____
4. Gastric ulcer w/o perforation or bleeding	_____
5. Hypertension, benign essential	_____
6. Rectal polyp	_____
7. Acute tonsillitis	_____
8. Acute cephalgia	_____
9. Nasal laceration w/o foreign body (first visit)	_____
10. Deviated septum	_____

Fig. 12.3 Coding exercise.

Performance Objective 12.4: Assigning Codes to Symptoms, Signs, and Abnormal Findings using ICD-10 codes.

Conditions: Student will study Chapter 18 (Symptoms, Signs and Abnormal Clinical and Laboratory Findings [R00–R99]) and the 10 listed on the instruction sheet in Fig. 12.4; then he or she will code each using the appropriate ICD-10-CM diagnosis code.

Supplies/Equipment: Pen, current ICD-10-CM manual, and instruction sheet (see Fig. 12.4)

Time Allowed: 30 minutes

Accuracy Needed to Pass: 90%

Procedural Steps	Points Earned	Comments
Evaluator: Note time began: _____		
1. Carefully read and study the instruction sheet in Fig. 12.4.		
2. Review the instructions given for coding health status and injuries.		
3. Using the most current ICD-10-CM manual, identify and underline each main term, then code each of the 10 diagnoses provided in Fig. 12.4. (30)		
4. Proofread your answers for accuracy.		
Optional: May deduct points for taking more time than allowed.		

Total Points = 30

Student's Score: _____

Evaluator: _____

Comments: _____

_____

_____

_____

_____

Instructions: (1) Determine the main term in each of the following diagnoses.
(2) Using the steps to accurate diagnostic coding, code each disease/condition to its greatest specificity.

(*Note:* Never code from the Index alone. Find the main term in the Index to Diseases, and then turn to the Tabular Section and code to the greatest specificity. Remember: ICD-10 Codes can have up to 7 characters.)

Diagnostic statement	ICD-10 Code
1. Drowsiness	_____
2. Low self-esteem	_____
3. Fever w/chills	_____
4. Elevated blood glucose level	_____
5. Anorexia	_____
6. Severe sepsis w/septic shock	_____
7. Heart murmur	_____
8. Aphagia	_____
9. Petechiae	_____
10. Facial droop	_____

Fig. 12.4 Coding exercise.

APPLICATION EXERCISES

Health Insurance Professional's Notebook

Create a section in your Health Insurance Professional's Notebook for help with diagnostic coding when you become employed. Include such things as:

- Guidelines to accurate diagnostic coding for both coding structures
- Coding examples
- Table of Conventions
- Informative websites
- Resources and references

ADDITIONAL CODING EXERCISES

Use the guidelines given in the text and the most current ICD-10-CM manual to code these diagnoses and conditions to their greatest level of specificity.

Exercise 1: ICD-10-CM

Acute gastritis without bleeding: _____

Right upper quadrant abdominal tenderness: _____

Foreign body in left ear: _____

Chronic hypertrophy of tonsils and adenoids: _____

Fibrocystic disease of breast (female): _____

Acute suppurative mastoiditis with subperiosteal abscess: _____

Recurrent direct left inguinal hernia with gangrene: _____

Acute upper respiratory infection with influenza: _____

Benign cyst of right breast: _____

Bunion of right great toe: _____

Exercise 2: ICD-10-CM

Nondisplaced abduction fracture anterior acetabulum, subsequent encounter with routine healing: _____

Bronchiectasis with acute bronchitis: _____

Acute bleeding peptic ulcer: _____

Influenza with gastroenteritis: _____

Acute cholecystitis with cholelithiasis and choledocholithiasis: _____

Meningitis due to *Salmonella* infection: _____

Dysphagia after unspecified cerebrovascular disease: _____

Alcohol abuse with alcohol-induced sleep disorder: _____

Displacement of heart valve prosthesis, initial encounter: _____

Intraoperative hemorrhage and hematoma of spleen complicating a procedure on the spleen: _____

Exercise 3: ICD-10-CM
Combination Codes for Conditions and Common Symptoms

Arteriosclerotic heart disease of native coronary artery w/unstable angina pectoris: _____

Crohn's disease of small intestine with fistula: _____

Toxic liver disease with chronic active hepatitis with ascites: _____

274

Combination Codes for Poisonings and the External Cause

Poisoning by aspirin, accidental (unintentional): _____

Poisoning by aspirin, intentional self-harm: _____

Poisoning by aspirin, undetermined: _____

Laterality (ICD-10 codes only)

Malignant neoplasm of upper-inner quadrant of left female breast: _____

Dermatochalasis of left lower eyelid: _____

Phlebitis and thrombophlebitis of superficial vessels of right lower extremity: _____

Webbed fingers, bilateral: _____

Exercise 4: ICD-10-CM

Pressure ulcer of right hip, stage III: _____

Drug or chemical induced diabetes mellitus with diabetic peripheral angiopathy with gangrene: _____

Perforation due to foreign body accidently left in body after surgical operation: _____

Laceration with foreign body of abdominal wall, right lower quadrant, with penetration into peritoneal cavity; initial encounter: _____

Displaced transverse fracture of shaft of humerus, right arm, initial encounter for closed fracture: _____

Bilateral inguinal hernia, with obstruction, without gangrene; recurrent: _____

Difficulty in walking, NEC: _____

Pain, unspecified: _____

Flaccid hemiplegia due to old cerebral infarction: _____

Residuals of previous severe burn, left wrist: _____

Exercise 5: ICD-10-CM

Palpitations: _____

Cocaine dependence, uncomplicated: _____

Right upper quadrant pain: _____

Anorexia nervosa, unspecified: _____

Calculus of kidney: _____

Presbyopia: _____

Type 1 diabetes mellitus without complication: _____

Mitral stenosis, congenital: _____

Chronic obstructive pulmonary disease with acute exacerbation: _____

Dehydration: _____

Chapter Checklist

Student Name: _____

Chapter Completion Date: _____

Evaluate your classroom performance. Complete the self-evaluation and submit it to your instructor. When your instructor returns this form to you, compare your self-evaluation with the evaluation completed by your instructor.

1.	Record	Your start time and date: _____
2.	Read	The assigned chapter in the text
3.	View	PowerPoint slides (if available)
4.	Complete	Exercises in the workbook as assigned
5.	Compare	Your answers to the answers posted on the bulletin board/website/handout
6.	Correct	Your answers
7.	Complete	All tests and required activities
8.	Read	Assigned readings (if any)
9.	Complete	Chapter performance objectives (competencies), if any
10.	Evaluate	Chapter performance and submit to your instructor
11.	Record	Your ending time and date: _____
12.	Move on	Begin next chapter as assigned

PERFORMANCE EVALUATION

Student Name: _____

Chapter Completion Date: _____

Evaluate your classroom performance. Compare this evaluation with the one provided by your instructor.

Skill	Student Self-Evaluation			Instructor Evaluation		
	Good	Average	Poor	Good	Average	Poor
Attendance/punctuality						
Personal appearance						
Applies effort						
Is self-motivated						
Is courteous						
Has positive attitude						
Completes assignments in timely manner						
Works well with others						

Student's Initials: _____

Date: _____

Points Possible: _____

Points Awarded: _____

Chapter Grade: _____

Instructor's Initials: _____

Date: _____

13 Procedural, Evaluation and Management, and HCPCS Coding

Current Procedural Terminology (CPT) is "a list of descriptive terms and identifying codes for reporting medical services and procedures that physicians perform. ... The purpose of CPT is to provide a uniform language that accurately describes medical, surgical, and diagnostic services, thereby serving as an effective means for reliable nationwide communication among physicians, patients, and third parties" (American Medical Association [AMA], 1992). "The only legal way to be paid for a service is to bill using the correct CPT code. The medical facility also must document that the level of service claimed was delivered. Failure to do so may be fraud" (American Academy of Child and Adolescent Psychiatry, 2007).

CPT codes describe medical or psychiatric procedures performed by physicians and other healthcare providers. The codes were developed by the Health Care Financing Administration (HCFA), now known as the Centers for Medicare and Medicaid Services (CMS), to assist in the assignment of reimbursement amounts to providers by Medicare carriers. More and more managed care and other insurance companies now base their reimbursements on the values established by HCFA.

In 2000, the CPT code set was designated by the Department of Health and Human Services as the national coding standard for physician and other healthcare professional services and procedures under the Health Insurance Portability and Accountability Act (HIPAA). This means that for all financial and administrative healthcare transaction sent electronically, the CPT code set will need to be used (*Current Procedural Terminology* [CPT®], AMA, 2010).

Chapter 13 provides students with the basics of CPT coding. The text identifies and explains the organization and structure of the CPT manual, as well as how procedures and services provided to patients treated in physicians' offices are transformed into valid procedural codes. After reading Chapter 13, students should have a basic understanding of CPT coding terminology and definitions. This text is not intended to prepare students for CPT certification; rather, it provides a foundation of the procedural coding process. After thoroughly reading and studying the chapter and completing the exercises and activities in the text and the workbook, students should be able to identify and execute the step-by-step process of assigning CPT, Evaluation and Management (E/M), or HCFA's Common Procedure Coding System (HCPCS) codes.

WORKBOOK CHAPTER OBJECTIVES

After completing the workbook activities for Chapter 13, the student should be able to:
1. Define the terms used in the chapter.
2. Answer the review questions according to the evaluation criteria set by the instructor.
3. Identify coding conventions and their meaning.
4. Make judgments or arrive at rational solutions to coding scenarios requiring critical thinking.
5. Use problem-solving skills (individually or in a group setting) to determine correct responses and outcomes in case studies and application exercises.
6. Apply the correct steps for accurate coding.
7. Assign the correct CPT and HCPCS codes to procedures and services.
8. Identify the correct use of modifiers.

DEFINING CHAPTER TERMS

Using the computer, students should type an accurate definition for each of the chapter terms listed. These definitions should be in the students' own words. When finished, students should compare their definitions with those listed in the glossary at the back of the textbook and correct any inaccuracies.

adjudication
category
Category II codes
Category III codes
chief complaint (cc)
code set
concurrent care
consultation
counseling
CPT-5 Project
critical care
crosswalk
emergency care
established patient
Evaluation and Management (E/M) codes
face-to-face time
HCFA Common Procedure Coding System (HCPCS)
HCPCS codes
Health Care Financing Administration (HCFA)
indented codes
inpatient
key components
Level I codes

Level II codes
Level III codes
main terms
modifiers
modifying terms
morbidity
mortality
new patient
observation
outpatient
Physicians' Current Procedural Terminology, 4th edition (CPT-4)
referral
section
see
special report
stand-alone code
subheading
subjective information
subsection
telehealth communication
unit/floor time

ASSESSMENT

Multiple Choice

Directions: In these questions and statements, choose the response that **best** answers or completes the stem and circle the letter that precedes it.

1. The manual containing codes used in reporting medical services and procedures performed by healthcare providers in the care and treatment of patients is the:
   a. HCPCS Level II
   b. ICD-10-CM
   c. CPT-4
   d. All of the above

2. CPT codes were developed by the:
   a. World Health Organization (WHO)
   b. AMA
   c. HCFA
   d. Department of Health and Human Services (HHS)

3. The CPT manual is published by the:
   a. AMA
   b. HCFA
   c. WHO
   d. HHS

4. A new CPT manual is published:
   a. Annually
   b. Semiannually
   c. Biannually
   d. Every 5 years

5. The first CPT was developed and published in:
   a. 1955
   b. 1966
   c. 1970
   d. 1977

6. The five-digit coding system replaced the four-digit system in the CPT edition published in:
   a. 1955
   b. 1966
   c. 1970
   d. 1977

7. The main body of the CPT manual is organized in:
   a. 4 sections
   b. 6 sections
   c. 10 sections
   d. 12 sections

8. The 5-digit CPT codes may be defined further by two additional digits to help explain an unusual circumstance associated with a service or procedure. These two digits are called:
   a. Modifiers
   b. Amendments
   c. Appendices
   d. CPT codes cannot have more than five digits

9. As with the ICD-10-CM, the CPT index is organized by:
   a. Disease process
   b. Anatomical sites
   c. Main terms
   d. Symptoms

10. A main term can stand alone, or it can be followed by up to _____ modifying term(s).
    a. One
    b. Two
    c. Three
    d. Four

11. To help determine the appropriateness and medical necessity of a service or procedure, a _____ should accompany the claim.
    a. Copy of the patient's health record
    b. Letter of explanation
    c. Special report
    d. Diagram

12. The narrative describing a procedure or service that contains the full description of the procedure without additional explanation is referred to as a(n):
    a. Complete code
    b. Unmodified code
    c. Descriptive code
    d. Stand-alone code

13. Procedures that do not contain the entire written description and refer to the common portion of the procedure listed in the preceding entry are coded with a(n):
    a. Modified code
    b. Indented code
    c. Unfinished code
    d. Incomplete code

14. CPT uses _____ to separate main and subordinate clauses in the code descriptions.
    a. A bullet
    b. Parentheses
    c. A triangle
    d. A semicolon

15. The most important thing to remember when using modifiers is that the health record must contain _____ to support the modifier.
    a. Adequate documentation
    b. Signatures of two physicians
    c. An operative report
    d. Proof of insurance coverage

16. Main terms in CPT-4 are organized by four primary classes of main entries. Which of these *is not* one of these primary classes?
    a. A condition
    b. An eponym
    c. An abbreviation
    d. An apparatus

17. The amount of time the physician spends on bedside care of the hospitalized patient and reviewing the health record and writing orders is called:
    a. Face-to-face time
    b. Unit floor time
    c. Counseling time
    d. Treatment time

18. The classification for a patient who is not sick enough to qualify for acute inpatient status but requires hospitalization for a brief time is referred to as:
    a. Outpatient status
    b. Observation status
    c. Unit floor time
    d. Nonemergency status

19. A procedure by which codes used for data in one database are translated into the codes of another database, allowing information to be shared among databases, is called:
    a. A crosswalk
    b. Database sharing
    c. Intervention
    d. Electronic recognition

20. HCPCS Level II codes are organized into _____ sections.
    a. 5
    b. 8
    c. 12
    d. 17

21. If Megan Cartwright was having an excision of an ovarian cyst, the main term would be:
    a. Excision
    b. Ovarian
    c. Cyst
    d. Either a or c

22. Which codes are designed to classify services provided by a healthcare provider and used primarily in outpatient settings?
    a. CPT-4
    b. E/M
    c. HCPCS
    d. Level III

23. The health insurance professional must determine three factors that would direct him or her to the proper category in the E/M coding section, which include all of these *except*:
    a. Place of service
    b. Type of service
    c. Time spent with patient
    d. Patient status

24. Contributing factors that affect the E/M coding level reported include all of these *except*:
    a. Counseling
    b. Coordination of care
    c. Nature of presenting problem
    d. Whether or not a modifier is used

25. _____ is the AMA's ongoing effort to improve the structure and processes of CPT codes to reflect today's coding demands as well as HIPAA challenges.
    a. The CPT-5 project
    b. HCPCS Level II
    c. The crosswalk design
    d. The Patient Affordable Care Act

True/False
Directions: Place a "T" in the blank preceding each of these statements if it is true; place an "F" if it is false.

_____ 1. Today, most managed care and other insurance companies base their reimbursements on the values established by the CMS.

_____ 2. If the correct CPT code is not known, a narrative description of the procedure or service rendered can be used for third-party claims.

_____ 3. Modifiers are listed in Appendix A at the back of the CPT manual.

_____ 4. Missing or incorrect modifiers are a common reason for claim denial.

_____ 5. If a Category III code is available and accurately describes the service provided, it should be used instead of an unlisted Category I code.

_____ 6. Modifier 99 can be used if the coder cannot find a five-digit CPT code that adequately describes the procedure performed.

_____ 7. There are two types of CPT codes: stand-alone and indented.

_____ 8. E/M codes are based on the complexity of the history, examination, or medical decision making performed during the visit.

_____ 9. A new patient is one who is new to the practice (regardless of service location) or one who has not received medical treatment by the healthcare provider or any other provider in that same office *within the past 3 years.*

_____ 10. Coding E/M services is based on the amount of time spent with the patient or his or her family.

_____ 11. Time is not considered a factor unless 75% of the encounter is spent in counseling.

_____ 12. Time is never a factor for emergency department visits.

_____ 13. All three key components (history, examination, and medical decision making) must be met or exceeded for new patients; only two must be met for established patients.

_____ 14. Hospital discharge services codes are used for reporting services provided on the final day of a multiple-day stay.

_____ 15. To qualify for the use of E/M codes 99281 through 99288, the facility must be available for immediate emergency care 24 hours a day for patients not on "observation status."

_____ 16. Critical care services can be provided only if the facility has an emergency department that operates 24 hours a day.

_____ 17. To use the critical care services codes properly, the physician must be constantly at the patient's bedside.

_____ 18. Time is the controlling factor for assigning the appropriate critical care code.

_____ 19. Modifiers are never used in E/M coding.

_____ 20. HCPCS Level II (national) codes are five-digit alphanumeric codes consisting of one alphabetic character (a letter between A and V) followed by three digits.

_____ 21. If there are CPT and HCPCS Level II codes for the service provided, the CMS requires that the HCPCS Level II code be used.

_____ 22. As with CPT-4, HCPCS Level II code sets contain modifiers; however, modifiers in HCPCS Level II are either alphabetic or alphanumeric.

_____ 23. HIPAA requires that procedure coding be standardized.

_____ 24. With the implementation of HIPAA, the CMS has required medical offices to eliminate any unapproved local procedure or modifier codes (Level III codes).

_____ 25. The AMA is in the process of developing CPT-5, which will totally change the procedural coding process.

Short Answer/Fill-in-the-Blank
Note: If space provided is not adequate, use a separate piece of blank paper.

1. Explain the purpose of CPT coding in your own words.

_____

_____

_____

2. Provide a brief outline of the purpose and development of the CPT system.

_____

_____

_____

_____

3. List and discuss the three levels of procedural coding.

_____

_____

_____

4. The health record must contain adequate documentation to support the use of _____.

5. Each main section of the CPT is preceded by _____ specific to that section.

6. Explain the purpose of Category III codes.

_____

_____

_____

7. List the appendices found in CPT and briefly describe what each contains.

_____

_____

_____

_____

_____

_____

_____

_____

_____

_____

_____

_____

8. Name and give an example of each of the four primary classes of main term entries.

_____

_____

_____

_____

9. Name the three ways a CPT code can be displayed. Include an example of each.

_____

_____

_____

10. If a "special report" accompanies a claim to explain unusual circumstances, list what should be included in this document.

_____

_____

_____

_____

_____

11. Explain the use and importance of a semicolon (;) in assigning a CPT code.

_____

_____

_____

12. Codes in the tabular section of CPT are formatted using four classifications. List and explain each of these.

_____

_____

_____

_____

13. List the six basic steps of CPT coding discussed in the textbook.

_____

_____

_____

_____

_____

_____

14. Distinguish between a "new" patient and an "established" patient.

_____

_____

_____

15. The range of codes for office or other outpatient services is _____ to _____ for new patients and _____ to _____ for established patients.

16. List the three factors that direct the health insurance professional to the proper category in the E/M coding section of CPT.

_____

_____

_____

17. In addition to determining each of the three factors listed in question 16, the health insurance professional must establish what level of service the patient received. Levels of service are based on three key components, which are:

_____

_____

_____

18. In addition to the three key components listed in question 17, there may be four contributing factors that affect the E/M coding level reported. These contributing factors are:

_____

_____

_____

_____

19. The first element to consider in assigning an E/M code is the level of patient history. Name the four levels of history taking.

_____

_____

_____

_____

20. How is the level of medical decision making determined, and what three elements must be considered?

_____

_____

_____

_____

21. In addition to the three key components in assigning an E/M code, contributing factors sometimes enter into the picture that help determine the extent of history, examination, and medical decision making necessary to treat the patient effectively. List and explain these contributing factors.

_____

_____

_____

22. Explain the difference between face-to-face time and unit floor time in the E/M coding process.

_____

_____

_____

_____

_____

_____

_____

Matching

Directions: Place the letter identifying the correct symbol in the blank in front of the numbered statements. (*Note:* Refer to symbols in Table 13.2 in the textbook. Not all symbols are used.)

_____ 1.	Code is new to the CPT book	a. *
_____ 2.	Description has been changed or modified	b. ●
		c. —
_____ 3.	Identifies changes in wording of new or revised codes	d. ▲
		e. +
_____ 4.	Add-on code	f. ►◄
_____ 5.	Identifies codes that include conscious (moderate) sedation	g. ⊘
		h. ⊙
_____ 6.	Modifier 51 exempt	

CRITICAL THINKING ACTIVITIES

A. In these scenarios, determine whether each patient is "new" or "established."
   1. Jessica Sidwell has an appointment at Broadmoor Medical Clinic today. She is new to the area, having recently moved to Milton from another state.
   2. Elwood Camp was seen at the hospital for a consultation 2 weeks ago. He is coming to the office today for a follow-up appointment.
   3. When Dr. Jones was attending a seminar in another city, Dr. Lucero treated Barbara Farris for acute sinusitis.
   4. Robert Fuller, who was seen by Dr. Jones 2 years ago for an eye infection, has an appointment today with Dr. Lucero. Robert has just returned from an 18-month tour of duty in Afghanistan.
   5. Martha Gibbs, who has a 10 AM appointment today, saw Dr. Lucero 5 years ago when she was a resident at Columbia University Clinic in Missouri.
   6. Jill Bennet has an appointment with Dr. Jones tomorrow for a consultation. She has not been seen at Broadmoor Medical Clinic before, but her primary care provider has forwarded her complete health record.

B. In these scenarios, determine whether the procedure or service should be classified as a "consultation" or a "referral."
   1. Dr. Jones has been treating Sylvia Potter for a skin condition. He has prescribed several medications, but the problem persists. Dr. Jones instructs Mrs. Potter to make an appointment with Dr. Fontaine, a renowned dermatologist at the University Clinic, for his opinion of the condition.
   2. Dr. Lucero has asked you to make an appointment for Zebulon Porter with a cardiologist for diagnostic tests to pinpoint the cause of Mr. Porter's cardiac symptoms.
   3. Ellen Tyson is being seen at Broadmoor Medical Clinic for gastrointestinal problems that do not respond to treatment. Dr. Lucero asks Dr. Benson, a psychiatrist, to evaluate Ms. Tyson to see if her symptoms might be psychosomatic.
   4. The emergency department physician on duty telephones Dr. Jones to evaluate a patient who has sustained a back injury as a result of an automobile accident. After Dr. Jones examines the patient, the patient is rushed to the operating room for immediate surgery.
   5. Dr. Lucero's patient, Lucas Bonnet, asks for an appointment with ophthalmologist Vincent Carter for a second opinion before eye surgery.

C. Underline the main terms in these procedures:
   Intertrochanteric femoral fracture (closed treatment)
   Removal of gallbladder calculi
   Lung, bullae excision
   Closed treatment of wrist dislocation
   Dilation of cervix
   Placement of upper gastrointestinal feeding tube
   Radiograph and fluoroscope of chest, four views
   Magnetic resonance imaging, lower spine
   Darrach procedure
   Automated CBC
   Electrosurgical removal, five skin tags

PROBLEM SOLVING/COLLABORATIVE (GROUP) ACTIVITIES

A. Underline the main term and code these procedures:

Puncture aspiration of breast cyst: _____

Diagnostic bronchoscopy with biopsy: _____

Pacemaker insertion with transvenous electrode, atrial: _____

Tonsillectomy and adenoidectomy (T&A), 12-year-old boy: _____

Removal of urethral diverticulum from female patient: _____

Therapeutic D&C, nonobstetric: _____

Biofeedback training: _____

Face-to-face psychotherapy (individual), 50 minutes: _____

B. Select the "new" patient office visit E/M codes using the key components listed.

1. Detailed history, detailed examination, low-complexity decision making: _____

2. Problem-focused history, problem-focused examination, straightforward decision making: _____

3. Comprehensive history, comprehensive examination, high-complexity decision making: _____

C. Select the "established" patient office visit E/M codes using the key components listed.

1. Detailed history, detailed examination, low-complexity decision making: _____

2. Comprehensive history, comprehensive examination, moderate-complexity decision making: _____

3. Detailed history, comprehensive examination, high-complexity decision making: _____

D. Explain the guidelines for reporting a "miscellaneous" procedure or service for which there is no listed CPT code.

E. You have received a denial from an insurance carrier because you, in error, used a deleted procedure code on the claim. How could you have prevented this from happening, and how can you find the correct code?

PROJECTS/DISCUSSION TOPICS

A. Your instructor will choose one or more of these topics to discuss in class or assign a topic to you as a project. Study Chapter 13 to be prepared for taking an active part in any or all of these issues:
   1. Why is it important to use the most recent CPT manual available?
   2. What role does CPT coding play in insurance reimbursement?
   3. Discuss the importance of adhering to accurate coding and billing guidelines.
   4. When are modifiers used, and how do they affect CPT coding?
   5. Discuss the proper use of "observation" codes.

B. Can 99218-99220 be reported for each day a patient is in observation? The codes state "per day" in the definition.

CASE STUDIES

In the Critical Thinking Activities for this workbook chapter, six scenarios were presented, and you had to determine whether the patient was new or established. Now, study these same six scenarios and code the procedures or services listed in each.

1. Jessica Sidwell has an appointment at Broadmoor Medical Clinic today. She is new to the area, having recently moved to Milton from another state.
   Initial new patient office visit Level II
   Intramuscular antibiotic injection

2. Elwood Camp was seen at the hospital for a consultation 2 weeks ago. He is coming to the office today for a follow-up appointment.
   Postoperative follow-up visit

3. When Dr. Jones was attending a seminar in another city, Dr. Lucero treated Barbara Farris for acute sinusitis.
   Established patient office visit Level II
   Removal of nasal polyp, simple

4. Robert Fuller, who was seen by Dr. Jones 2 years ago for an eye infection, has an appointment today with Dr. Lucero. Robert has just returned from an 18-month tour of duty in Afghanistan. Because it had been 2 years since Robert had been to the office, Dr. Lucero performed a complete physical examination.
   Established patient office visit Level III
   Comprehensive eye examination
   Removal of foreign body from right eye (external/superficial)

5. Martha Gibbs, who has a 10 AM appointment today, saw Dr. Lucero 5 years ago when she was a resident at Columbia University Clinic in Missouri.
   New patient office visit Level III
   Pap smear
   Lipid panel
   Electrocardiogram (12 leads)
   Occult blood fecal test

6. Jill Bennet has an appointment with Dr. Jones tomorrow for a consultation. She has not been seen at Broadmoor Medical Clinic before, but her primary care provider has forwarded her complete health record. Jill has been experiencing problems with her periods (heavy bleeding, bleeding between periods, and severe cramping).
   Initial visit new patient Level III
   Transvaginal ultrasound
   Vaginal colposcopy with biopsy

INTERNET EXPLORATION

A. Log on to the AMA website and peruse the links on CPT coding. Be prepared for an activity or exercise at your instructor's discretion.

B. The websites listed here are just a few of the many that provide information for further education if you are interested in becoming a certified coder:
   - http://www.aapc.com
   - http://www.ahima.org/certification
   - http://physicianswebsites.com/CMBS-Certification.html
   - http://www.cms.gov/MedHCPCSGenInfo/20_HCPCS_Coding_Questions.asp

   If any of these URLs are no longer active, use appropriate search words to find similar websites that provide important information on these topics.

C. Visit http://www.cms.gov/ and use the search words "CPT-4 Coding" to explore some of the pertinent topics regarding CPT-4 and/or HCPCS coding.

PERFORMANCE OBJECTIVES

Performance Objective 13.1: Coding Procedures and Services

Conditions: Student will identify the main term in each of 10 procedural events by underlining it and then correctly code these same procedures.

Supplies/Equipment: Pen, current CPT manual, and list of procedures to code

Time Allowed: 30 minutes

Accuracy Needed to Pass: 90%

Procedural Steps	Points Earned	Comments
Evaluator: Note time began: _____		
Colonoscopy with biopsy		
Chest x-ray, single view, frontal		
Lipid panel		
HDL cholesterol		
Strep test, rapid		
ECG with interpretation		
Simple suture (face), local anesthetic		
Bilateral mammography		
Destruction, flat wart		
Partial splenectomy		

Total Points = 20 (2 points each)

Student's Score: _____

Evaluator: _____

Comments: _____

_____

_____

_____

_____

Performance Objective 13.2: Coding Office Visits (E/M Codes)

Conditions: Student will study the scenarios in Box 13.1 and code each encounter using E/M codes from the CPT manual.

Supplies/Equipment: Pen, current CPT manual, and instruction sheet in Box 13.1

Time Allowed: 30 minutes

Accuracy Needed to Pass: 90%

Procedural Steps	Points Earned	Comments
Evaluator: Note time began: _____		
1. Carefully read and study the case studies in Box 13.1.		
2. Correctly identify the proper E/M code for each of these scenarios:		
Scenario 1:		
Scenario 2:		
Scenario 3:		
Scenario 4:		
Scenario 5:		
Scenario 6:		
Optional: May deduct points for taking more time than allowed.		

Total Points = 30 (5 points each)

Student's Score: _____

Evaluator: _____

Comments: _____

_____

_____

_____

_____

Box 13.1

1. Heidi Andrews, an 8-year-old girl, presents as a new patient to Broadmoor Medical Clinic with a severe skin rash. History and examination are problem focused; decision making is straightforward.
2. Forrest Gunther, an established patient with a history of chronic sinusitis, presents with sinus drainage, sore throat, severe nasal congestion, cough, and fever of 100.1°F. History and examination are problem focused; medical decision making is low complexity.
3. Elena Rodriguez presents with a benign lesion on her right leg. Although this patient has not been seen in the clinic before, she says she has had the mole for several years. The problem is low to moderate severity, and Dr. Jones spends 20 minutes face to face with Ms. Rodriguez.
4. Loris Hiller, an 82-year-old man, comes to the clinic for a follow-up examination. He has well-controlled diabetes but has other health problems including diabetic retinopathy, hypertension, glaucoma, and chronic obstructive pulmonary disease. History and examination are detailed, with moderate-complexity medical decision making. Dr. Lucero spends 25 minutes with Mr. Hiller.
5. Melinsa Delarosa, a 55-year-old woman, was admitted for observation of chest pains to Broadmoor Medical Center and discharged the same day. The key components are comprehensive history and examination with moderate-complexity medical decision making.
6. Dr. Jones admits 15-month-old Brittany Lanz to Broadmoor Medical Center. Brittany has been experiencing recurring episodes of respiratory distress with greenish-yellow nasal discharge, cough with wheezing, and fever of 103.6°F. Her mother reports a decrease in appetite and irritability with intermittent ear pulling. A comprehensive history is taken with a complete multisystem examination. Because of multiple diagnoses and management options plus an excessive amount of data to be reviewed in the health record, the medical decision making is high complexity.

Performance Objective 13.3: Locating HCPCS Codes

Conditions: Student will code 10 procedures, services, or supplies listed.
Supplies/Equipment: Pen, and current HCPCS (CPT Level II codes) manual
Time Allowed: 30 minutes
Accuracy Needed to Pass: 90%

Procedural Steps	Points Earned	Comments
Evaluator: Note time began: _____		
1. 2-mL sterile syringe with needle		
2. Nonemergency transport (taxi)		
3. Diaphragm for contraceptive use		
4. Acetaminophen injection, 10 mg		
5. Standard wheelchair with footrests		
6. Ampicillin injection, 500 mg		
7. Ostomy pouch, closed with barrier and filter		
8. Custom fabricated thoracic rib belt		
9. Spenco molded foot insert, removable		
10. 1 unit plasma, fresh frozen (donor retested)		
11. Proofread your answers for accuracy.		
Optional: May deduct points for taking more time than allowed.		

Total Points = 20 (2 points each)

Student's Score: _____

Evaluator: _____

Comments: _____

_____

_____

_____

_____

Performance Objective 13.4: Choosing Modifiers

Conditions: Student will identify the correct modifier to use in each of the scenarios given in Box 13.2.
Supplies/Equipment: Pen or typewriter, current CPT manual, and scenarios listed in Box 13.2
Time Allowed: 30 minutes
Accuracy Needed to Pass: 90%

Procedural Steps	Points Earned	Comments
Evaluator: Note time began: _____		
1. Carefully read and study the scenarios in Box 13.2.		
2. Correctly identify the proper modifier to use for each of these scenarios:		
Scenario 1:		
Scenario 2:		
Scenario 3:		
Scenario 4:		
Scenario 5:		
Scenario 6:		
Proofread your answers for accuracy.		
Optional: May deduct points for taking more time than allowed.		

Total Points = 30 (5 points each)

Student's Score: _____

Evaluator: _____

Comments: _____

_____

_____

_____

_____

Box 13.2

1. When Teresa Hardy underwent her hysterectomy, complications occurred during the surgical procedure. Typically, the procedure lasts about 1 ½ hours; however, Teresa's lasted nearly 3 hours.

2. Performing a cystoscopy on an adult normally would not require general anesthesia; however, for 3-year-old Benjamin Field, Dr. Lucero determined that a general anesthetic would be best.

3. Dr. Jones removed a ruptured appendix from a patient and provided a general anesthetic for the procedure. Listing separate charges for each of the services would be appropriate; the health insurance professional would code as follows: 44960—appendectomy, ruptured appendix. The code for a surgeon administering his or her own anesthetic for the procedure (44960) would require a modifier.

4. The bilateral modifier is restricted to surgical procedures only (CPT codes 10040–69990). It is not required for radiology procedure codes or diagnostic procedure codes. Procedures now are assumed to be unilateral unless they are always performed bilaterally or are otherwise noted in CPT. The most commonly accepted method of reporting bilateral procedures is to list the procedure twice and add the correct modifier.

5. Certain complex surgical procedures require the skills of more than two surgeons. A good example is the surgical team that implants an artificial heart. The physicians performing the surgery usually have different skills or specialties. Each member of the team would add a modifier to the procedures he or she performed as part of the surgical team.

6. A patient is brought to the hospital with internal hemorrhaging that is repaired surgically. Three days after surgery, the patient begins hemorrhaging again and the surgeon must perform the same repair again. If a different physician performed the second repair, he or she would use a different modifier.

Health Insurance Professional's Notebook

Create a section in your Health Insurance Professional's Notebook for help with procedural coding when you become employed. Include such things as:

- Guidelines to accurate procedural coding
- Coding examples
- List of CPT manual appendices and their contents
- CPT manual sections and their code ranges
- Informative websites
- Resources and references

ADDITIONAL CODING EXERCISES

Using the guidelines given in the text and the most current CPT manual, code these procedures, services, or supplies.

Exercise 1
Procedure: Surgery Section

_____ Removal of 25 skin tags

_____ Partial removal of the spleen

_____ Radical cervical lymphadenectomy

_____ Excision of benign tumor of the mediastinum

_____ Incision and drainage of a simple lymph node abscess

_____ Flexible sigmoidoscopy with three biopsies

_____ Colonoscopy with removal of polyp by a snare

_____ Exploratory laparotomy, exploratory celiotomy

_____ Repair of an initial incarcerated inguinal hernia in a 5 ½-year-old

_____ Complete vasectomy

_____ Reversal of urethral anastomosis

_____ Anterior segment of the left eye, emboli removal

_____ Removal of left eye, muscles attached to implant

_____ Destruction of 0.4-cm malignant lesion of the neck

_____ Suture of sciatic nerve

Exercise 2
Procedure: Radiology, Pathology, and Laboratory Sections

_____ Bilateral mammography

_____ Radiological examination of mastoids, two views

_____ Chest x-ray single view, frontal

_____ Complete hip x-ray study, two views

_____ Ultrasound of the chest using B-scan

_____ Fetal profile, biophysical

_____ Teletherapy isodose plan, simple

_____ Automated urinalysis without microscopy

_____ Gases, blood pH only

Code these using one of the six surgical pathology codes in the CPT manual:

_____ The specimen is a uterus, tubes, and ovaries. The procedure was an abdominal hysterectomy for ovarian cancer (Level VI).

_____ The specimen is a portion of the lung. The procedure was a left lower lobe wedge resection (Level VI).

_____ The specimen is the prostate. The procedure was a transurethral resection of the prostate (Level IV).

Exercise 3
Procedure: Medicine Section

_____ Routine electrocardiogram with 12 leads, with interpretation and report

_____ Cardiac catheterization on the right side of the heart

_____ Pulmonary stress test, simple

_____ Direct nasal mucous membrane test

_____ Awake and drowsy electroencephalogram and photic stimulation in clinic

_____ Range of motion measurement and report on both legs

_____ Chemotherapy administered subcutaneously

_____ Initial psychiatric interview examination

_____ Acid reflux test of the esophagus with nasal catheter pH electrode placement, recording, analysis, and interpretation

_____ Fitting of contact lens for treatment of cataract, including the lens

_____ Nasopharyngoscopy with evaluation

_____ Hemodialysis with a single physician evaluation

_____ Oral polio vaccine

Exercise 4
Procedure: Integumentary System

_____ Destruction, flat wart

_____ Layer closure of skin wound, > 0.30 cm, trunk

_____ Repair nail bed

_____ Mastectomy, partial

Procedure: Musculoskeletal System

_____ Injection, ganglion cyst

_____ Treatment of closed patella dislocation without anesthesia

_____ Injection of small joint bursa

_____ Biopsy, bone, trocar, or needle superficial

298

Procedure: Hemic/Lymphatic/Diaphragm (38100–39599)

_____ Repair, esophageal/diaphragmatic hernia

_____ Partial splenectomy

_____ Excision, two deep cervical nodes

Procedure: Radiology/Pathology

_____ Upper gastrointestinal x-ray study with films and KUB

_____ Ultrasound, pregnant uterus after first trimester

_____ Routine urinalysis with microscopy

_____ Colorimetric hemoglobin

Chapter Checklist

Student Name: _____

Chapter Completion Date: _____

Evaluate your classroom performance. Complete the self-evaluation and submit it to your instructor. When your instructor returns this form to you, compare your self-evaluation with the evaluation completed by your instructor.

1.	Record	Your start time and date: _____
2.	Read	The assigned chapter in the textbook
3.	View	PowerPoint slides (if available)
4.	Complete	Exercises in the workbook as assigned
5.	Compare	Your answers to the answers posted on the bulletin board, website, or handout
6.	Correct	Your answers
7.	Complete	All tests and required activities
8.	Read	Assigned readings (if any)
9.	Complete	Chapter performance objectives (competencies), if any
10.	Evaluate	Chapter performance and submit to your instructor
11.	Record	Your ending time and date: _____
12.	Move on	Begin next chapter as assigned

PERFORMANCE EVALUATION

Student Name: _____

Chapter Completion Date: _____

Evaluate your classroom performance. Compare this evaluation with the one provided by your instructor.

Skill	Student Self-Evaluation			Instructor Evaluation		
	Good	Average	Poor	Good	Average	Poor
Attendance/punctuality						
Personal appearance						
Applies effort						
Is self-motivated						
Is courteous						
Has positive attitude						
Completes assignments in timely manner						
Works well with others						

Student's Initials: _____

Date: _____

Points Possible: _____

Points Awarded: _____

Chapter Grade: _____

Instructor's Initials: _____

Date: _____

14 | The Patient

In Chapter 14, we learned about the importance of patient needs and expectations. Patients need to be recognized and treated as individuals by all members of the healthcare team. Patients want to be continuously informed about their illness and condition. An atmosphere of respect for the individual patient focuses on quality of life, involves the patient in medical decisions, treats the patient with dignity, and respects a patient's autonomy. Patients have indicated that they feel vulnerable and powerless in the face of illness, and proper treatment and coordination of their care help to ease those feelings.

Chapter 14 also looked at future trends in patient care, specifically that patients are "consumers" of healthcare, and, as consumers, they have a right to expect quality care. Patient advocacy begins with the relationship between the patient and the physician.

A wide scope of patient topics was presented in Chapter 14, including billing policies and practices. The activities and exercises in this accompanying workbook chapter will expand your knowledge of the important relationship between the patient and the healthcare team and help develop a better understanding of the topics presented in Chapter 14.

WORKBOOK CHAPTER OBJECTIVES

After completing the workbook activities for Chapter 14, the student should be able to:
1. Define the terms used in the chapter.
2. Answer the review questions according to the evaluation criteria set by the instructor.
3. Use problem-solving skills (individually or in a group setting) to determine correct responses and outcomes in case studies and application exercises.
4. Work in a group setting to resolve scenarios dealing with credit and collection policies.
5. Generate suitable collection techniques (e.g., telephone conversations and letters).
6. Create a table of pertinent laws and acts that apply to collection and credit.
7. Explore the Internet to learn more about the topics addressed in Chapter 14.

DEFINING CHAPTER TERMS

Using the computer, students should type an accurate definition for each of the chapter terms listed. These definitions should be in the students' own words. When finished, students should compare their definitions with those listed in the glossary at the back of the textbook and correct any inaccuracies.

accounts receivable
alternate billing cycle
assignment of benefits
billing cycle
collection agency
collection ratio
daily journal
defendant
de-identified
disbursements journal
Equal Credit Opportunity Act
Fair Credit Billing Act (FCBA)
Fair Credit Reporting Act
Fair Debt Collection Practices Act
general journal

general ledger
HIPAA-covered entities
meaningful use
"one-write" systems
patient information form
patient ledger
payroll journal
plaintiff
protected health information (PHI)
self-pay patient
small claims litigation
surrogates
treatment, payment, or healthcare operations (TPO)
Truth in Lending Act

Multiple Choice

Directions: In the questions and statements presented, choose the response that **best** answers or completes the stem by circling the letter that precedes it.

1. Creating a good patient-staff relationship begins when:
   a. The patient arrives at the medical facility
   b. The patient is in the examination room
   c. The patient telephones for an appointment
   d. The patient encounter has been completed

2. The healthcare staff can find out what their patients' expectations are by:
   a. Writing a letter
   b. Asking questions
   c. Having them fill out forms
   d. Taking a survey

3. The services offered by a medical facility usually cannot be felt or seen, which means they:
   a. Are intangible
   b. Are not important
   c. Cannot be documented
   d. Cannot be billed

4. Most physicians prefer to leave the subject of fees up to their:
   a. Nurse
   b. Accountant
   c. Reception staff
   d. Health insurance professional

5. Today's healthcare consumers use the Internet for all of these *except*:
   a. Scheduling appointments
   b. Acquiring information about physicians
   c. Learning how certain procedures are performed
   d. Direct patient–physician consultations

6. Data that are explicitly linked to a particular individual (including data items that reasonably could be expected to allow individual identification) are referred to as:
   a. Protected health information
   b. HIPAA-explicit information
   c. Individually identifiable health information
   d. Both a and c

7. An arrangement by which a patient requests that his or her health insurance benefit payments be made directly to a physician or hospital is called a(n):
   a. Release of information
   b. Discharge of authority
   c. Power of attorney
   d. Assignment of benefits

8. Although healthcare practitioners are dedicated to the health and well-being of their patients, for most, their ultimate goal is:
   a. Research
   b. Making a profit
   c. Keeping up on new medical technologies
   d. Publishing articles in prestigious journals

304

9. The total amount of fees collected divided by the total amount charged provides the practice with a(n):
   a. Profit
   b. Billing ratio
   c. Collection ratio
   d. Accounts receivable balance

10. A patient's name, age, address, telephone number, Social Security number, and employer information are generally referred to as:
    a. Demographics
    b. Vital statistics
    c. De-identified data
    d. All of the above

11. When a medical facility uses patient billing software, it is *crucial* to:
    a. Input data correctly
    b. Keep the equipment clean
    c. Make weekly backups
    d. Use state-of-the-art electronic equipment

12. Most medical offices send out statements periodically, which is referred to as a:
    a. Collection practice
    b. Statement control
    c. Billing cycle
    d. Mailing

13. Patients who have inadequate health insurance coverage or no insurance at all are called:
    a. Self-pay patients
    b. Deadbeats
    c. Indigent
    d. Red-flaggers

14. When no insurance is listed on a patient information form, the health insurance professional should:
    a. Alert the physician
    b. Ask the patient to leave
    c. Ask the patient to pay up front
    d. Inquire as to why no insurance is listed

15. An installment payment plan of more than four payments falls under:
    a. HIPAA regulations
    b. The Fair Credit Billing Act
    c. The Equal Credit Opportunity Act
    d. The Federal Truth in Lending Act of 1968, Regulation Z

16. The act that deals primarily with credit reports issued by credit reporting agencies is called:
    a. The Fair Credit Reporting Act
    b. The Fair Credit Billing Act
    c. The Equal Credit Opportunity Act
    d. The Federal Truth in Lending Act of 1968, Regulation Z

17. An organization that obtains or arranges for payment of money owed to a third party is referred to as a:
    a. Legal aid society
    b. Small claims association
    c. Collection agency
    d. Certified public account (CPA) group

18. The process available to individuals or businesses to recover legitimate debts through the court system without using expensive legal advisors is known as:
    a. Adjudication
    b. Small claims litigation
    c. Appellate court
    d. Grievance

19. In a small claims suit, the party initiating the action is referred to as the:
    a. Plaintiff
    b. Defendant
    c. Bailiff
    d. Attorney

20. The party being sued is the:
    a. Plaintiff
    b. Defendant
    c. Bailiff
    d. Attorney

21. It is important to know that a patient's written authorization is not required if the patient's information is used for:
    a. TPO
    b. Coding
    c. EMRs
    d. Education

22. Which of these is *not* considered a patient "identifier"?
    a. Name
    b. Social Security number
    c. Diagnosis
    d. Address

23. Which of these entities has made "minor" changes in the paper CMS-1500 claim form?
    a. HHS
    b. CMS
    c. HIPAA
    d. NUCC

24. Which of these is *not* typically used for accurate business accounting practices?
    a. Disbursements journal
    b. General ledger
    c. Payroll register
    d. Insurance claims aging report

25. Most healthcare offices report that collection calls are most successful between:
    a. 7 AM and 9 AM
    b. 5 PM and 7 PM
    c. Noon and 2 PM
    d. 10 AM and 2 PM

True/False

Directions: Place a "T" in the blank preceding each of these statements if it is true; place an "F" if it is false.

_____ 1. Patient expectations are the same from office to office.

_____ 2. Besides being brief and of high quality, paperwork in a medical office should be relevant to the reason the patient is there.

_____ 3. Patients need to be tolerant of long waits because the physician's time is worth more than their own.

306

_____ 4. If the reception area is empty when the patient enters, he or she may think the healthcare provider is second-rate.

_____ 5. Patients must realize and accept the fact that partition walls are thin in many medical facilities, and private conversations can be overheard.

_____ 6. Most patients typically have no idea what their medical care and treatment should cost before they make an appointment.

_____ 7. Today's healthcare consumers expect the cost of their healthcare to be addressed up front.

_____ 8. It is a trend in today's fast-paced world for people to believe that their time is just as valuable as their healthcare provider's time.

_____ 9. Members of the healthcare team should discuss their personal lives with patients to promote good provider–patient relationships.

_____ 10. Identifiable medical information includes medical records, medical billing records, any clinical or research databases, and tissue bank samples.

_____ 11. "Covered entities" can transfer protected health information to noncovered entities (those that do not come under HIPAA rules) without violating HIPAA.

_____ 12. HIPAA gives patients the right to access their medical information and to know to whom the covered entity has disclosed this information.

_____ 13. Patients have the right to obtain copies of their protected health information from their physicians or health plans unless the information is likely to endanger their lives or the lives of other people.

_____ 14. Patients have the right to correct or amend their medical records.

_____ 15. Covered entities can release de-identified health information without patient authorization.

_____ 16. Most patients appreciate having fee and billing information presented clearly and matter-of-factly but in a pleasant and courteous manner.

_____ 17. Experts consider the most effective payment policy is for the front desk staff to request payment when the patient–provider encounter is concluded.

_____ 18. Computerized patient billing software typically includes accounts receivable, insurance billing, and practice management modules.

_____ 19. The most effective way to collect money is to establish a formal financial policy that is clear to patients and the medical staff and to enforce it.

_____ 20. By law, medical facilities are not allowed to extend credit.

_____ 21. Under most state laws, full payment for medical services is due and payable at the time the service is provided.

_____ 22. Regarding collection and credit, it is mandatory that every patient be treated equally.

_____ 23. It is often not cost-effective to use small claims litigation for past due accounts that are less than $30.

_____ 24. To use the small claims process, the practice must retain an attorney.

_____ 25. Professional collection agencies typically retain 50% of collected fees.

Short Answer

Note: If space provided is not adequate, use a separate piece of blank paper.

1. The text discussed "surrogates" that patients might look for in a medical office. List at least four of these common surrogates.

_____

_____

_____

_____

2. List three successful online patient-centered topics.

_____

_____

_____

3. It is a trend for patients to be viewed as "consumers" in today's healthcare world. Explain this phenomenon.

_____

_____

_____

_____

4. The text lists five consumer essentials that experts believe should be mandatory for any medical facility wanting to provide patient-centered service. These are:

_____

_____

_____

_____

_____

5. HIPAA states that specific "covered entities" must comply with HIPAA rules for any health or medical information of identifiable individuals. Identify these covered entities.

_____

_____

_____

6. List the elements that a HIPAA-compliant release of information must include.

_____

_____

_____

_____

7. Compare an electronic patient accounting system to the previously popular "pegboard" system.

_____

_____

_____

_____

_____

8. Briefly describe an EMR and explain why you think healthcare practices should (or should not) switch from paper records to EMRs.

_____

_____

_____

_____

_____

Matching

Directions: Place the letter identifying the correct choice in the blank in front of the numbered statements. (**Note:** Not all choices are used.)

_____ 1. A chronological record of all patient transactions, including previous balances, charges, payments, and current daily balances

_____ 2. A listing of all expenses paid out to vendors, such as building rent, office supplies, and salaries

_____ 3. A separate record some offices keep for wages and salaries

_____ 4. A chronological listing of all transactions, considered the most basic of all office records

_____ 5. The "core" of a practice's financial records

_____ 6. A chronological accounting of activities of a particular patient (or family), including all charges and payments

_____ 7. The entire grouping of patient ledgers

a. accounts receivable
b. general ledger
c. patient ledger
d. payroll journal
e. accounts payable
f. general journal
g. disbursements journal
h. chronological journal
i. core journal
j. activities journal
k. daily journal

CRITICAL THINKING ACTIVITIES

A. This statement recently appeared in the *Health Day News:* "Patients who have good relationships with their physicians tend to be more satisfied with their care and have better results." Write a critical thinking paragraph discussing whether or not you agree with this statement; explain why or why not.

_____

_____

_____

_____

_____

_____

309

B. Lindell Holmes, a former patient at Broadmoor Medical Clinic, has not made a payment on his outstanding account for more than 90 days. His account was turned over to the Milton County Collection Agency on 10/07/20XX. Two weeks later, Mr. Holmes comes to the clinic and pays his bill in full with money order #003665UPS. Assuming that the collection agency keeps 50% of all collections, correctly post this payment on the ledger card in Fig. 14.1.

DOB: 03/22/51
Self-pay

STATEMENT

BROADMOOR MEDICAL CLINIC
4353 Pine Ridge Drive
Milton, XY 12345-0001
Telephone: 555-656-7890

LINDELL R. HOLMES
4216 WEST PINE AV
MILTON, XY 12345

DATE 20XX	PROFESSIONAL SERVICE DESCRIPTION	CHARGE	CREDITS PAYMENTS	ADJUSTMENTS	CURRENT BALANCE
6/09	99203 New Pt Exam	135 00			135 00
6/10	94620 ROA-CASH	185 00	132 00		188 00
7/10	Phone call				
8/10	Col. Letter-cert				

Due and payable within 10 days.   Pay last amount in balance column ⬆

Fig. 14.1 Ledger card.

C. Assume that Broadmoor Medical Clinic does not use a collection agency for delinquent accounts and on 10/07/20XX filed a small claims suit at the local county courthouse on Mr. Holmes. The filing fee was $30, and the Milton County Sheriff's Department charged $25 for serving the papers to Mr. Holmes on 10/13. Using the ledger card in Fig. 14.2, post these charges to Mr. Holmes' account.

DOB: 03/22/51
Self-pay

STATEMENT

BROADMOOR MEDICAL CLINIC
4353 Pine Ridge Drive
Milton, XY 12345-0001
Telephone: 555-656-7890

LINDELL R. HOLMES
4216 WEST PINE AV
MILTON, XY 12345

| DATE 20XX | PROFESSIONAL SERVICE DESCRIPTION | CHARGE | CREDITS | | CURRENT BALANCE |
			PAYMENTS	ADJUSTMENTS	
6/09	99203 New Pt Exam	135 00			135 00
6/10	94620 ROA-CASH	185 00	132 00		188 00
7/10	Phone call				
8/10	Col. Letter-cert				

Due and payable within 10 days.   Pay last amount in balance column ⇧

Fig. 14.2 Ledger card.

PROBLEM SOLVING/COLLABORATIVE (GROUP) ACTIVITIES

A. Create a page for Broadmoor Medical Clinic's Policy Manual outlining a payment and collection policy.

B. Compose an outline for a conversation you would use for collecting delinquent accounts using the telephone. Follow the policy you generated in the previous exercise and remember to be courteous but firm. Also, make sure you do not violate any collection laws or consumers' rights.

C. Set up a payment plan for a self-pay patient who owes $850. Make certain that you follow the policy you generated in Exercise A and the rules outlined in the Federal Truth in Lending Act of 1968, Regulation Z.

PROJECTS/DISCUSSION TOPICS

A. Generate a table of all of the pertinent laws and acts discussed in Chapter 14 that address credit and collection, along with the date they were enacted and a brief description of what each addresses. Use library references and the Internet to complete this assignment, if necessary.

B. Patient "identifiers":
   1. Create a comprehensive list of potential identifiers that can link information to a particular individual.

   2. Explain how a patient's health record can be de-identified.

C. A topic that has long been controversial is who owns patients' medical records. Research this topic (using the library or applicable search words on the Internet or both) and write a one-page essay of your findings for class discussion. You should take into consideration the HIPAA rules when writing your paper.

D. Research your area to discover if billing services are available and what assistance they offer to medical facilities such as Broadmoor Medical Clinic.

CASE STUDIES

A. When Emily Fortune's appointment is concluded on February 7, 20XX, you hand her an encounter form listing the fees, which total $265. Mrs. Fortune does have insurance, but her policy has a $2500 deductible; her carrier will pay nothing toward the fees generated on this date. She advises you that because her condition restricts her ability to perform her job, she cannot pay the entire bill right now, but she can pay $50 a month. Review the credit policy you created for Broadmoor's Policy Manual. Is Mrs. Fortune's monthly payment in line with this policy? If not, how should the payment plan be revised so that it meets the stipulations outlined in the Policy Manual?

B. LaDon Williams is a self-pay patient at Broadmoor. He has not paid on his outstanding balance ($300) for 2 months. During a telephone conversation, Mr. Williams agrees to come to the Clinic and discuss a credit plan. He informs the reception staff that he can afford to pay only $10 a month on his delinquent account. The reception staff refuses to accept the payment, informing Mr. Williams that the entire bill must be paid at once or his account will be turned over for collection. Can this situation possibly create a problem for Broadmoor Medical Clinic? If so, explain.

INTERNET EXPLORATION

A. Log on to the Internet. Using "find doctors" or similar search words, determine how much information is available on the Internet for today's healthcare consumers.

B. Using search words, such as "patients as consumers," explore the Internet in search of information and thoughts on this subject.

C. To learn more about how to maximize patient collections, search the Internet using the appropriate search words.

D. Explore the Internet for information on how to file a small claims suit in your state.

PERFORMANCE OBJECTIVES

Performance Objective 14.1: Compose a Patient Termination Letter

Conditions: Student will compose a letter terminating a patient's care because of nonpayment of fees, as discussed in the scenario in Box 14.1.

Supplies/Equipment: Pen or computer, textbook, paper, and information in Box 14.1

Time Allowed: 30 minutes

Accuracy Needed to Pass: 90%

Procedural Steps	Points Earned	Comments
Evaluator: Note time began: _____		
Read the scenario in Box 14.1 and compose a letter of termination; remember to follow all of the legal requirements discussed in the text.		
1. Format (15)		
Date and inside address		
Subject line		
Salutation		
Body		
Complimentary close and signature		
References and enclosure lines		
Special notations		
2. Content (brief, but contains all necessary information; courteous; and offers alternative care) (25)		

Total Points = 40

Student's Score: _____

Evaluator: _____

Comments: _____

_____

_____

_____

_____

Box 14.1

Patricia Henderson, 1111 Spruce Avenue, Milton, XY 12345, owes Broadmoor Medical Clinic $465 for professional services rendered beginning in April 2013 through June 2014. Mrs. Henderson has not made any payments since September 2014, and all letters and telephone calls have proved unsuccessful in collecting this account. Dr. Jones has instructed you to send Mrs. Henderson a letter informing her that he can no longer treat her for her chronic asthma because of her refusal to pay her bill.

Performance Objective 14.2: Composing a Generic Collection Form Letter

Conditions: Student will compose a series of three "generic" form letters to keep on file as a template for sending to patients who are delinquent on their payments. Refer to the examples in the textbook for assistance in this exercise.

Supplies/Equipment: Pen or computer, textbook, and paper

Time Allowed: 30 minutes

Accuracy Needed to Pass: 90%

Procedural Steps	Points Earned	Comments
Evaluator: Note time began: _____		
Compose a "generic" collection form letter.		
1. Format (15 points × 3)		
Date and inside address		
Subject line		
Salutation		
Body		
Complimentary close and signature		
References and enclosure lines		
Special notations		
2. Content (20 points × 3)		
Opening paragraph		
Main content paragraph		
Closing paragraph with expectations		

Total Points = 105

Student's Score: _____

Evaluator: _____

Comments: _____

_____

_____

_____

_____

Health Insurance Professional's Notebook

Generate a section in your notebook for resources to aid in patient services and collections, such as:

- Informative websites
- Pertinent HIPAA information
- List of laws (and their explanation) that apply to credit and collection
- Samples of letters dealing with:
    - Collections
    - Termination of patients
- Information on billing services and collection agencies

Chapter Checklist

Student Name: _____

Chapter Completion Date: _____

Evaluate your classroom performance. Complete the self-evaluation and submit it to your instructor. When your instructor returns this form to you, compare your self-evaluation with the evaluation completed by your instructor.

1.	Record	Your start time and date: _____
2.	Read	The assigned chapter in the textbook
3.	View	PowerPoint slides (if available)
4.	Complete	Exercises in the workbook as assigned
5.	Compare	Your answers to the answers posted on the bulletin board, website, or handout
6.	Correct	Your answers
7.	Complete	All tests and required activities
8.	Read	Assigned readings (if any)
9.	Complete	Chapter performance objectives (competencies), if any
10.	Evaluate	Chapter performance and submit to your instructor
11.	Record	Your ending time and date: _____
12.	Move on	Begin next chapter as assigned

PERFORMANCE EVALUATION

Student Name: _____

Chapter Completion Date: _____

Evaluate your classroom performance. Compare this evaluation with the one provided by your instructor.

Skill	Student Self-Evaluation			Instructor Evaluation		
	Good	Average	Poor	Good	Average	Poor
Attendance/punctuality						
Personal appearance						
Applies effort						
Is self-motivated						
Is courteous						
Has positive attitude						
Completes assignments in timely manner						
Works well with others						

Student's Initials: _____   **Instructor's Initials:** _____

Date: _____   **Date:** _____

Points Possible: _____

Points Awarded: _____

Chapter Grade: _____

15 Keys to Successful Claims Management

Processing health insurance claims can be a tedious task. When Medicare and Medicaid are involved, the Department of Health and Human Services mandates that most claims be settled in a timely manner—typically within 28 days. To keep the claims process humming, health insurance professionals must know and keep up to date on the guidelines of many different third-party payers, with the goal of filing "clean claims" and filtering out those that will not successfully complete the process before they enter the system. The exercises and activities in this workbook chapter will help to hone your knowledge and ability to complete claims forms accurately, efficiently, and in a timely manner.

The process for completing the CMS-1500 claim form was discussed in Chapter 5, and the general guidelines for correctly filling out the 33 blocks of the form can be found on both the Evolve site and in Appendix B in the back of the textbook. Reviewing this chapter will refresh your memory and provide assistance in completing these exercises.

WORKBOOK CHAPTER OBJECTIVES

After completing the workbook activities for Chapter 15, the student should be able to:
1. Define the terms used in the chapter.
2. Answer the review questions according to the evaluation criteria set by the instructor.
3. Use problem-solving skills (individually or in a group setting) to determine correct responses and outcomes in case studies and application exercises.
4. Work in a group setting to resolve scenarios dealing with office functions and duties of the health insurance professional.
5. Interpret the information contained on an explanation of benefits (EOB).
6. Determine why insurers deny payment of specific medical procedures.
7. Establish the primary carrier for patients with dual coverage.
8. Compose applicable appeal letters for patients.

DEFINING CHAPTER TERMS

Using the computer, students should type an accurate definition for each of the chapter terms listed. These definitions should be in the students' own words. When finished, students should compare their definitions with those listed in the glossary at the back of the textbook and correct any inaccuracies.

adjudication process
appeal
birthday rule
charge-to-collection ratio
clean claim
coordination of benefits (COB)
correct code initiative
downcoding

employer identification number (EIN)
explanation of benefits (EOB)
insurance claims register (log)
Medicare secondary payer (MSP) claims
National provider identifier (NPI)
real-time claims adjudication (RTCA)
secondary claim
suspension file

319

Multiple Choice

Directions: In the questions and statements presented, choose the response that **best** answers and completes the stem and circle the letter that precedes it.

1. The claims process begins when:
   a. The patient–provider encounter is concluded
   b. The CMS-1500 form has been completed and submitted
   c. The patient first contacts the office for an appointment
   d. The patient's record is placed on the health insurance professional's desk

2. In most cases, the health insurance professional should reverify patient information:
   a. Monthly
   b. At least once a year
   c. Each time the patient visits the office
   d. It is not necessary to reverify patient information

3. In the case of a minor child of a divorced couple who is covered under both parents' group healthcare plans, the health insurance professional should:
   a. Determine which carrier is primary
   b. Have the patient fill out two patient information forms
   c. Submit CMS-1500 forms to both carriers simultaneously
   d. Check with the office manager to avoid submitting a "dirty" claim

4. Many medical practices include a section (often positioned at the bottom of the form) for the patient to sign an:
   a. Authorization to release information
   b. Agreement to pay the bill in full
   c. Authorization to pay with a credit card
   d. Authorization to use a personal check

5. Services that typically require preauthorization or precertification include:
   a. Laboratory tests
   b. Emergency department services
   c. Routine "wellness" examinations
   d. Inpatient hospitalization

6. After a paper claim is completed, to help reduce claims rejection and delay, it is good practice *first* to have the claim:
   a. Signed
   b. Proofread
   c. Photocopied
   d. Recorded on the insurance claim log

7. The most important process in the healthcare insurance cycle is:
   a. Affixing the provider's NPI
   b. Submitting a clean claim
   c. Acquiring the patient's release of information
   d. Completing all 33 blocks in the CMS-1500 form

8. The number that is assigned by the Internal Revenue Service (IRS) and used as the employer identifier standard for all electronic healthcare transactions is the:
   a. Group number
   b. Social Security number (SSN)
   c. Provider identification number (PIN)
   d. Employer identification number (EIN)

9. After the claim has been received by a third-party payer, it is reviewed, and the carrier makes payment decisions. This process is formally referred to as:
   a. Adjudication
   b. Judgment ruling
   c. Claims processing
   d. Decision-making

10. When the insurance carrier receives a paper claim, it is dated and the claim is processed through a(n):
   a. Visual imaging tomographer (VIT)
   b. Optical character recognition (OCR) scanner
   c. Character verification regulator (CVR)
   d. Computerized claim optimizer (CCO)

11. A series of files set up chronologically and labeled according to the number of days since a claim was submitted is commonly referred to as a(n):
   a. Tracking file
   b. Insurance claims register
   c. General ledger file
   d. Suspension file

12. A columnar form on which insurance claims are tracked is a(n):
   a. Tracking file
   b. Suspension file
   c. General ledger file
   d. Insurance claims register

13. The document sent by the insurance carrier to the provider and patient explaining how the claim was adjudicated is called a(n):
   a. Insurance claims register
   b. Adjudication document
   c. Explanation of Benefits
   d. Payment tracking form

14. The key to knowing how much of the claim was paid, how much was not, and why is documented on the:
   a. EOB
   b. EIN
   c. ROA
   d. PIN

15. When a carrier assigns a substitute code because a claim was submitted with outdated, deleted, or nonexistent CPT codes, it is called:
   a. Fraud
   b. Upcoding
   c. Downcoding
   d. Crosswalking

16. *Ideally,* insurance claims should be submitted to the insurance carrier within:
   a. 30 days
   b. 60 days
   c. 90 days
   d. 1 year

17. If there is any question as to time limits for filing claims, the health insurance professional should contact the:
   a. Department of Health and Human Services (HHS)
   b. Office manager
   c. Physician
   d. Carrier

18. The insurance company that pays after the primary carrier is referred to as the:
    a. Subsequent payer
    b. Secondary insurer
    c. Preferred provider
    d. Health maintenance organization

19. In the case of dual coverage, if it is not immediately obvious which payer is primary, the health insurance professional should first ask:
    a. The patient
    b. The employer
    c. The office manager
    d. The insurance carrier

20. Complete fields 9, 9a, and 9d on the CMS-1500 claim form if "YES" appears in:
    a. Block 1a
    b. Block 4
    c. Block 11d
    d. Block 27

21. If a patient and spouse (or parent) are covered under two separate group policies, it results in what is commonly referred to as:
    a. Double coverage
    b. Coordination of benefits
    c. Primary versus secondary coverage
    d. A patient cannot be covered under two separate group policies

22. Claims that are submitted to another insurance company *before* they are submitted to Medicare are called:
    a. Medicare Secondary Payer claims
    b. Coordination of benefits claims
    c. Payer of last resort claims
    d. Crossover claims

23. The process of calling for a review of a decision made by a third-party carrier is referred to as a(n):
    a. Appeal
    b. Claims review
    c. Adjudication
    d. Correct coding edit

24. The Medicare appeal process has _____ levels.
    a. Three
    b. Four
    c. Five
    d. Six

25. The health insurance professional should be familiar with the CMS-1500 paper claim process because:
    a. The NUCC recommends it.
    b. It is a HIPAA mandate.
    c. Not all providers submit claims electronically.
    d. The CMS-1500 form must be used for Medicare claims.

True/False

Directions: Place a "T" in the blank preceding each of these statements if it is true; place an "F" if it is false.

_____ 1. Ultimately, it is the patient's responsibility to know when and how to notify the insurance company for preauthorization or precertification.

_____ 2. Medicare (fee-for-service) does not need prior authorization to provide covered services.

_____ 3. It is the health insurance professional's responsibility to document appropriate comments in the patient's medical record that pertain to his or her health.

322

_____ 4. One of the main changes in the revised CMS-1500 (02/12) claim form is the expansion from 4 diagnostic codes to 12 in Block 21.

_____ 5. All major government payers have the same guidelines for completing the CMS-1500 claim form.

_____ 6. The medical practice should have a mechanism in place for tracking claims.

_____ 7. Claims follow-up does not warrant high priority in a busy medical office.

_____ 8. When dealing with Medicare and Medicaid, claims inquiries must be in writing.

_____ 9. The third-party payer sends an EOB only if a payment accompanies the document.

_____ 10. EOBs can be in electronic or paper format.

_____ 11. When an insurance claim is denied, the health insurance professional cannot pursue the claim further.

_____ 12. Often, if a claim is reduced or rejected, the problem lies with the provider's office.

_____ 13. Coding accurately and knowing which coding systems payers use help avoid payment errors on claims.

_____ 14. If the claims adjuster changes a valid procedure code that was submitted on the claim, the health insurance professional must accept the change.

_____ 15. Correct code initiative edits are intended to reduce overpayments that result from improper coding.

_____ 16. All participating (PAR) providers are allowed to bill the patient for any balance the insurance carrier does not pay.

_____ 17. The provider cannot waive Medicare copayments unless financial hardship has been established and documented.

_____ 18. All third-party payers have a 30-day time limit for claims to be submitted if they are to be considered for payment.

_____ 19. Government payers usually will pay a claim even if the time limit for claim submission has been exceeded.

_____ 20. The time limit for filing appeals varies from carrier to carrier.

_____ 21. When a patient has other insurance coverage primary to Medicare, the other insurer's payment information must be included on the Medicare claim.

_____ 22. The total amount of money collected divided by the total amount charged is referred to as the _collection ratio_.

_____ 23. HIPAA requires all payers to use the applicable healthcare claims status category codes and claim status codes.

_____ 24. One way of optimizing the billing and claims process is to ask patients to wait to pay until they receive a statement in the mail.

_____ 25. If all efforts of appeal are exhausted without success, a remaining option is to contact the state insurance commissioner's office.

Short Answer

Note: If space provided is not adequate, use a separate piece of blank paper.

1. List the six keys to successful claims processing.

_____

_____

_____

_____

_____

_____

2. Explain the rationale for photocopying the front and the back of a patient's health insurance identification card.

_____

_____

3. If any attachments accompany a claim, list the information that should appear on each document.

_____

_____

_____

4. Explain in detail what the health insurance professional should do when a claims error is discovered that could result, or already has resulted, in inaccurate reimbursement.

_____

_____

_____

5. List six items typically found on an EOB (remittance advice [RA]).

_____

_____

_____

_____

_____

_____

6. List six things that influence how often medical facilities submit insurance claims.

_____

_____

_____

_____

_____

_____

7. List two important things the health insurance professional should do when a coordination of benefits situation exists.

_____

_____

8. List and explain the basic rules for appealing a claim.

_____

_____

_____

CRITICAL THINKING ACTIVITIES

A. A major U.S. university conducted an experiment in which patients went online and answered a series of questions about their health history before their medical encounter. The purpose of this study was to "assess the feasibility and reliability of a web-based, self-administered, patient assessment system compared with a standard, interviewer-administered approach." Discuss the pros and cons of such a system.

B. Explain the rules regarding preauthorization and precertification and list the types of services and procedures that typically require it.

C. Write a short paragraph on the importance of documentation in a patient's health record.

PROBLEM SOLVING/COLLABORATIVE (GROUP) ACTIVITIES

A. Create a flowchart diagramming the steps a paper claim goes through from the time the patient concludes his or her healthcare encounter until the payment is posted to the provider's billing system.

B. Generate a page for Broadmoor Medical Clinic's office policy manual for a nonautomated tracking system for healthcare claims. You may use either the suspension file system or the log system.

C. Fig. 15.1 shows a sample EOB. The blank boxes are numbered 1 through 10. Write a complete description of what each box explains.

1. _____

2. _____

3. _____

4. _____

5. _____

6. _____

7. _____

8. _____

9. _____

10. _____

325

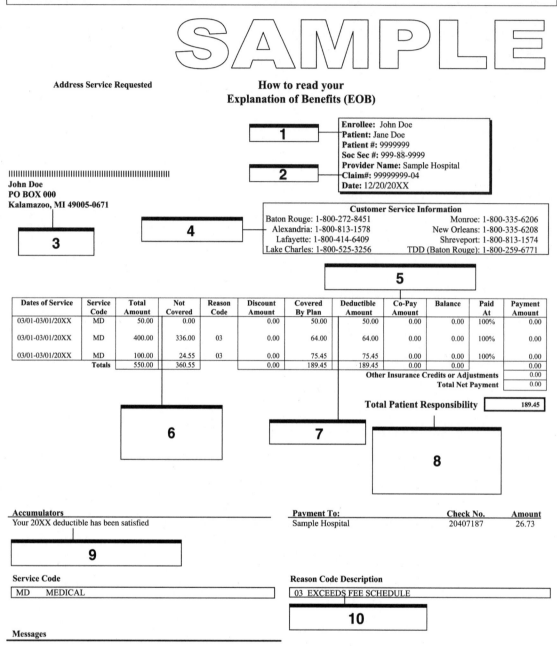

New Explanation of Benefits Form
This is a sample of our new Explanation of Benefits form, along with descriptions of various sections. This will help plan members and providers understand how benefits are paid.

SAMPLE

Address Service Requested

How to read your
Explanation of Benefits (EOB)

	1	**Enrollee:** John Doe
		Patient: Jane Doe
		Patient #: 9999999
		Soc Sec #: 999-88-9999
		Provider Name: Sample Hospital
	2	**Claim#:** 99999999-04
		Date: 12/20/20XX

|||||||||||||
John Doe
PO BOX 000
Kalamazoo, MI 49005-0671

3

4

Customer Service Information

Baton Rouge: 1-800-272-8451	Monroe: 1-800-335-6206
Alexandria: 1-800-813-1578	New Orleans: 1-800-335-6208
Lafayette: 1-800-414-6409	Shreveport: 1-800-813-1574
Lake Charles: 1-800-525-3256	TDD (Baton Rouge): 1-800-259-6771

5

Dates of Service	Service Code	Total Amount	Not Covered	Reason Code	Discount Amount	Covered By Plan	Deductible Amount	Co-Pay Amount	Balance	Paid At	Payment Amount
03/01-03/01/20XX	MD	50.00	0.00		0.00	50.00	50.00	0.00	0.00	100%	0.00
03/01-03/01/20XX	MD	400.00	336.00	03	0.00	64.00	64.00	0.00	0.00	100%	0.00
03/01-03/01/20XX	MD	100.00	24.55	03	0.00	75.45	75.45	0.00	0.00	100%	0.00
Totals		550.00	360.55		0.00	189.45	189.45	0.00	0.00		0.00

Other Insurance Credits or Adjustments 0.00
Total Net Payment 0.00

Total Patient Responsibility 189.45

6

7

8

Accumulators
Your 20XX deductible has been satisfied

9

Payment To:	**Check No.**	**Amount**
Sample Hospital	20407187	26.73

Service Code

MD	MEDICAL

Reason Code Description

03	EXCEEDS FEE SCHEDULE

10

Messages

Fig. 15.1 Sample explanation of benefits form.

Complete one or more of these projects and topics as your instructor indicates.

A. Join a class discussion on what can be done to avoid errors on CMS-1500 forms.

B. Share experiences with the class regarding errors in claims or billing that you, or family members, may have experienced and how they were resolved.

C. Reread the "Imagine This" scenario about Mr. Benson and Dr. Peters in the textbook (p. 354). Discuss how Dr. Peters's health insurance professional might have helped Mr. Benson resolve this problem.

D. Compile a table listing the major payers along with their time limits for submitting claims.

CASE STUDIES

A. Fig. 15.2 shows an insurance ID card. After studying the card, answer these questions.

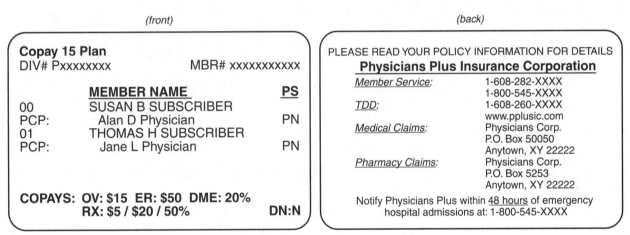

Fig. 15.2 Insurance ID card for S. Subscriber.

1. Who is the subscriber?
2. Do the subscriber and the dependent have the same primary care provider (PCP)?
3. If yes, what is their PCP's name? If no, list the subscriber and the dependent along with the name of each member's PCP.
4. If Thomas had an office visit for which he was charged $75, how much should he pay at the time of the service?
5. Susan was in an accident and was treated in the emergency department and released on the same day. The charges for this encounter totaled $2354. What was Susan's share?
6. Susan was confined to a wheelchair for 6 weeks after her accident. The cost of the wheelchair was $896. How much of this charge did Physicians Plus Insurance Corporation pay?
7. Susan was given a prescription for a pain medication. If the pharmacist gave her the generic form of the drug, the cost would be $26.50; the cost of the brand name would be $67. What would Susan's savings be if she accepted the generic drug?
8. Susan's accident occurred at 7:43 PM on 10/14/20XX, and she was treated in the emergency department on the same date (she was not admitted as an inpatient from the emergency department). She did not report the accident to Physicians Plus until 4 PM on 10/17/20XX. Will Physicians Plus pay this claim?

327

B. Wanda Fortune's ledger card is shown in Fig. 15.3; Fig. 15.4 shows an EOB from her insurance carrier (TRICARE). Post the information from the EOB onto Ms. Fortune's ledger card. (Assume that the TRICARE payment was received on 8/01/20XX.)

Note: Ms. Fortune's cost share is 25% of the TRICARE-approved amount.

TRICARE
SPONSOR: George M.
SS#   321-44-5555
DOB   4/16/77

STATEMENT

BROADMOOR MEDICAL CLINIC
4353 Pine Ridge Drive
Milton, XY 12345-0001
Telephone: 555-656-7890

BENEFICIARY:
Wanda Mae
SS# 321-44-6600
DOB 11/02/80

GEORGE M. FORTUNE
566 LONGMEADOW
MILTON, XY 12345

DATE 20XX	PROFESSIONAL SERVICE DESCRIPTION	CHARGE		CREDITS		CURRENT BALANCE	
				PAYMENTS	ADJUSTMENTS		
7/08	OV EST (99213)	45	00			45	00
"	Comp Met Pane (80053)	20	00			65	00
"	Auto Hemo (85018)	12	00			77	00
7/09	TRICARE Submitted						

Due and payable within 10 days.   Pay last amount in balance column ⇧

Fig. 15.3 Ledger card for Wanda (George) Fortune.

TRICARE EXPLANATION OF BENEFITS

This is a statement of the action taken on your TRICARE Claim.
Keep this notice for your records.

Prime Contractor

Date of Notice:	August 02, 20XX
Sponsor SSN:	321-44-5555
Sponsor Name:	George M. Fortune
Beneficiary Name:	Wanda Mae Fortune

Benefits were payable to:

Wanda Mae Fortune
566 Longmeadow
Milton, XY 12345

BROADMOOR MEDICAL CLINIC
4353 PINE RIDGE DRIVE
MILTON XY 12345-0001

Claim Number: 919533693-00-00

Services Provided By Date of Services		Services Provided		Amount Billed	TRICARE Approved	See Remarks
PROVIDER OF MEDICAL CARE						
07/08/20XX	1	Office/outpatient visit, est	(99213)	$ 45.00	$ 38.92	1
07/08/20XX	1	Comprehen metabolic panel	(80053)	20.00	19.33	1
07/08/20XX	1	Automated hemogram	(85018)	12.00	12.00	1
Totals:				**$ 77.00**	**$ 70.25**	

Claim Summary		Beneficiary Liability Summary		Benefit Period Summary		
Amount billed:	77.00	Deductible	0.00	**Fiscal Year Beginning:** October 01, 20XX		
TRICARE Approved:	70.25	Copayment:	0.00		Individual	Family
Non-Covered: 14*	6.75	Cost Share	17.56	Deductible:	150.00	150.00
Paid by Beneficiary:	0.00			Catastrophic Cap:		
Other Insurance:	0.00			**Enrollment Year Beginning:**		
Paid to Provider:	52.69			**December 01, 20XX**		
Paid to Beneficiary:	0.00				Individual	Family
Check Number:				POS Deductible:	300.00	600.00
				Prime Cap:		856.32

Fig. 15.4 TRICARE explanation of benefits for Fortune.

C. Joann Carlyle was seen by Todd Hamblin, a dermatologist at Broadmoor Medical Clinic, for removal of a xanthoma growth beneath each of her eyes. After the procedure, Dr. Hamblin instructed Evelyn Tanner, his health insurance professional, to bill the procedures as follows:

Excision lesion, right cheek	11442	$430
Excision lesion, left cheek	11442-59	$430
Intermediate repair	12051	$720
TOTAL		$1580

Fig. 15.5 illustrates how Evelyn completed Block 24 of the CMS-1500 form. Assume that Ms. Carlyle had met her deductible for the year, and Dr. Hamblin is a PAR provider for Ms. Carlyle's insurance carrier. Her coinsurance was 90/10 for outpatient hospital surgical procedures; however, the insurance carrier paid only $711 (90% of one excision and 90% of one repair) and denied the second procedure and repair.

| 24. A. DATE(S) OF SERVICE From | | | To | | | B. PLACE OF SERVICE | C. EMG | D. PROCEDURES, SERVICES, OR SUPPLIES (Explain Unusual Circumstances) CPT/HCPCS | | MODIFIER | | E. DIAGNOSIS POINTER | F. $ CHARGES | G. DAYS OR UNITS | H. EPSDT Family Plan | I. ID. QUAL. | J. RENDERING PROVIDER ID. # | |
MM	DD	YY	MM	DD	YY													
01	12	XX	01	12	XX	22		11442			A		430 00	1		NPI	009229011	
01	12	XX	01	12	XX	22		12051			A		360 00	1		NPI	009229011	
01	12	XX	01	12	XX	22		11442			A		430 00	1		NPI	009229011	
01	12	XX	01	12	XX	22		12051			A		360 00	1		NPI	009229011	
																NPI		
																NPI		

25. FEDERAL TAX I.D. NUMBER	SSN EIN	26. PATIENT'S ACCOUNT NO.	27. ACCEPT ASSIGNMENT? (For govt. claims, see back)	28. TOTAL CHARGE	29. AMOUNT PAID	30. Rsvd for NUCC Use
421898989	☐ ☒	052599	☒ YES ☐ NO	$ 1580 00	$	$

Fig. 15.5 Block 24 of CMS-1500 form for Ms. Carlyle.

1. Why were the second excision and repair denied?
2. What, if anything, can Evelyn do to collect the insurance payment for the second procedure and repair?
3. If Evelyn submits a corrected claim, how should she fill out Block 24?
4. If Evelyn does nothing and sends a statement to Ms. Carlyle for the balance, what recourse, if any, does Ms. Carlyle have?

INTERNET EXPLORATION

A. Using the Internet, search the words "Understanding an EOB" (or similar words) and explore various websites that offer information on how to interpret and understand an EOB.

B. Denial of claims due to "downcoding" is relatively common for many healthcare providers. To learn about what problems can result from downcoding, use the Internet to search for applicable articles discussing this problematic practice, such as "How to Avoid Downcoding and Payment Denials" at http://www.medscape.com/viewarticle/408362. If you cannot find this article, use the search word "downcoding" to find alternative articles on this topic.

C. The Internet has a wealth of information for filing appeals—especially appeals for Medicare claims. Search the Internet (using the medicare.gov and the Centers for Medicare and Medicaid Services websites or search words such as "filing a Medicare appeal") to learn more about this process.

Performance Objective 15.1: Determining Primary Coverage

Conditions: Student will study the information in Fig. 15.6, determine the primary carrier, and complete a claim using the information in Patient Record No. 052567.

Supplies/Equipment: Pen, Patient Record No. 052567, and CMS-1500 claim form

Time Allowed: 50 minutes

Accuracy Needed to Pass: 90%

Procedural Steps	Points Earned	Comments
Evaluator: Note time began: _____		
1. Carefully read and study Patient Record No. 052567 in Fig. 15.6.		
2. Determine the primary carrier. (10)		
3. Correctly complete *all* blocks required for the appropriate claim. (65)		
4. Proofread the claim for accuracy.		
Optional: May deduct points for taking more time than allowed.		

Total Points = 75

Student's Score: _____

Evaluator: _____

Comments: _____

_____

_____

_____

_____

Performance Objective 15-1 – Determining Primary Coverage

Broadmoor Medical Clinic	Clinic EIN# 42-1898989
4353 Pine Ridge Drive	Dr. Robert L. Jones NPI 1234567890
Milton, XY 12345-0001	Dr. Marilou Lucero NPI 2907511822
Clinic NPI X100XX1000	
Telephone: 555-656-7890	Date claims one day after encounter

Patient/Insurance Information

Truman Ross Beckler   DOB: 08/29/1946
430 Cedar Drive
Middletown, XT 12345   PH 555-672-4207
555-452-0334   SS # 321-44-5511

Medicare   321445511X
Unix Benefits Inc.   198442000LJ

Vera T. Beckler   DOB 05/02/1950
Employer: ALCAT Industries

Billing Information

Record No. 052567

07/08/20XX	99213	$145.00
07/08/20XX	93000	60.00
07/08/20XX	85025	22.00

Diagnosis: Epigastric pain
ICD-10 Code: R10.13

Supervising (DQ) Physician: Robert L. Jones, M.D.

Notes: Mr. Beckler is retired and has both Medicare Parts A and B. He also has full healthcare coverage under his wife's employer group health plan (Unix Benefits Inc.)

Notes: Assume the date of current onset of illness was the same day of the encounter. Date the primary claim one day after the encounter and date the secondary claim one day after the primary payer's EOB is received.

Fig. 15.6 Patient record information for Beckler.

Performance Objective 15.2: Interpret EOB, Post Payment to Ledger Card, and File Secondary Claim

Conditions: Student will interpret the EOB in Fig. 15.7, post the payment to the ledger card in Fig. 15.8, and file a secondary CMS-1500 claim.

Supplies/Equipment: Patient Record No. 052567, EOB (see Fig. 15.7), ledger card (see Fig. 15.8), and CMS-1500 claim form

Time Allowed: 50 minutes

Accuracy Needed to Pass: 90%

Procedural Steps	Points Earned	Comments
Evaluator: Note time began: _____		
1. Carefully study the UNIX EOB.		
2. Determine the correct payment to post to patient's ledger card. (15)		
3. Prepare a claim for the secondary carrier. Complete *all* blocks required for secondary claims. (65)		
4. Proofread the claim for accuracy.		
5. Note name of document that must accompany secondary claims. (5)		
Optional: May deduct points for taking more time than allowed.		

Total Points = 85

Student's Score: _____

Evaluator: _____

Comments: _____

_____

_____

_____

_____

EXPLANATION OF BENEFITS

UNIX Benefits Inc.
1000 Alameda Blvd.
San Jose CA 98877
800-222-33-4444
800-222-33-4545 (FAX)

Insured's Name: Vera T. Beckler
UNIX Member # 198442000LJ

Date: 07/20/20XX

Patient Name: Truman R. Beckler
430 Cedar Drive
Middletown XT 12345

Provider: Broadmoor Medical Clinic
R. L. Jones NPI 1234567890
Claim No. 98885050333-XX
Check No. UNIX2034422

(1) Date of Service	(2) CPT Code	(3) Total Charges	(4) Allowable Charges	(5) Applied to Deductible	(6) Co-Pay	(7) Total Benefit	(8) Reason Code(s)
07/08/20XX	99213	145.00	120.00	50.00	10.00	60.00	01A/01C
07/08/20XX	93000	60.00	45.00	--	--	45.00	02B
07/08/20XX	85025	22.00	18.50	--	--	18.50	02B
TOTALS		**227.00**	**183.50**	**50.00**	**10.00**	**123.50**	

Reason Code(s) Description:

01A – Amount in Column 3 exceeds UNIX fee schedule
01C – Amount in Column 5 has been applied to annual deductible
02B – UNIX pays this procedure/service at 100%

NOTES:

Payment has been sent directly to your provider
Annual deductible has been satisfied for year 20XX

THIS IS NOT A BILL – SAVE THIS COPY FOR YOUR RECORDS

Fig. 15.7 Explanation of benefits for Beckler.

Truman DOB 08/29/1946
Medicare 321445511X

Vera DOB 05/02/1950
Emp: AL-CAT Industries
UNIX Benefits Inc.
198442000LJ

STATEMENT

BROADMOOR MEDICAL CLINIC
4353 Pine Ridge Drive
Milton, XY 12345-0001
Telephone: 555-656-7890

PH 555-672-4207

TRUMAN ROSS BECKLER
430 CEDAR DRIVE
MIDDLETOWN XT 12345

DATE 20XX	PROFESSIONAL SERVICE DESCRIPTION	CHARGE		CREDITS		CURRENT BALANCE	
				PAYMENTS	ADJUSTMENTS		
3/16	Vera OV 99212	125	00	12 50		112	50
3/17	Unix Claim						
3/30	Unix CK 2031944			100 00	12 50	-0-	
7/08	Truman 99213	145	00			145	00
"	Truman 93000	60	00			205	00
"	Truman 85025	22	00			227	00
7/09	Unix Claim						

Due and payable within 10 days.   Pay last amount in balance column ⬆

Fig. 15.8 Ledger card for Beckler.

Chapter **15 Keys to Successful Claims Management**

Performance Objective 15.3: Composing an Appeal Letter
Scenario
Plastic surgeon Everett Bartholomew performed a bilateral blepharoplasty on 66-year-old Janine Frieze on April 27, 20XX. Before the procedure, you (his health insurance professional) telephoned National Mutual Health Care, Ms. Frieze's insurance carrier, for preauthorization. Susan Peterson of National Mutual provided authorization number 303885030 for Ms. Frieze's blepharoplasty; however, when the EOB was received for this claim (#767678000CG), benefits were denied because the insurance carrier determined the procedure to be "not medically necessary." In his documentation in the health record, Dr. Bartholomew states that the eyelids were "obstructing the patient's vision."

Note: National Mutual's address is PO Box 45446A, Princeton, XY 23456. Address it to the attention of Susan Peterson, Claims Department. Ms. Frieze's date of birth is 09/26/1947, and her SSN is 444-00-1199.

Conditions: Using the information in the scenario, compose a letter to National Mutual Health Care, appealing their decision to not pay for Janine Frieze's blepharoplasty. Explain why you think the procedure should be covered. Note any documentation supporting your case.

Supplies/Equipment: Pen or computer and paper
Time Allowed: 50 minutes
Accuracy Needed to Pass: 90%

Procedural Steps	Points Earned	Comments
Evaluator: Note time began: _____		
1. Carefully read the scenario.		
2. Compose a letter appealing National Mutual's decision.		
3. Letter Format (12)		
Date and inside address		
Attention line		
Subject line		
Salutation		
Complimentary close and signature		
Reference and enclosure lines		
4. Content (30)		
Opening paragraph		
Main content paragraph		
Closing paragraph		
5. Proofread the letter for accuracy.		
Optional: May deduct points for taking more time than allowed.		

Total Points = 42

Student's Score: _____

Evaluator: _____

Comments: _____

_____

_____

APPLICATION EXERCISES

Health Insurance Professional's Notebook

Assemble information and example forms for the Health Insurance Professional's Notebook regarding claims, such as:

- Sample EOBs and RAs along with explanations for interpretation
- Templates for filing secondary claims
- Flowcharts showing how claims proceed through the adjudication process
- Sample appeal letters and forms
- Chart of major payers and their time limits for submitting claims
- Steps for submitting Medicare appeals
- Forms for submitting Medicare appeals

Chapter Checklist

Student Name: _____

Chapter Completion Date: _____

Evaluate your classroom performance. Complete the self-evaluation and submit it to your instructor. When your instructor returns this form to you, compare your self-evaluation with the evaluation completed by your instructor.

1.	Record	Your start time and date: _____
2.	Read	The assigned chapter in the textbook
3.	View	PowerPoint slides (if available)
4.	Complete	Exercises in the workbook as assigned
5.	Compare	Your answers with the answers posted on the bulletin board, website, or handout
6.	Correct	Your answers
7.	Complete	All tests and required activities
8.	Read	Assigned readings (if any)
9.	Complete	Chapter performance objectives (competencies), if any
10.	Evaluate	Chapter performance and submit to your instructor
11.	Record	Your ending time and date: _____
12.	Move on	Begin next chapter as assigned

PERFORMANCE EVALUATION

Student Name: _____

Chapter Completion Date: _____

Evaluate your classroom performance. Complete this evaluation with the one provided by your instructor.

Skill	Student Self-Evaluation			Instructor Evaluation		
	Good	Average	Poor	Good	Average	Poor
Attendance/punctuality						
Personal appearance						
Applies effort						
Is self-motivated						
Is courteous						
Has positive attitude						
Completes assignments in timely manner						
Works well with others						

Student's Initials: _____

Date: _____

Points Possible: _____

Points Awarded: _____

Chapter Grade: _____

Instructor's Initials: _____

Date: _____

Chapter **15 Keys to Successful Claims Management**

16 The Role of Computers in Health Insurance

Chapter 16 discusses how the 21st century has brought the power of automation and the Internet to the medical office—specifically through electronic billing and insurance claims processing. The electronic claims process may sound complicated, but it is relatively simple. Instead of sending insurance claims to third-party carriers through the mail, the same information is transmitted electronically (in a matter of seconds) by computer over telephone or broadband lines. First, the information is input into a computer using special software. Next, the computer transmits the insurance information in the form of a claim to the third-party carrier directly or via a clearinghouse. The clearinghouse checks the data for errors and arranges it in a particular format required by the insurance carrier. The carrier processes the claim and mails the provider (or, in some cases, the patient) a reimbursement check, EOB, or both. The electronic claims submission process is faster than the paper method. Reimbursement is often received in the provider's office within 7 to 14 days as opposed to the 30 to 60 days it takes for payment of a paper claim. According to the American Medical Association, electronic claim processing has been shown to reduce claim rejection rates from 30% to 2%.

WORKBOOK CHAPTER OBJECTIVES

After completing the workbook activities for Chapter 16, the student should be able to:
1. Define the terms used in the chapter.
2. Answer the review questions according to the evaluation criteria set by the instructor.
3. Attain logical conclusions (or answers) by analyzing and evaluating given information and scenarios.
4. Use problem-solving skills (individually or in a group setting) to determine valid responses and outcomes in case studies and application exercises.
5. Actively participate in group discussions.
6. Interpret and resolve situations presented in case studies.
7. Complete performance objectives within the criteria determined by the instructor.
8. Perform the necessary steps for unbiased self-evaluation and understanding of material presented in the workbook.

DEFINING CHAPTER TERMS

Using the computer, students should type an accurate definition for each of the chapter terms listed. These definitions should be in the students' own words. When finished, students should compare their definitions with those listed in the glossary at the back of the textbook and correct any inaccuracies.

Administrative Simplification and Compliance Act (ASCA)
billing service
clearinghouse
code sets
combination records
digital imaging hybrid
direct data entry (DDE)
electronic claims clearinghouse
electronic data interchange (EDI)
electronic funds transfer (EFT)
electronic media claim (EMC)
electronic medical record (EMR)

electronic remittance advice (ERA)
enrollment process
evidence-based practice (EBP)
identifiers
meaningful use
privacy standards
security standards
small provider of services
small supplier
telehealth
telemedicine
unusual circumstances

341

Multiple Choice

Directions: In the questions and statements presented, choose the response that **best** answers or completes the stem and circle the letter that precedes it.

1. Specific areas of administrative simplification addressed by HIPAA include all of these *except:*
   a. EDI
   b. Accreditation
   c. Code sets
   d. Specific identifiers

2. The organization created to reform health insurance and simplify the healthcare administrative processes is known as:
   a. CMS
   b. HCFA
   c. HIPAA
   d. DHS

3. The electronic transfer of information in a standard format between two entities is known as:
   a. EDI
   b. PHI
   c. DHS
   d. ICD

4. The numbers used in the administration of healthcare to distinguish individual providers, health plans, employers, and patients are called:
   a. Standards
   b. Security codes
   c. Code sets
   d. Identifiers

5. To send claims electronically, the medical practice needs:
   a. A computer
   b. A modem
   c. HIPAA-compliant software
   d. All of the above

6. If a medical practice chooses to submit claims electronically to an insurance carrier, it must go through a(n):
   a. Internal audit
   b. Background check
   c. Enrollment process
   d. Appeals process

7. A business entity that receives claims from several medical facilities, consolidates these claims, and transmits them to various insurance carriers is called a(n):
   a. Electronic data interchange (EDI) transmitter
   b. Claims clearinghouse
   c. Fiscal intermediary (FI)
   d. Claims consolidation firm

8. The system wherein data representing money are moved electronically between accounts or organizations is called:
   a. Direct data entry (DDE)
   b. Electronic funds transfer (EFT)
   c. Electronic medical record (EMR)
   d. Electronic remittance advice (ERA)

9. An electronic file wherein patients' health information is stored in a computer system is called:
   a. Direct data entry (DDE)
   b. Electronic funds transfer (EFT)
   c. Electronic medical record (EMR)
   d. Electronic remittance advice (ERA)

10. One of the most significant activities of the healthcare industry is:
    a. Information management
    b. Inventory management
    c. Office management
    d. Drug management

11. One of the major disadvantages of EMRs is:
    a. Language
    b. Cost
    c. Training staff
    d. Keeping hardware and software up to date

12. Submitting claims directly to an insurance carrier is referred to as:
    a. Direct data entry (DDE)
    b. Electronic funds transfer (EFT)
    c. Electronic medical record (EMR)
    d. Electronic remittance advice (ERA)

13. If the practice submits claims primarily to one carrier, it may be advisable to use:
    a. A clearinghouse
    b. An FI
    c. DDE
    d. ERA

14. The ultimate goal in healthcare is to establish an EMR system that is:
    a. Cheap
    b. Hacker-proof
    c. Intercommunicative
    d. Unrestricted

15. The acronym for the organization enacted by Congress to improve the administration of Medicare by taking advantage of the efficiencies gained through electronic claim submission is:
    a. CMS (formerly HCFA)
    b. HIPAA
    c. ASCA
    d. HHS

16. The code set currently used for physician diagnoses is:
    a. NDC
    b. CPT-4
    c. ICD-10-PCS
    d. ICD-10-CM

17. The record-keeping method in which some documents are stored electronically and some are kept in paper form is referred to as:
    a. Combination records
    b. Blended registers
    c. Sequenced accounts
    d. Digital imaging hybrids

18. If the goal of a healthcare office is to change to a completely electronic medical record system, a _____ may be a good choice.
    a. Digital imaging hybrid
    b. Combination record
    c. Blended register account
    d. Sequenced register account

19. Disadvantages to EMRs include all of these *except:*
    a. Cost
    b. Security breaches
    c. Transfer time
    d. Lack of software available

20. To qualify for Medicare/Medicaid's monetary incentives to put EMRs into operation, providers must demonstrate _____ EMRs.
    a. A significant need for
    b. Meaningful use of
    c. Adequate patient load for
    d. That they can afford

True/False

Directions: Place a "T" in the blank preceding each of these statements if it is true; place an "F" if it is false.

_____ 1. Federal regulations now mandate that all healthcare information that is electronically transmitted follow specific rules and guidelines to provide security and protection for PHI.

_____ 2. The Administrative Simplification and Compliance Act (ASCA) requires health plans and healthcare clearinghouses to use certain standard transaction formats and code sets for the electronic transmission of health information.

_____ 3. ASCA made it compulsory for all Medicare claims to be submitted electronically effective October 16, 2003, without exception.

_____ 4. ASCA's "rule" does not require any other transactions (changes, adjustments, or appeals to the initial claim) to be submitted electronically.

_____ 5. Claims submitted via DDE are considered to be electronic claims for purposes of the "rule."

_____ 6. The biggest obstacle to getting set up for electronic claims processing is the time that it takes for approval from various federal and state agencies.

_____ 7. The move from paper to electronic submissions will result in significant savings for all medical providers.

_____ 8. ASCA's "rule" is applicable only to providers, practitioners, and suppliers who submit claims under Part A or Part B of Medicare.

_____ 9. ERA payments can be posted automatically to patient accounts.

_____ 10. Experts predict that computerized medical records can improve the quality of patient care.

_____ 11. The first step for providers to accomplish "meaningful use" is to invest in a certified EMR system.

_____ 12. A *small provider of services* is a medical facility (e.g., a hospital or skilled nursing facility) with fewer than 25 full-time equivalent (FTE) employees.

_____ 13. A *small supplier* is a physician, practitioner, facility, or supplier with fewer than 10 FTEs.

_____ 14. Physicians who did not adopt an EMR by 2015 were penalized 10% of Medicare payments, increasing incrementally to 25% by the end of the program.

_____ 15. EMR is a system wherein data representing money are moved electronically between accounts or organizations.

Short Answer/Fill-in-the-Blank

1. Name four ways computers are commonly used in today's medical offices.

_____

_____

_____

_____

2. List and explain the five specific areas of administrative simplification addressed by HIPAA.

_____

_____

_____

_____

_____

3. Explain the process of EDI in your own words.

_____

_____

_____

4. List the four essential elements of EDI.

_____

_____

_____

_____

5. Discuss the benefits of EDI.

_____

_____

_____

6. There are essentially two ways to submit claims electronically. Name them and briefly explain each process.

_____

_____

7. Explain how a clearinghouse works.

_____

_____

_____

8. Discuss the pros and cons of DDE compared with using an electronic claims clearinghouse.

_____

_____

_____

9. Name the two types of EMR "hybrids" and provide a brief explanation of both.

_____

_____

10. List three potential issues professionals face when changing to an EMR system.

_____

_____

_____

11. List and discuss the exceptions to the electronic claims submission requirement under ASCA's "rule."

_____

_____

_____

12. List the various components typically contained in an EMR system.

_____

_____

_____

CRITICAL THINKING ACTIVITIES

A. Write a paragraph (250–300 words) on the effect of computers on health insurance.

B. The textbook discusses EDI. In its most basic definition, EDI is the replacement of paper-based patient health records with electronic equivalents. How does HIPAA fit into this picture as far as the benefits of EDI are concerned?

C. Some experts say that EMRs will cut healthcare costs. Do you agree? Why or why not?

D. In your own opinion, what do you think the future holds for EMRs?

PROBLEM-SOLVING/COLLABORATIVE (GROUP) ACTIVITIES

A. Broadmoor Medical Clinic is planning to computerize its office, and the office manager has asked you to research necessary hardware to switch from paper to electronic claim submission. Generate a list of state-of-the-art hardware necessary for this conversion. The hardware components should have expansion capabilities for anticipated clinic growth. Also, decide whether the clinic should use a clearinghouse or direct claims submission. (**Note:** The clinic submits claims to all major carriers.) Use the Internet for your research or interview local medical office personnel for this activity.

B. Along with the hardware necessary for computerization, Broadmoor Medical Clinic will need a high-quality patient accounting software program. Currently, the patient load at Broadmoor is 1000 patients and 10 physicians. Research possible software that would be suitable for the clinic. Use the Internet or interview local medical facility personnel.

PROJECTS/DISCUSSION TOPICS

A. Join a class discussion on:
   - Advantages and disadvantages of EMRs
   - Privacy concerns of EMRs

B. Looking at both sides:
   1. A study found that approximately 25% of patient charts are unavailable when patients come to a medical office for an appointment. That means the healthcare provider does not have the patient's medical history or treatment regimen available during the patient visit, and information from the encounter will have to be entered into the chart later—if ever.
   2. EMRs are one of the most promising developments in medical cost control, patient care, and patient privacy. Ironically, their inability to eliminate the need for supplemental paper charts has been one reason that less than 5% of physicians use them.

C. What kinds of adjustments would health insurance professionals have to make when converting from paper records to EMRs?

D. Compose a page for Broadmoor's Policy Manual for the steps necessary to submit claims electronically. You can choose the clearinghouse method or DDE.

CASE STUDIES

A. Study the sample remittance advice (RA) in Fig. 16.1 and answer these questions:
  1. How many claims are on this RA?
  2. What was the total amount billed to Medicare?
  3. Of the amount on Benny Fischer's second claim, how much did Medicare pay?
  4. By what method were these claims paid?
  5. What was the total amount of the payment?
  6. Were there any crossover claims?
  7. If so, which patients had their claim crossed over?
  8. What was the total amount applied to patients' deductibles?
  9. What does the code "PR" mean?
 10. How much of I.M. Hurt's charge is he responsible for?

Provider Block	
Broadmoor Medical Clinic	Clinic EIN # 42-1898989
4353 Pine Ridge Drive	Dr. Robert L. Jones NPI 1234567890
Milton, XY 12345-0001	Dr. Marilou Lucero NPI 2907511822
Clinic NPI X100XX1000	Date claims 1 day after examination
Telephone: 555-656-7890	
Fax: 555-656-7899	Number of computers in clinic: 15
E-mail: broadmoorFP	

```
PROVIDENCE MEDICARE SERVICES
600 EAST PARK DRIVE                                    MEDICARE REMITTANCE NOTICE
SOUTHPARK, YZ 17111-2777

BROADMOOR MEDICAL CLINIC                               PROVIDER #: 1234567890
4353 PINE RIDGE DRIVE                                  PAGE #: 1 OF 1
MILTON, XY 12345-0001                                  DATE: 04/28/XX
555-656-7890                                           CHECK/EFT #: 0003300442
```

****

****

PERF PROV	SERV DATE	POS	NOS	PROC	MODS	BILLED	ALLOWED	DEDUCT	COINS	GRP/RC	AMT	PROV PD

NAME FISCHER, BENNY   HIC 222665555A   ACNT   FISC 6123133-01   ICN 0202199306840   ASG Y   MOA MA01

123456ABC	0225	0225XX	11	1	99213		66.00	49.83	0.34	9.97	CO-42	16.17	39.52
PT RESP	10.31			CLAIM TOTALS		66.00	49.83	0.34	9.97		16.17	
										NET	39.52	

NAME FISCHER, BENNY   HIC 222665555A   ACNT   FISC 6123133-01   ICN 0202199306850 ASG Y MOA MA01 MA07

| 123456ABC | 0117 | 0117XX | 11 | 1 | 99213 | | 66.00 | 49.83 | 0.00 | 9.97 | CO-42 | 16.17 | 39.86 |
| PT RESP | 9.97 | | | CLAIM TOTALS | | 66.00 | 49.83 | 0.00 | 9.97 | | 16.17 | 39.86 |

CLAIM INFORMATION FORWARDED TO: STATE OF XY MEDICAID   NET   39.86

NAME HURT, I.M.   HIC 512357683A   ACNT   HURT5-329   ICN 0202199306860   ASG Y   MOA MA01

123456ABC	0117	0117XX	11	1	90659		25.00	3.32	0.00	0.00	CO-42	21.68	3.32
123456ABC	0117	0117XX	11	1	G0008		10.00	4.46	0.00	0.00	CO-42	5.54	4.46
PT RESP	0.00			CLAIM TOTALS		35.00	7.78	0.00	0.00		27.22	7.78
										NET	7.78	

NAME MARLOWE, PHILIP   HIC 033448165A   ACNT   MARLO861-316-   ICN 0202199306870 ASG Y MOA MA01 MA07

| 123456ABC | 0209 | 0209XX | 11 | 1 | 99213 | | 66.00 | 49.83 | 0.00 | 9.97 | CO-42 | 16.17 | 39.86 |
| PT RESP | 9.97 | | | CLAIM TOTALS | | 66.00 | 49.83 | 0.00 | 9.97 | | 16.17 | 39.86 |

CLAIM INFORMATION FORWARDED TO: STATE OF XY MEDICAID   NET   39.86

NAME RAP, JACK   HIC 113778916A   ACNT   RAP33-721   ICN 0202199306880 ASG Y MOA MA01 MA07

123456ABC	0314	0314XX	11	1	99213		66.00	49.83	0.00	9.97	CO-42	16.17	39.86
123456ABC	0314	0314XX	11	1	82962		10.00	4.37	0.00	0.00	CO-42	5.63	4.37
123456ABC	0314	0314XX	11	1	94760		12.00	0.00	0.00	0.00	CO-B15	12.00	0.00
REM: M80												
PT RESP	9.97			CLAIM TOTALS		88.00	54.20	0.00	9.97		33.80	44.23
										NET	44.23	

TOTALS:	# of CLAIMS	BILLED AMT	ALLOWED AMT	DEDUCT AMT	COINS RC AMT.	TOTAL AMT	PROV PD ADJ AMT	PROV AMT	CHECK AMT
	5	321.00	211.47	0.34	39.88	109.53	171.25	.00	171.25

GROUP CODES:

PR	Patient Responsibility
CO	Contractual Obligation
OA	Other Adjustment

PT RESP	Patient responsibility is the unpaid amount for which the patient is liable and includes the patient responsibility for all of the details.
CLAIM TOTALS: **BILLED AMT**	The total billed amount.
ALLOWED AMT	The total allowed amount.
DEDUCTIBLE	The total amount applied to the deductible.
COINSURANCE	The total amount of coinsurance.
GRP/RC AMT	The GRP/RC amount is the difference between the billed amount and the allowed amount.
PROV PD	The actual payment amount paid to the provider for the service.

Fig. 16.1 Providence Medicare remittance advice.

B. Fig. 16.2 is a printout of an electronic page from a company that offers direct claims submission. Using the information from the Broadmoor Medical Clinic provider block (p. 340), complete the questionnaire. In the "Information Requested" box, provide a detailed description of the information desired.

Electronic Contact:
To contact **Direct Technology** electronically, simply fill out the form below and click *submit*.

* = Required field

Name: _____ *

Company: _____

Address: _____

City: _____

State: [N/A ▼]

ZIP: _____

Phone: _____

Fax: _____

E-mail Address: _____ *

Specialty: [--Select From List-- ▼] *

Product of interest: [--Select From List-- ▼] *

How did you hear about us: [--Select From List-- ▼] *

Other: specify _____

Timeframe for Purchase [-Please Select- ▼]

# of Providers in Practice [ ] *   # of Computers in Practice [ ] *

How do you prefer to be contacted [Select ▼] * Best time to call [ ]

Information requested:

_____

[Submit] [Reset]

Address Contact:
Direct Technology
1110 Sylvan Heights
Harper, XY 11233
directtech@support.com

Phone Contact:
Phone: (555) 488-8100
Toll-Free : (800) 233-0321
FAX: (555) 488-7737

Fig. 16.2 Printout of electronic contact form.

A. Log on to the Internet and, using the search words "electronic medical records," research what the "experts" have to say about the subject.

B. Search the Internet using the search words "computers in health insurance" and learn how computers benefit the health insurance process. This weblink is one example: http://www.ehow.com/list_7240917_uses-computers-insurance.html.

C. Visit this website for a relevant "quizlet": http://quizlet.com/4242020/role-of-computers-in-health-insurance-ch16-flash-cards.

Performance Objective 16.1: Composing an Email Message

Conditions: Student will compose an email to Dr. Beatrice Fisher requesting the health records for patient Miriam P. Cover (BD 09/18/1956), who has recently moved to Milton. Mrs. Cover has an appointment on March 7, 20XX, with Dr. Jones for continued treatment of her diabetes. Dr. Fisher's email address is bfisher@uihospclinic.net. Mrs. Cover should get a copy of the message at mpcover@hotmail.com.

Supplies/Equipment: Pen or computer, paper, and email screen duplicated in Fig. 16.3

Time Allowed: 20 minutes

Accuracy Needed to Pass: 90%

Procedural Steps	Points Earned	Comments
Evaluator: Note time began: _____		
1. Carefully read the instructions given for Performance Objective 16.1.		
2. Enter the email address of Dr. Fisher in the correct space. (5)		
3. Enter the email address of Mrs. Cover in the correct space. (5)		
4. Enter the applicable subject for the message. (5)		
5. Compose a brief message as outlined in the instructions. (10)		
6. Close with your name and the clinic's name, address, and a phone number. (5)		
Optional: May deduct points for taking more time than allowed.		

Total Points = 30

Student's Score: _____

Evaluator: _____

Comments: _____

_____

_____

_____

_____

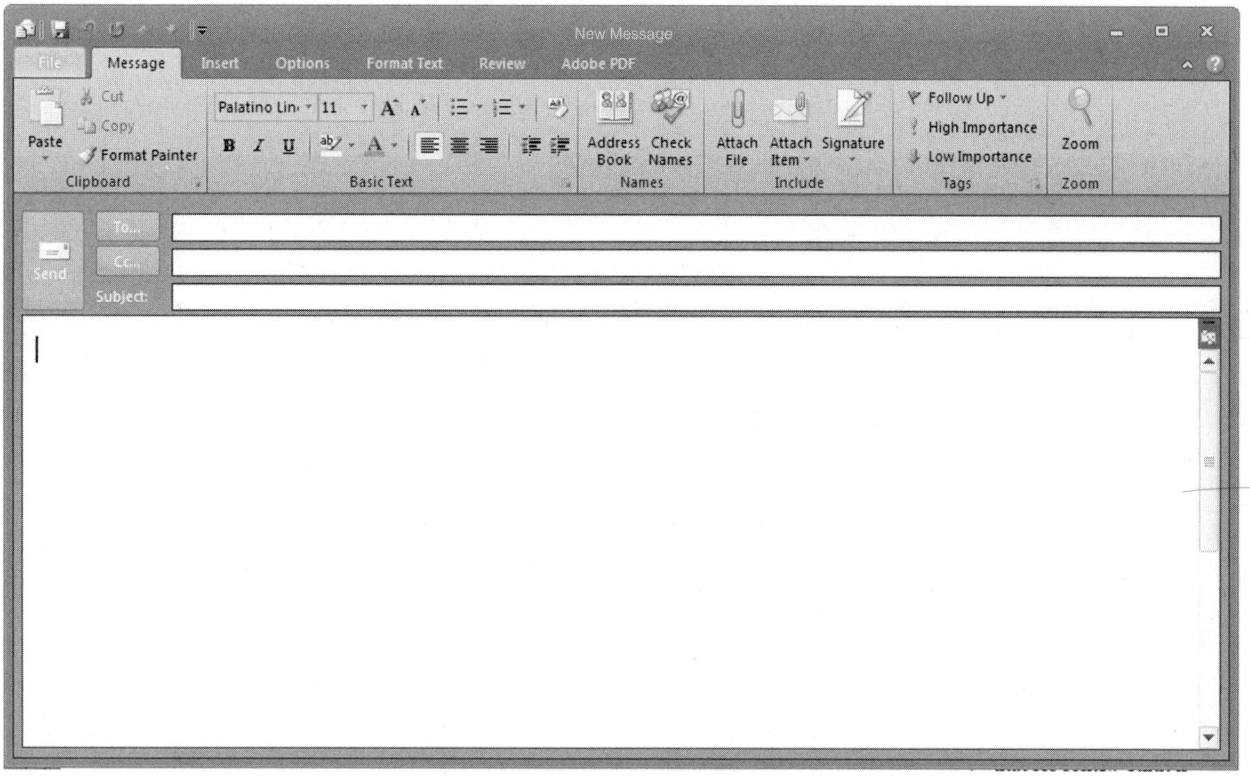

Fig. 16.3 Duplication of email screen.

Performance Objective 16.2: Completing an ETF/ERA Enrollment Form

Conditions: Student will complete the EFT/ERA enrollment form shown in Fig. 16.4 using Broadmoor Clinic's information. Direct Technology is the practice management vendor; Curt Jones is the vendor contact name. Claim Connect is the clearinghouse you'll be using with user ID # 292927444. EFT will be to a checking account at the Milton National Bank.

Supplies/Equipment: Pen or computer and paper, and EFT/ERA enrollment form (see Fig. 16.4)

Time Allowed: 30 minutes

Accuracy Needed to Pass: 90%

Procedural Steps	Points Earned	Comments
Evaluator: Note time began: _____		
1. Carefully read the instructions given for Performance Objective 16.2.		
2. Complete the applicable blanks on the EFT/ERA enrollment form using the information provided. (25)		
Optional: May deduct points for taking more time than allowed.		

Total Points = 25

Student's Score: _____

Evaluator: _____

Comments: _____

_____

_____

_____

_____

Electronic Funds Transfer / Electronic Remittance Advice Enrollment Form

Please read all information carefully. Check the appropriate box for this request.
ENROLL IN: ☐ *EFT* ☐ *ERA* *Note: you may enroll in EFT and / or ERA*

Complete the following information, please type or print:

Practice Name _____ Practice Tax ID (TIN)_____

Practice Address _____

Practice Management Vendor _____

Vendor Contact Name_____ Vendor Phone _____

Vendor E-mail Address_____ Approved Vendor/ Clearinghouse _____

Authorized Signature / Date _____

---

1. Electronic Fund Transfer (EFT) – New Enrollment

_____Enroll in EFT   Effective date (Internal Use Only) _____

Do you require payments to be deposited into multiple bank accounts? Yes____ No_____

Do you require payments to be deposited into checking and/or savings account?   Checking_____ Savings_____

New EFT enrollment or changes to existing EFT banking information will trigger a new EFT pre-note validation period. The EFT pre-note validation period will run for 10 days from the effective date. You will be notified of banking issues; otherwise, production will start on day 11.

Request cancellation of EFT as of: _____

NOTE:
You must include a voided check or savings account deposit slip with this enrollment form for your request to be considered. Providers are responsible for notifying Elipse if the above banking information changes.

---

2. Electronic Remittance Advice (ERA) – New Enrollments (only available when registered with Dentalxchange via ClaimConnect). Enrollment in ERA will also eliminate production of paper Explanation of Benefit (EOB) within 60 days of activation.

Enroll in ERA _____   Effective Date (Internal Use Only) _____

ClaimConnect User ID _____   Request Cancellation of ERA as of: _____

ELIPSE INSURANCE CO.
1446 Fortune Lane
Morning Sun, XY 23456
Phone 555-333-4444

Fig. 16.4 Electronic funds transfer form.

Performance Objective 16.3: Completing a Direct Deposit Authorization Form

Conditions: Student will complete the direct deposit authorization form for Broadmoor Medical Clinic shown in Fig. 16.5 using the clinic information acquired to date. Banking information is provided in Box 16.1.

Supplies/Equipment: Pen or computer and paper, and instructions (see Box 16.1)

Time Allowed: 50 minutes

Accuracy Needed to Pass: 90%

Procedural Steps	Points Earned	Comments
Evaluator: Note time began: _____		
1. Carefully read the instructions given for Performance Objective 16.3.		
2. Complete the applicable blanks on the direct deposit enrollment form using the information provided in Box 16.1. (35)		
Optional: May deduct points for taking more time than allowed.		

Total Points = 35

Student's Score: _____

Evaluator: _____

Comments: _____

_____

_____

_____

_____

Box 16.1

Bank Name: Milton National Bank
Address: 8610 Park Plaza, Milton, XY 12345
Routing No.: 00898870-5216-14
Account No.: 606-445-1
Account Type: Checking

Authorization for Direct Deposit
Enrollment, Change, and Cancellation Authorization

Please read all of the information on this form carefully.
Authorization Information. Check the appropriate box for this authorization.

☐ ENROLL in Direct Deposit   ☐ CHANGE to Direct Deposit   ☐ CANCEL previous authorization

---

Provider Information
Please print. Complete all of the information below, including your tax identification number (TIN).

PROVIDER INFORMATION

Name(s) _____   Required for Processing: TIN ___ ___ - ___ ___ ___ ___ ___ ___ ___

Street _____   City _____   State _____   Zip _____

Business Telephone Number (___) _____

E-Mail Address: _____

Account Information
Complete this section for direct payments to either your checking or savings account.

BANK NAME: _____   ADDRESS: _____
BANK ID (first 8 digits of the routing number): ___ ___ ___ ___ ___ ___ ___ ___
BANK SCD (self-checking digit–the last digit of the routing number): ___
ACCOUNT NUMBER: _____   ACCOUNT TYPE: Savings ☐ or Checking ☐

TO BE COMPLETED for each additional bank account

BANK NAME: _____   ADDRESS: _____
BANK ID (first 8 digits of the routing number): ___ ___ ___ ___ ___ ___ ___ ___
BANK SCD (self-checking digit–the last digit of the routing number): ___
ACCOUNT NUMBER: _____   ACCOUNT TYPE: Savings ☐ or Checking ☐

TO BE COMPLETED for each additional bank account

BANK NAME: _____   ADDRESS: _____
BANK ID (first 8 digits of the routing number): ___ ___ ___ ___ ___ ___ ___ ___
BANK SCD (self-checking digit–the last digit of the routing number): ___
ACCOUNT NUMBER: _____   ACCOUNT TYPE: Savings ☐ or Checking ☐

Authorization Agreement for Direct Deposit of Benefits Payments. Read the authorization and sign your name below.

I hereby authorize the Company to initiate credit entries to the account(s) at the bank(s) listed above for all benefits payments. This agreement will remain in effect until I notify Company of the desire to cancel or change this service or until Company notifies me that this service has been terminated. I understand that I must allow reasonable time for my instructions to be executed. If Company credits more money than the correct benefit amount to the account due to duplicate electronic funds transfers (where "duplicate" is defined as multiple electronic funds transfers received for the same services rendered, the same membership, and the same dates of service) or erroneous electronic funds transfers (where erroneous is defined as complete electronic funds transfers received in error), I authorize Company to withdraw the over payment. I authorize and request the bank listed above to accept any credit entries by Aetna to such account and to credit the same to such account.

Please Print Name _____   **Date** _____

Authorized Signature _____

Provider Network Authorization _____   **Date** _____

Fig. 16.5 Direct deposit form.

Health Insurance Professional's Notebook

Assemble information and example forms for the Health Insurance Professional's Notebook regarding:

- Examples of forms and completion instructions for EFT and RMA enrollment
- Names and telephone numbers of reputable hardware and software dealers
- Informational brochures on patient accounting software
- Sample ERAs and instructions on how to interpret each
- Information, resources, and websites on EMRs

Chapter Checklist

Student Name: _____

Chapter Completion Date: _____

Evaluate your classroom performance. Complete the self-evaluation and submit it to your instructor. When your instructor returns this form to you, compare your self-evaluation with the evaluation completed by your instructor.

1.	Record	Your start time and date: _____
2.	Read	The assigned chapter in the textbook
3.	View	PowerPoint slides (if available)
4.	Complete	Exercises in the workbook as assigned
5.	Compare	Your answers to the answers posted on the bulletin board, website, or handout
6.	Correct	Your answers
7.	Complete	All tests and required activities
8.	Read	Assigned readings (if any)
9.	Complete	Chapter performance objectives (competencies), if any
10.	Evaluate	Chapter performance and submit to your instructor
11.	Record	Your ending time and date: _____
12.	Move on	Begin next chapter as assigned

PERFORMANCE EVALUATION

Student Name: _____

Chapter Completion Date: _____

Evaluate your classroom performance. Compare this evaluation with the one provided by your instructor.

Skill	Student Self-Evaluation			Instructor Evaluation		
	Good	Average	Poor	Good	Average	Poor
Attendance/punctuality						
Personal appearance						
Applies effort						
Is self-motivated						
Is courteous						
Has positive attitude						
Completes assignments in timely manner						
Works well with others						

Student's Initials: _____

Date: _____

Points Possible: _____

Points Awarded: _____

Chapter Grade: _____

Instructor's Initials: _____

Date: _____

In this chapter, you were introduced to topics that are considered more advanced. Your instructor may or may not include this chapter in the course curriculum because it delves more into the area of health information management as opposed to that of health insurance professionals. Some of the subject matter presented may prove to be confusing and, at best, challenging, but do not become discouraged. Chapter 17 is intended to give students an overview of what a career path to becoming a health information technician (HIT) or a health information management (HIM) specialist involves. These are considered more advanced careers for which students may become certified and typically involve up to 4 years of college. Usually, an HIT or an HIM specialist is employed by hospitals rather than by physician offices or clinics, and employment responsibilities may differ considerably from those of a health insurance professional in a medical office. If the information presented in Chapter 17 piques your interest and you think you may want to pursue a career in HIM, discuss this with your instructor or your student advisor.

WORKBOOK CHAPTER OBJECTIVES

After completing the workbook activities for Chapter 17, the student should be able to:
1. Define the terms used in the chapter.
2. Answer the review questions according to the evaluation criteria set by the instructor.
3. Use problem-solving skills (individually or in a group setting) to determine correct responses and outcomes in case studies and application exercises.
4. Interpret a variety of aging reports.
5. Research the Internet to locate information to understand given topics better.
6. Complete performance objectives according to the criteria determined by the instructor.
7. Perform the necessary steps for unbiased self-evaluation and understanding of material presented in the workbook.

DEFINING CHAPTER TERMS

Using the computer, students should type an accurate definition for each of the chapter terms listed. These definitions should be in the students' own words. When finished, students should compare their definitions with those listed in the glossary at the back of the textbook and correct any inaccuracies.

accounts receivable aging report
activities of daily living (ADLs)
ambulatory payment classifications (APCs)
average length of stay (ALOS)
business associate
capitation
case mix adjustment
comorbidities
contractual write-off
conversion factor (CF)
cost outliers
covered entity
diagnosis-related group (DRG)
discounted fee-for-service
disproportionate share
DRG grouper
fee-for-service (FFS)
geographical practice cost index (GPCI)
home health PPS

inpatient prospective payment system (IPPS)
inpatient psychiatric facility PPS
inpatient rehabilitation facility (IRF) PPS
labor component
long-term care hospital (LTCH) PPS
managed care organizations (MCOs)
nonlabor component
outpatient prospective payment system (OPPS)
packaging
peer review organization (PRO)
per diem rates
principal diagnosis
prospective payment system (PPS)
reimbursement
relative value scale (RVS)
relative weight (RW)
resource-based relative value scale (RBRVS)
resource utilization groups (RUGs)
secondary diagnosis

361

short-stay outlier
skilled nursing facility (SNF) PPS
standardized amount

Tax Equity and Fiscal Responsibility Act (TEFRA)
usual, customary, and reasonable (UCR)
value-based payment modifier (VBPM)

ASSESSMENT

Multiple Choice

Directions: In the questions and statements presented, choose the response that **best** answers or completes the stem and circle the letter that precedes it.

1. Payment to the insured (or his or her provider) for a covered expense or loss experienced by or on behalf of the insured is referred to as:
   a. Coverage
   b. Copayment
   c. Deductible(s)
   d. Reimbursement

2. A system of payment whereby the provider charges a specific fee for each service rendered and is paid that fee by the patient or by the patient's insurance carrier is called:
   a. Capitation
   b. Fee-for-service
   c. Discounted fee-for-service
   d. Prospective payment system (PPS)

3. Medicare's system for reimbursing Part A inpatient hospital costs is called:
   a. Capitation
   b. Fee-for-service
   c. Discounted fee-for-service
   d. Prospective payment system (PPS)

4. The amount of payment in the PPS is determined by the assigned:
   a. Capitation amount
   b. Diagnosis-related group (DRG)
   c. Usual, customary, and reasonable (UCR) fee
   d. Either b or c

5. A common method of paying physicians in health maintenance organizations is:
   a. UCR
   b. PPS
   c. Capitation
   d. Fee-for-service

6. PPS for acute hospital care for Medicare patients was mandated by:
   a. Centers for Medicare and Medicaid Services (CMS) in 1980
   b. Department of Health and Human Services (HHS) in 1981
   c. Social Security Amendments of 1983
   d. All of the above

7. The method of determining Medicare's reimbursement for services based on establishing a standard unit value for medical and surgical procedures is:
   a. PPS
   b. RVS
   c. DRG
   d. APC

8. Patients whose hospital stays are either considerably longer or considerably shorter than average are referred to as:
   a. Cost outliers
   b. Case mix patients
   c. Per diem patients
   d. Atypical patients

9. In the _____, payments for services are determined by the resource costs needed to provide them rather than actual charges.
   a. HCPCS system
   b. Fee-for-service system
   c. Relative value scale (RVS)
   d. Resource-based relative value scale (RBRVS)

10. The key piece of information in determining the DRG classification is the patient's:
    a. Chief complaint
    b. Primary diagnosis
    c. Principal diagnosis
    d. Underlying symptoms

11. Also taken into consideration in determining the DRG is the patient's _____ and any additional operations and procedures done when in the hospital.
    a. Gender
    b. Ethnicity
    c. Previous medical history
    d. Principal procedure

12. A computer software program that takes the coded information and identifies the patient's DRG category is a:
    a. Decoder
    b. Digitalized coder
    c. DRG identifier
    d. DRG grouper

13. A service classification system designed to explain the amount and type of resources used in an outpatient encounter is:
    a. DRG
    b. ALOS
    c. APCs
    d. PPS

14. Ambulatory payment classifications are made up of the coding and classification of services provided to the patient based on the:
    a. ICD coding system
    b. CPT Level I coding system
    c. HCPCS Level II coding system
    d. Both b and c

15. The basic idea of the resource utilization groups (RUGs) is to calculate payments according to severity and level of care in:
    a. Outpatient clinics
    b. Acute care hospitals
    c. Skilled nursing facilities
    d. Long-term care facilities

16. A factor used by Medicare to adjust for variance in operating costs of medical practices located in different parts of the United States is the:
    a. GPCI
    b. ANSII
    c. RBRVS
    d. VBPM

363

17. Calculating DRG payments involves a formula in which the DRG weight is multiplied by a _____,
    a figure representing the average cost per case for all Medicare cases during the year.
    a. Cost outlier
    b. Labor component
    c. Standardized amount
    d. Disproportionate share

18. Under Medicare's PPS, long-term care hospitals (LTCHs) generally treat patients who require hospital-level care for
    an average of:
    a. 10 days
    b. 15 days
    c. 25 days
    d. There is no limit with long-term care.

19. An adjustment to the federal payment rate for LTCH stays that are considerably shorter than the average length of
    stay for an LTC-DRG is called a(n):
    a. Minimum-stay adjuster
    b. Short-stay outlier
    c. GPCI
    d. ALOS

20. Under the Home Health PPS, an adjustment for the health condition and service needs of the beneficiary is referred
    to as the:
    a. Geographical price cost index
    b. Average length of stay
    c. Case mix adjustment
    d. Activities of daily living (ADLs)

21. An organization typically composed of physicians and other healthcare professionals who are paid by the federal
    government to evaluate the services provided by other practitioners and to monitor the quality of patient care is called:
    a. PPS
    b. HIPAA
    c. PRO
    d. CMS

22. If an agreement does not exist between the provider and the insurance carrier to accept the payer's allowed amount
    as payment in full, the provider can bill the patient for the outstanding amount, which is referred to as:
    a. Contractual write-offs
    b. Prospective payment
    c. Balance billing
    d. Patient equity

23. Under PPS, reimbursements for each hospital are adjusted for differences in all of these *except:*
    a. Area wages
    b. Teaching activity
    c. Provider's specialty
    d. Care to the poor

24. Similar to the RVS, the components of the RBRVS include all of these *except:*
    a. Patient diagnosis
    b. Amount of physician work
    c. Practice expense
    d. Professional liability expense

25. When the healthcare provider has signed an agreement with a third party not to bill for any charges remaining after
    all required payments have been made, it is called:
    a. An accounts receivable write-off
    b. A predetermined deduction
    c. Balance billing
    d. A contractual write-off

364

True/False

Directions: Place a "T" in the blank preceding the numbered statement if it is true; place an "F" if it is false.

_____ 1. Medicare patients are not included in the PPS system.

_____ 2. Prospective payment rates are set at a level intended to cover operating costs for treating a typical inpatient in a given DRG.

_____ 3. Under Medicare's PPS, hospitals are paid a set fee for treating patients in a single DRG category, regardless of the actual cost of care for the individual.

_____ 4. The established payment rate for all services that a patient in an acute care hospital receives during an entire stay is based on a predetermined payment level that is selected on the basis of averages.

_____ 5. The biggest challenge in developing an RVS-based payment schedule was patient diversity.

_____ 6. The Affordable Care Act eliminated patient cost-sharing requirements (coinsurance and deductible) for most Medicare-covered preventive services.

_____ 7. DRGs are used for reimbursement in the PPS of the Medicare and Medicaid healthcare insurance systems.

_____ 8. DRGs adopted by CMS are defined by diagnosis and procedure codes used in the coding manuals.

_____ 9. A patient's DRG categorization depends on the coding and classification of the patient's medical information using only the CPT coding system.

_____ 10. Each DRG is assigned a relative weight (RW) and an average length of stay (ALOS).

_____ 11. When patients are admitted to either a residential healthcare facility or a nursing home, physicians are required to prepare a written plan of care for treatment.

_____ 12. Activities of daily living are behaviors related strictly to mental health.

_____ 13. Medicare payment rules are established by Congress.

_____ 14. The Medicare program is administered mainly at the local and regional level by private insurance companies that contract with CMS to handle day-to-day billing and payment matters.

_____ 15. One of the chief objectives in creating the PPS was to monitor the quality of hospital services for Medicare beneficiaries.

_____ 16. Being a successful health insurance professional stops with knowing how to complete and submit insurance claims.

_____ 17. CMS uses the same PPS for reimbursement to acute inpatient hospitals, hospital outpatient services, and skilled nursing facilities.

_____ 18. Not all peer review organizations (PROs) deal with healthcare.

_____ 19. Non-PARs not accepting assignment can charge beneficiaries no more than 115% of the Medicare allowance.

_____ 20. Contractual write-offs and bad-debt write-offs are basically the same.

_____ 21. A computerized practice management system can alleviate potential administrative problems a healthcare practice may encounter in complying with the HIPAA Privacy Rule.

_____ 22. The HHS mandates that all medical facilities use the same format for submitting electronic health transactions.

_____ 23. The VBPM applies only to physician payments under the Medicare PFS.

_____ 24. Many different patient accounting systems are available today that are capable of performing comparable patient accounting functions.

_____ 25. If a medical practice contracts with a "business associate," the practice should ensure that the agreement includes certain protections defined by HIPAA.

Short Answer

Note: If space provided is not adequate, use a separate piece of blank paper.

1. List and explain Medicare's three primary reimbursement systems.

_____

_____

_____

2. List and discuss Congress' four chief objectives in creating the PPS.

_____

_____

_____

_____

3. List the factors on which the DRG inpatient classification system is based.

_____

_____

_____

4. Explain, in your own words, what a "cost outlier" is.

_____

_____

5. List the three components that make up a relative value unit (RVU).

_____

_____

_____

6. List the three components of the RBRVS system.

_____

_____

_____

7. When calculating DRG payment, the DRG "weight" is multiplied by the "standardized amount," which is the sum of what two factors?

_____

_____

8. Explain how payment is calculated for a CPT code under the RVU system.

_____

_____

9. Explain what a PRO is and discuss its basic responsibilities.

_____

_____

10. Congress required the HHS to contract with PROs to monitor specific healthcare functions. List these functions.

_____

_____

_____

11. List at least five of the seven system functions that most of today's patient accounting systems are capable of performing.

_____

_____

_____

_____

_____

12. List at least five capabilities that medical billing software systems typically have built into them.

_____

_____

_____

_____

_____

13. Explain the purpose of an accounts receivable aging report.

_____

_____

_____

14. What types of firms come under the umbrella of "covered entity"?

_____

_____

_____

15. List four advantages gained when a healthcare facility uses HIPAA-compliant software.

_____

_____

_____

_____

CRITICAL THINKING ACTIVITIES

A. Abby Silverton works as a health insurance professional in a small, rural clinic. In addition to Abby, the medical team includes a physician's assistant, a part-time nurse, and a medical assistant. The average yearly patient load is roughly 70 local patients—mostly elderly. The clinic is currently using the "pegboard" system of patient accounting. Prepare an outline for Abby to present at the next staff meeting discussing the advantages and disadvantages of switching to a computerized patient accounting system.

B. The Flexner Report is said by some to be the most important event in the history of American medical education. Research this topic and write a critical thinking essay on the focus points of this document and its effect on a health insurance professional.

C. Enough cannot be said about the importance of documentation in medical records. There is a common saying, "If it isn't documented, it didn't happen." Generate a one-page essay on this subject and how it affects a health insurance professional.

PROBLEM-SOLVING/COLLABORATIVE (GROUP) ACTIVITIES

A. Generate a group discussion debating whether or not a health insurance professional would benefit by becoming knowledgeable about computer hardware and participate in the selection of patient accounting systems.

B. Convene a "brainstorming" session in which each group member participates in researching and developing a "wish list" of features and functions of the "ideal" patient billing system for Broadmoor Medical Clinic. Consulting with a local medical facility may be advantageous.

C. Assemble a "fact-finding" group or partnership and investigate educational opportunities in the field of health information technology.

CASE STUDIES

A. One of the standard reports generated by most patient accounting software programs is the accounts receivable aging report. Study the example in Table 17.1 in this workbook and answer these questions.
   1. What percentage of the total dollar amounts on this page are current?
   2. What percentage of the total dollar amounts on this page are more than 30 days old?
   3. What percentage of the total dollar amounts on this page are more than 60 days old?
   4. What percentage of the total dollar amounts on this page are more than 120 days old?

Note: Round up to the nearest whole percentage.

Table 17.1 Aging Report

Broadmoor Medical Clinic Accounts Receivable Aging Report					
Name	**Current**	**>30 Days**	**>60 Days**	**>90 Days**	**>120 Days**
Abel, Paul		419.50			
Allen, Tricia			860.25		
Asner, Robert			90.00		
Benson, Ted			155.50		
Boles, Frieda					334.19
Bumgardner, Leona				11.60	
Callison, Tanner		120.00			
Colby, Ruth		85.00			
Cullen, Vincent			456.30		
Dawson, Cynthia	190.00				
Daymeri, Tao	211.90				
Ditmer, Pauline				142.35	
Dolby, Nelda				96.80	
Dunison, Arthur					1211.42
Edwards, Lois	77.00				
Efflinger, Dorothy		62.50			
Ekdale, Wesley		175.22			
Eversmeier, Theo				200.00	
Page Totals	*478.90*	*862.22*	*1562.05*	*450.75*	*1545.61*

B. Fig. 17.1 is a sample page from an insurance claims aging report. Study it and then, on a separate piece of paper, list the information that can be abstracted from this report.

BROADMOOR MEDICAL CLINIC
4353 PINE RIDGE DRIVE
MILTON XY 12345-0001

INSURANCE AGING SUMMARY

Date of Service	Procedure	Current 0 - 30	Past 31 - 60	Past 61 - 90	Past 91 - 120	Past 121 ⟶	Total Balance
Aetna (AET00)						Erik (602)333-3333	
SIMTA000 Tanus J Simpson						SSN:	
Claim: 1 Initial Billing Date: 12/3/20XX		Last Billing Date: 10/30/20XX		Policy: GG93-GXTA		Group: 99999	
12/3/20XX	43220	275.00					275.00
12/3/20XX	71040	50.00					50.00
12/3/20XX	81000	11.00					11.00
12/3/20XX	99213	50.00					50.00
	Claim Totals:	386.00	0.00	0.00	0.00	0.00	386.00
Claim: 15 Initial Billing Date: 10/30/20XX		Last Billing Date: 10/30/20XX		Policy: GG93-GXTA		Group: 99999	
10/25/20XX	99213	60.00					60.00
10/25/20XX	90707	10.00					10.00
	Claim Totals:	70.00	0.00	0.00	0.00	0.00	70.00
	Insurance Totals:	456.00	0.00	0.00	0.00	0.00	456.00
Cigna (CIG00)						Bill S. Preston 234-5678	
BRIJA000 Jay Brimley						SSN:	
Claim: 16 Initial Billing Date: 10/26/20XX		Last Billing Date: 10/26/20XX		Policy: 98547377		Group: 12d	
3/25/20XX	99214	55.00					55.00
3/25/20XX	97260	30.00					30.00
	Claim Totals:	85.00	0.00	0.00	0.00	0.00	85.00
	Insurance Totals:	85.00	0.00	0.00	0.00	0.00	85.00
US Tricare (US000)							
YOUMI000 Michael C Youngblood						SSN:	
Claim: 17 Initial Billing Date: 10/26/20XX		Last Billing Date: 10/26/20XX		Policy: USAA236678		Group: 25BB	
8/22/20XX	99213	60.00					60.00
8/22/20XX	97128	15.00					15.00
8/22/20XX	97010	10.00					10.00
	Claim Totals:	85.00	0.00	0.00	0.00	0.00	85.00
	Insurance Totals:	85.00	0.00	0.00	0.00	0.00	85.00
	Report Aging Totals	$626.00	$0.00	$0.00	$0.00	$0.00	$626.00
	Percent of Aging Total	100.0%	0.0%	0.0%	0.0%	0.0%	100.0%

Printed on 11/01/20XX 1:59 pm

*This report is being aged by the last billing date

Fig. 17.1 Insurance aging summary.

C. Table 17.2 is an example of an insurance aging report from a different software program. What does this report tell you?

Table 17.2	Insurance Company Aging Summary				
	Current	**30–59 Days**	**60–89 Days**	**90–119 Days**	**≥120 Days**
Personal	$27,806.24	$24,820.84	$16,045.36	$9647.64	$21,824.05
American	$898.00	$0.00	$125.00	$0.00	$0.00
Anthrose	$4637.00	$812.00	$1250.00	$333.00	$45.00
BayShore	$80.00	$0.00	$0.00	$0.00	$0.00
Bayshore Life	$2414.00	$212.00	$40.00	$865.00	$40.00
Catalina	$3604.00	$1546.00	$889.00	$282.00	$26.40
CIGNA	$68.00	$0.00	$60.00	$40.00	$0.00
Central Benefits	$12,647.00	$3103.00	$1100.54	$743.20	$1105.40
Dover Med	$87.00	$0.00	$0.00	$0.00	$90.00
Empire	$135.00	$0.00	$0.00	$0.00	$0.00
MetLife	$110.00	$0.00	$0.00	$0.00	$0.00
Provident	$0.00	$0.00	$32.00	$0.00	$0.00
Salem Health	$4242.70	$2099.70	$638.00	$416.00	$1010.10
United HC	$6237.00	$1087.68	$666.44	$65.00	$77.00
Total	*$86,328.84*	*$45,782.81*	*$27,276.03*	*$23,198.23*	*$36,155.51*

D. Table 17.3 is an insurance report summary that provides still another type of information. How does this report differ from the one in Fig. 17.1? How does this report differ from the one in Table 17.2? Write your answers in the space provided or on a separate piece of paper.

Table 17.3 Insurance Company Reimbursement Report: Summary

From: 01/01/XX	To: 12/31/XX		Generated on 01/11/XX
Code	Procedure/Group Name	Units	Charged
99213	Office Visit Expanded Focus	11,956	$616,720
99212	Office Visit Problem Focused	1,613	$ 49,662
99054	Office Visit Sundays and Holidays	889	$ 8,890
[many lines deleted]			
	Office Visits	15,496	$702,368
99392	Well Child 1–4 years	2,744	$150,920
99391	Well Child younger than 1 year	2,386	$124,072
99393	Well Child 5–11 years	1,042	$ 61,435
[many lines deleted]			
	Well Child Visits	7,516	$428,389

INTERNET EXPLORATION

A. Use the Internet to research the Tax Equity and Fiscal Responsibility Act (TEFRA).

B. Use the Internet to research appropriate search words to locate information and updates on these systems:
  ■ Medicare's IPPS
  ■ APCs
  ■ OPPS

C. There is a growing demand for qualified applicants in the health information management field. Research the Internet using http://www.healthmanagementcareers.org to learn more about this dynamic and growing field in healthcare.

Note: If this URL is unavailable, use appropriate search words to locate more detailed information on this subject.

PERFORMANCE OBJECTIVES

The Performance Objectives in Chapter 17 are designed to provide you with additional learning opportunities and reinforcement in the knowledge and understanding of the various types of reimbursement systems used in physicians' offices, clinics, and healthcare facilities, such as hospitals, skilled nursing facilities, rehabilitation facilities, and other institutional-type care facilities.

Performance Objective 17.1: Explaining Common Reimbursement Types

Conditions: Student will write a short paragraph explaining these reimbursement types: fee-for-service, discounted fee-for-service, PPS, capitation, and per diem.

Supplies/Equipment: Computer with word processing software, printer, and paper

Time Allowed: 30 minutes

Accuracy Needed to Pass: 90%

Procedural Steps	Points Earned	Comments
Evaluator: Note time began: _____		
1. Student explained the FFS payment system satisfactorily. (20)		
2. Student explained the discounted FFS payment system satisfactorily. (20)		
3. Student explained the PPS satisfactorily. (20)		
4. Student explained the capitation payment system satisfactorily. (20)		
5. Student explained the per diem payment system satisfactorily. (20)		

Total Points = 100

Student's Score: _____

Evaluator: _____

Comments: _____

_____

_____

_____

_____

373

Performance Objective 17.2: Defining DRGs, APCs, and RUGs

Conditions: Student will state what the abbreviations DRG, APC, and RUG stand for, write a brief definition of each, and explain where and how they are used in healthcare facilities.

Supplies/Equipment: Computer with word processing software, printer, and paper

Time Allowed: 30 minutes

Accuracy Needed to Pass: 85%

Procedural Steps	Points Earned	Comments
Evaluator: Note time began: _____		
1. Student provided an accurate and adequate explanation of DRGs. (20)		
2. Student provided an accurate and adequate explanation of APCs. (20)		
3. Student provided an accurate and adequate explanation of RUGs. (20)		

Total Points = 60

Student's Score: _____

Evaluator: _____

Comments: _____

_____

_____

_____

_____

Performance Objective 17.3: Understanding Computerized Patient Accounting Systems

Conditions: Describe a typical computerized patient accounting system, including the seven basic functions that this type of software is capable of performing.

Supplies/Equipment: Computer with word processing software, printer, and paper

Time Allowed: 30 minutes

Accuracy Needed to Pass: 85%

Procedural Steps	Points Earned	Comments
Evaluator: Note time began: _____		
1. Student provided an accurate, satisfactory description of a patient accounting system. (20)		
2. Student correctly identified the seven basic functions of this type of software. (20)		
3. Student demonstrated proficiency in writing and grammar skills. (20)		

Total Points = 60

Student's Score: _____

Evaluator: _____

Comments: _____

_____

_____

_____

_____

Health Insurance Professional's Notebook

1. Collect pertinent examples of documents discussed in this chapter, such as:
   - Electronic remittance advices
   - Aging and other practice reports

2. Include websites for information on:
   - Continuing education for health insurance professionals
   - Certification possibilities
   - Keeping current

Chapter Checklist

Student Name: _____

Chapter Completion Date: _____

Evaluate your classroom performance. Complete the self-evaluation and submit it to your instructor. When your instructor returns this form to you, compare your self-evaluation with the evaluation completed by your instructor.

1.	Record	Your start time and date: _____
2.	Read	The assigned chapter in the textbook
3.	View	PowerPoint slides (if available)
4.	Complete	Exercises in the workbook as assigned
5.	Compare	Your answers to the answers posted on the bulletin board, website, or handout
6.	Correct	Your answers
7.	Complete	All tests and required activities
8.	Read	Assigned readings (if any)
9.	Complete	Chapter performance objectives (competencies), if any
10.	Evaluate	Chapter performance and submit to your instructor
11.	Record	Your ending time and date: _____
12.	Move on	Begin next chapter as assigned

Student Name: _____

Chapter Completion Date: _____

Evaluate your classroom performance. Compare this evaluation with the one provided by your instructor.

Skill	Student Self-Evaluation			Instructor Evaluation		
	Good	**Average**	**Poor**	**Good**	**Average**	**Poor**
Attendance/punctuality						
Personal appearance						
Applies effort						
Is self-motivated						
Is courteous						
Has positive attitude						
Completes assignments in timely manner						
Works well with others						

Student's Initials: _____

Date: _____

Points Possible: _____

Points Awarded: _____

Chapter Grade: _____

Instructor's Initials: _____

Date: _____

18 Hospital Billing and the UB-04

As the title indicates, Unit V presents an alternate step, and the general trend of the material takes the student to a more challenging level. In this chapter, we left the physician's office and branched out into institutional healthcare—the hospital. As mentioned in the text, it would take an entire volume to include all of the information necessary to cover every aspect of hospital billing adequately. Just basic information is included to give students a "taste" of what this area of healthcare entails. If it piques the student's interest, he or she might want to explore opportunities for enrollment in a health information technology (HIT) or health information management (HIM) program.

The focus of Chapter 18 is on the hospital billing and coding process, which typically follows these steps: First, patients are registered. During the encounter, all medical care (and supplies) provided during their stay is documented in their medical record, which can be paper or electronic, along with the cost of each that is billable to a patient's account. At the end of the inpatient hospitalization or outpatient visit, charges are entered in the facility's patient accounting system. This information is then used to prepare insurance claims and patients' bills. Because the HIPAA-AS act has mandated that all Medicare claims be submitted electronically, with few exceptions, electronic claims submission is expanded in Chapter 18. Although the UB-04 is the universal paper form used for submitting hospital claims, the 837I electronic equivalent to the paper claim is also discussed.

The activities in this workbook chapter have been developed to supplement the material presented in Chapter 18 in the text in hopes of providing students with an opportunity for a better grasp of what is involved in hospital billing.

Because the federal government mandated that all payers and providers adopt the ICD-10 coding system by October 1, 2015, Chapter 18 includes diagnostic and procedural coding information and guidelines for only the ICD-10. ICD-10-CM is now used for reporting diagnoses in all health treatment facilities, both inpatient and outpatient, and ICD-10-PCS is used for reporting hospital inpatient procedures.

As mentioned in Chapter 18 of the textbook, it is strongly recommended that students check the Centers for Medicare and Medicaid Services (CMS) website periodically at http://cms.gov/icd10/ to keep abreast of changes and/or updates to the ICD-10 coding system.

(It is important to remember that CPT-4/HCPCS codes are still used for coding procedures and services in physicians' offices and outpatient facilities.)

WORKBOOK CHAPTER OBJECTIVES

After completing the workbook activities for Chapter 18, the student should be able to:
1. Define the terms used in the chapter.
2. Answer the review questions according to the evaluation criteria set by the instructor.
3. Use problem-solving skills (individually or in a group setting) to determine correct responses and outcomes in case studies and application exercises.
4. Identify the correct diagnostic codes from a series of case studies.
5. Engage in critical thinking techniques to solve case studies.
6. Use the Internet to locate information to understand given topics better.
7. Complete performance objectives according to the criteria determined by the instructor.
8. Perform the necessary steps for unbiased self-evaluation and understanding of material presented in the workbook.

DEFINING CHAPTER TERMS

Using the computer, students should type an accurate definition for each of the chapter terms listed. These definitions should be in the students' own words. When finished, students should compare their definitions with those listed in the glossary at the back of the textbook and correct any inaccuracies.

72-hour rule
accreditation
Accreditation Association for Ambulatory Health Care
  (AAAHC)

activities of daily living (ADLs)
acute care
acute care facility
acute condition

379

ambulatory payment classifications (APCs)
ambulatory surgery center (ASC)
benefit period
billing compliance
Blue Cross and Blue Shield member hospitals
case mix
charge description master (CDM)
clinic
coding compliance
cost sharing
covered entity
critical access hospital (CAH)
Defense Enrollment Eligibility Reporting System (DEERS)
diagnosis-related group (DRG)
electronic claims submission (ECS)
electronic medical record (EMR)
electronic remittance advice (ERA)
Emergency Medical Treatment and Labor Act (EMTLA)
emergent medical condition
exacerbation
form locators
for-profit hospitals
general hospital
governance
grouper software
health information management (HIM) system
home health agency
hospice
hospital information system (HIS)
hospital outpatient prospective payment system (HOPPS)
informed consent
integrated delivery system (IDS)
intermediate care facility

The Joint Commission
licensed independent practitioner
long-term care facility
medical ethics
Medicare Severity (MS) DRG system
Medicare Severity-Adjusted (DRG) system
multiaxial structure
National Committee for Quality Assurance (NCQA)
National Correct Coding Initiative (NCCI)
National Uniform Billing Committee (NUBC)
nonavailability statement (NAS)
outliers
outpatient prospective payment system (OPPS)
palliative care
pass-through
patient centric
Patient Protection and Affordable Care Act (PPACA)
per diems
present on admission (POA)
pricing transparency
principal diagnosis
prospective payment system (PPS)
quality improvement organizations (QIOs)
Registered Health Information Technician (RHIT)
respite care
secondary diagnosis
skilled nursing facility (SNF)
subacute care facility
subrogation
surrogate
swing bed
transaction set
UB-04
Utilization Review Accreditation Commission (URAC)
vertically integrated hospitals

ASSESSMENT

Multiple Choice

Directions: In the questions and statements presented, choose the response that **best** answers or completes the stem by circling the letter that precedes it.

1. The construction of today's modern hospital is regulated by:
   a. Federal and state laws
   b. State health department policies
   c. City ordinances
   d. All of the above

2. Today's hospitals mainly offer:
   a. Private and semiprivate rooms
   b. Four-bed room options
   c. Wards with up to 30 beds
   d. All of the above

3. Hospitals that provide all levels of care are referred to as:
   a. Megacomplexes
   b. Total care facilities
   c. Inpatient/outpatient centers
   d. Vertically integrated hospitals

4. A popular designation given to today's healthcare patients is:
   a. Users
   b. Clients
   c. Customers
   d. Consumers

5. A single building or campus, typically having a large number of beds, specialized facilities for various medical care types, and an emergency department, is called a:
   a. Clinic
   b. General hospital
   c. Preferred provider organization
   d. Health maintenance organization (HMO)

6. A medical facility smaller than a hospital is typically referred to as a(n):
   a. Clinic
   b. General hospital
   c. For-profit facility
   d. Outpatient facility

7. A healthcare facility that is equipped and staffed to respond immediately to critical situations and provide continuous care to patients with "worst-case" scenarios is a(n):
   a. Acute care facility
   b. Extended care facility
   c. Designated trauma center
   d. Community emergency center

8. A facility designed for patients who have had acute events as a result of an illness, injury, or exacerbation of a disease process is a(n):
   a. Acute care hospital
   b. Subacute care facility
   c. Skilled nursing facility (SNF)
   d. Long-term care facility

9. The type of facility in which patients have the advantage of constant access to nursing care as they move toward recovery and return to their home is a(n):
   a. Acute care hospital
   b. Subacute care facility
   c. Skilled nursing facility
   d. Long-term care facility

10. A facility that is licensed or approved under state or local law that is primarily engaged in providing experienced nursing care and related services is a(n):
    a. Acute care hospital
    b. Subacute care facility
    c. Skilled nursing facility
    d. Long-term care facility

11. Temporary relief for an individual providing healthcare to a family member is commonly called:
    a. Hospice
    b. Respite care
    c. Interval relief
    d. Adult daycare

12. The type of care facility provided for adults who are chronically ill or disabled and are no longer able to manage in independent living situations is referred to as:
    a. Hospice
    b. Respite care
    c. Home healthcare
    d. Long-term care

13. The acronym for the federal act that ensures public access to emergency services regardless of ability to pay is:
    a. NUBC
    b. COBRA
    c. EMTLA
    d. AAAHC

14. The voluntary process through which an organization is able to measure the quality of its services and performance against nationally recognized standards is called:
    a. Accreditation
    b. Certification
    c. Credentialing
    d. Validation

15. The independent, nonprofit organization that performs quality-oriented accreditation reviews on HMOs and similar types of managed care plans is:
    a. NCQA
    b. NUBC
    c. AAAHC
    d. AOA/COCA

16. The acronym for the organization formed in 1979 to assist ambulatory healthcare organizations improve the quality of care provided to patients is the:
    a. NCQA
    b. URAC
    c. AAAHC
    d. AOA/COCA

17. The independent, nonprofit organization that promotes continuous improvement in the quality and efficiency of healthcare delivery through the establishment of standards, education, and communication is the:
    a. NCQA
    b. URAC
    c. AAAHC
    d. NUBC

18. How any organization is run, in its simplest definition, is referred to as:
    a. Accreditation
    b. Governance
    c. Compliance
    d. Ethics

19. Moral principles that govern the practice of medicine by physicians and other healthcare practitioners are commonly referred to as medical:
    a. Ethics
    b. Etiquette
    c. Protocol
    d. Courtesy

20. Medicare hospital claims are processed by contracted nongovernment organizations or agencies that are commonly referred to as:
    a. Medicare administrative contractors (MACs)
    b. Fiscal intermediaries
    c. Medicare carriers
    d. All of the above

21. Medicare Part A pays toward:
    a. Hospital charges
    b. Physician charges
    c. Long-term healthcare
    d. All of the above

22. Medicare's acute care payment system is called the:
    a. Prospective payment system (PPS)
    b. Cost-sharing system
    c. Per-diem structure
    d. DEERS

23. The abbreviation for an inpatient hospital coding system that groups related diagnoses and their associated medical/surgical treatment is referred to as:
    a. APCs
    b. DRGs
    c. ASCs
    d. CMS

24. Many Medicaid programs adjust payments to reflect such things as patient demographics, diagnostic and treatment information, and total charges, which is referred to as:
    a. A per-diem structure
    b. A swing-bed configuration
    c. A case mix
    d. Cost sharing

25. If a military treatment facility is unavailable, TRICARE patients, in many cases, must obtain a:
    a. Military waiver
    b. Preauthorization statement
    c. Statement of authenticity
    d. Nonavailability statement (NAS)

26. Most third-party payers' reimbursement rates are subject to change:
    a. Quarterly
    b. Semiannually
    c. Annually
    d. Biannually

27. Most hospitals in the United States contract with Blue Cross and Blue Shield and are referred to as:
    a. Member hospitals
    b. Cost outliers
    c. Swing-bed hospitals
    d. Acute care hospitals

28. The designated spaces on the UB-04 are called:
    a. Blocks
    b. Data elements
    c. Form locators
    d. Code indicators

29. The universal claim form for current use in inpatient hospital claims is the:
    a. CMS-1500
    b. UB-82
    c. UB-92
    d. UB-04

30. The process by which a patient can participate in choices about his or her healthcare is commonly referred to as:
    a. Informed consent
    b. Preauthorization
    c. Governance
    d. Registration

31. An individual who has the legal authority to speak on a patient's behalf is called a:
    a. Volunteer
    b. Fiscal intermediary
    c. Covered entity
    d. Surrogate

32. The manual currently used for inpatient diagnostic coding is the:
    a. CPT-4
    b. HCPCS
    c. ICD-10-CM
    d. ICD-10-PCS

33. The manual that is now used for inpatient procedural coding is the:
    a. CPT-4
    b. HCPCS
    c. ICD-10-CM
    d. ICD-10-PCS

34. Coders must distinguish key elements or words in the patient's hospital health record that identify the:
    a. Prime diagnosis
    b. Primary diagnosis
    c. Principal diagnosis
    d. Chief diagnosis

35. The electronic equivalent to the UB-04 paper claim form is called the:
    a. 837I
    b. CMS-1500
    c. CMS-1450
    d. HCFA-1500

36. The overall data stream of the electronic UB-04 file is known as a(n):
    a. Segment
    b. 997 file
    c. Transaction set
    d. Element layout

37. The total number of codes in the ICD-10-PCS system is approximately:
    a. 4800
    b. 12,500
    c. 52,000
    d. 87,000

38. "That condition established after study to be chiefly responsible for occasioning the admission of the patient to the hospital for care" defines the:
    a. Primary diagnosis
    b. Principal diagnosis
    c. Discharge diagnosis
    d. First-listed diagnosis

39. The payment system implemented in 2000 and used by the Centers for Medicare and Medicaid Services (CMS) to reimburse for hospital outpatient services is called the:
    a. Ambulatory payment classification system
    b. Hospital outpatient prospective payment system
    c. Registered health payment system
    d. Vertically integrated payment system

40. OPPS (or HOPPS) allows for temporary payment of new technologies, drugs, devices, and biologics for which no ambulatory payment classification (APC) payment rate is available, which is called:
    a. Rubrics
    b. Outliers
    c. Pass-throughs
    d. Crosswalks

41. A computer application interface commonly used in hospitals to send and retrieve data for grouping, editing, and reimbursement outcomes is called the:
    a. Case mix
    b. Pass-through
    c. Charge description master
    d. Grouper software system

42. Identify the program implemented by CMS in 1996 to control improper coding that leads to inappropriate increased payment for healthcare services.
    a. National Correct Coding Initiative
    b. Outpatient Code Editor
    c. MS-DRG grouper
    d. Charge description master

43. Inpatient acute care hospitals that that are paid under the DRG payment system are required to report a specific indicator for every diagnosis on inpatient acute care hospital claims called:
    a. Present on admission (POA)
    b. The 72-hour rule
    c. Charge description master
    d. Form locator

44. Identify the congressional act that stipulates that hospitals cannot charge uninsured patients more for the same treatment than what those with health insurance are billed.
    a. Emergency Medical Treatment and Labor Act
    b. The Affordable Care Act
    c. Care Improvement Initiative
    d. Billing Compliance Act

45. The process of verifying that the diagnoses and procedure codes used on claims comply with all current coding guidelines and rules is called:
    a. Governance
    b. Accreditation
    c. Coding compliance
    d. Pricing transparency

46. According to the textbook, the implementation date for the ICD-10 coding system is:
    a. June 1, 2015
    b. September 30, 2015
    c. October 1, 2015
    d. October 1, 2016

47. ICD-10-PCS codes are composed of _____ characters:
    a. 3
    b. 7
    c. 5 to 8
    d. 10

48. Regardless of the coding system used, diagnosis codes must be supported by:
    a. Medical documentation
    b. At least one modifier
    c. Two physicians
    d. The hospital grouper software

385

49. Which of these statements *is* true about the characters that make up ICD-10-PCS codes?
    a. Each character can be alphabetical (not case-sensitive) or numeric.
    b. Only 0 through 9 are valid numerical values.
    c. Letters O and I are not valid values.
    d. All of the above

50. Identify the number of significant procedures other than the principal procedure that may be reported on the UB-04 claim form.
    a. 5
    b. 7
    c. 10
    d. 15

True/False

Directions: Place a "T" in the blank preceding the numbered statement if it is true; place an "F" if it is false.

_____ 1. Clinics generally provide outpatient services only.

_____ 2. Ambulatory surgery centers (ASCs) are facilities at which surgeries are performed that do not require hospital admission.

_____ 3. An ASC treats patients who already have seen a healthcare provider and patients who have not.

_____ 4. Because ASC patients are not formally admitted to the hospital, ASCs are among the more loosely regulated healthcare facilities.

_____ 5. A subacute care facility provides a level of maintenance care at which there is no urgent or life-threatening condition that requires medical treatment.

_____ 6. A nursing home can qualify as an SNF.

_____ 7. Licensed hospitals must provide care within the minimum health and safety standards established by state rules and regulations.

_____ 8. All hospitals *must* seek accreditation by nationally recognized accrediting agencies.

_____ 9. Critical Access Hospitals are certified under a different set of Medicare Conditions of Participation (CoP) that are more flexible than those of acute care hospitals.

_____ 10. Privacy and confidentiality issues are not as important in hospitals compared with physicians' offices.

_____ 11. The HIPAA Privacy Rule is not intended to prohibit providers from talking to other providers and to their patients.

_____ 12. Each state's Medicaid program determines the method it uses to pay for hospital inpatient services.

_____ 13. An NAS is necessary for all outpatient procedures.

_____ 14. Inpatient TRICARE payments are calculated using the same PPS as Medicare.

_____ 15. Most third-party payers require preauthorization for inpatient hospitalization and some outpatient procedures and diagnostic testing.

_____ 16. Most private insurers negotiate contracts with facilities regarding hospital inpatient payment methods on a month-to-month basis.

_____ 17. The hospital billing process begins when the patient is discharged from the facility.

_____ 18. The "principal diagnosis" is defined as the condition determined after study to be chiefly responsible for the patient's admission to the hospital.

_____ 19. In ICD-10 coding, some body system categories include codes for nonspecific conditions, which should be ignored.

_____ 20. Transaction Standard Version 5010 accommodates the proposed new ICD-10 code sets.

_____ 21. CPT-4/HCPCS codes are used only in physicians' offices and outpatient clinics.

386

_____ 22. The 72-hour rule states that all diagnostic services provided for Medicare patients within 72 hours of the hospital admission must be billed separately from inpatient charges.

_____ 23. APC is the grouping system that the CMS developed for facility reimbursement of hospital outpatient services.

_____ 24. The primary goal of the Affordable Care Act is to provide free healthcare to all American citizens.

_____ 25. Hospitals submitting claims electronically can use any format available.

_____ 26. The accrediting body for many allied health education programs is CAAHEP.

_____ 27. The law requires electronic processing of all documents between the healthcare provider and the insurance carrier, without exception.

_____ 28. Secondary conditions are either comorbidities or complications, frequently referred to as "*CCs.*"

_____ 29. Like ICD-10-CM codes, ICD-10-PCS codes contain seven characters, which can be numbers or letters and are based on the type of procedure performed, the approach, the body part, and other characteristics.

_____ 30. Each character in the structure of an ICD-10-PCS code must be alphabetic.

Short Answer

Note: If space provided is not adequate, use a separate piece of blank paper.

1. Discuss the function of today's modern hospital.

_____

_____

_____

2. List and discuss emerging issues in healthcare.

_____

_____

_____

3. Discuss and evaluate the accreditation process for assessment and certification of hospitals and other institutional healthcare facilities.

_____

_____

_____

4. Explain EMTLA and what function it serves.

_____

_____

5. Define a "covered entity" and list the three types of organizations that fall under this classification.

_____

_____

_____

6. List the basic principles of medical ethics.

_____

_____

_____

7. Informed consent is the process by which a fully informed patient can participate in choices about his or her health-care and typically includes a discussion of certain elements. List these elements.

_____

_____

_____

_____

8. Name the major hospital payers and tell how a health insurance professional can acquire the most recent guidelines for submitting claims.

_____

_____

_____

9. Explain the concept of "present on admission" and how it affects billing.

_____

_____

_____

10. List the four methods by which Blue Cross and Blue Shield's fees for facility services are established.

_____

_____

_____

_____

11. Discuss the basic function of the National Uniform Billing Committee.

_____

_____

_____

12. Describe a charge description master (CDM).

_____

_____

_____

13. List five advantages of ECS.

_____

_____

_____

_____

14. If more than one diagnosis meets the criteria for principal diagnosis, what should the coder do?

_____

_____

15. What is the purpose of the National Correct Coding Initiative?

_____

_____

16. List and explain the two important rules adopted by the HHS in 2009.

_____

17. How does the APC system work?

_____

_____

18. Hospital staff members should inform patients of their rights and responsibilities. Name four responsibilities that patients are obligated to perform.

_____

_____

_____

_____

19. Name six exceptions to the HIPAA electronic claims submission requirement.

_____

_____

_____

_____

_____

_____

20. List five functions that a typical HIM computerized system can handle.

_____

_____

_____

_____

_____

21. ICD-10-PCS codes have a "multiaxial" structure. Explain what this means.

_____

_____

22. The Hospital Value-Based Purchasing (VBP) program is a CMS initiative established by the Affordable Care Act (ACA) of 2010. What does it do?

_____

_____

23. What is the main intent of the Patient Protection and Affordable Care Act (PPACA)?

_____

_____

24. Both the 8371 and the UB-04 require the use of codes maintained by the NUBC. Provide four examples of these codes.

_____

_____

_____

_____

CRITICAL THINKING ACTIVITIES

A. Brittany Weston was asked by a former coworker how hospital billing differs from that performed in the small, two-physician office they previously had worked in together. Assume you are Brittany. Create a dialogue or a critical thinking paragraph of how you might explain these differences.

B. The text discusses two basic payment systems: (1) Medicare's PPS, using diagnosis-related groups for inpatient hospitalization, and (2) the outpatient prospective payment system (OPPS), using APCs. Compare and contrast these two payment systems.

390

C. Experts say that two of the most common hospital billing problems are (1) receiving incorrect insurance information; and (2) failing to acquire the necessary preauthorization or precertification. How might these problems be avoided or minimized?

D. How might the "emerging issues" discussed in Chapter 18 affect today's hospitals?

PROJECTS/DISCUSSION TOPICS

A. Create a chart or a bulletin board display showing the various types of healthcare facilities and the nature of care provided in each.

B. Your group will be assigned a specific healthcare profession common to today's modern hospitals such as a medical records technician, a registered health information technician, a hospital coding specialist, or a hospital claims specialist. Use the Internet or other available reference sources to find out what the scope of practice is, what courses and training you would need, the necessary certification or credentialing, and any other information that would be helpful to get started and succeed on this career path.

C. Discuss the process of accreditation and why it is important for hospitals to be accredited.

D. Generate a one-page patient handout for inpatients outlining Broadmoor Medical Center's billing policies. You may use the Internet to locate sample policies by existing facilities, if desired, or visit a local hospital.

E. Discuss the difference between "primary" (now referred to as the "first-listed" diagnosis) and "principal" diagnoses.

F. Locate a comprehensive health insurance policy (from the Internet, from a local insurance company such as Blue Cross and Blue Shield, or from your own policy), and outline its hospital inpatient coverage.

G. Examine the two rules—X12 Version 5010 and ICD-10-CM—and actively participate in a discussion of how they will affect hospital coding.

CASE STUDIES

A. Maria Franklin saw Dr. Lucero at Broadmoor Medical Clinic on 10/03/20XX for complaints of nausea, vomiting, and diarrhea. Dr. Lucero documented the condition in Ms. Franklin's health record as *probable gastroenteritis*. We learned in Chapter 12, however, that in this scenario, the health insurance professional would code the nausea, vomiting, and diarrhea but *not* the gastroenteritis because it is described as *probable* and is not yet confirmed. The diagnosis on the CMS-1500 form would be the symptoms rather than probable gastroenteritis. Dr. Lucero subsequently admits Maria to the hospital. For inpatient facility billing, coding of signs or symptoms (especially as the principal diagnosis) is not a routine practice because many payers would not pay for or would question inpatient admissions coded with signs and symptoms only. What would the health insurance professional use as the principal diagnosis on the UB-04? Discuss.

B. Hillas Archer, who is having an outpatient hernia repair at Broadmoor Medical Center, also has diabetes and coronary artery disease. What is the principal diagnosis? Should Mr. Archer's diabetes and coronary artery disease also be coded on the UB-04? Discuss.

C. Fig. 18.1 is a sample statement from Community General Hospital. There are 12 numbered areas on the form. John Doe's father is in your office asking for an explanation of the bill. Explain the information in each of these 12 areas to him.

1. _____
2. _____
3. _____
4. _____
5. _____
6. _____
7. _____
8. _____
9. _____
10. _____
11. _____
12. _____

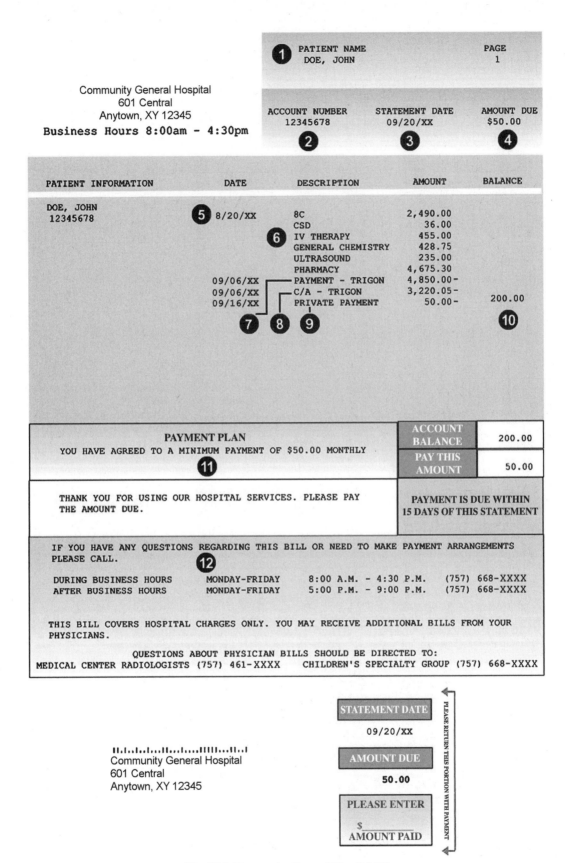

Fig. 18.1 Community General Hospital bill.

D. In the sample statement shown in Fig. 18.2, explain each of the 16 entries to an inquiring patient. (**Suggestion:** Use a classmate to play the role of an "inquiring patient.")

Sample of Physician Bill

PATIENT NAME
STATEMENT SAMPLE

① ACCOUNT NO.
43056123

BILLING DATE
12/18/XX

PATIENT/GUARANTOR

STATEMENT SAMPLE
539 MAIN LN
OAKLEY, CA 94561

② PLEASE
PAY THIS ➤ 36.00
AMOUNT

③ AMOUNT PAID _____

PLEASE REFER TO THE BACK OF THIS PAGE FOR OTHER IMPORTANT INFORMATION
PLEASE RETURN TOP PORTION ONLY

Ⅴ DETACH HERE   DETACH HERE Ⅴ

DATE OF SERVICE	INVOICE NUMBER	DEPT> PHYSICIAN: REFERRING MD SERVICE / BILLING ACTIVITY	REF#	AMOUNT	PATIENT BALANCE
④	**⑤**	**⑥** **⑦** **⑧**	**⑩**	**⑫**	**⑬**
	8000290	NEUROLOGICAL SURGERY>BERGER:CAMPA			
11/15/XX	**⑨**	OUTPATIENT-ESTABLISHED-LEVEL 4	99214	211.00	
	⑪	INSURANCE PAYMENT 12/13/XX		150.00CR	
		CONTRACTUAL ADJUSTMENT AMT		25.00CR	
		...Patient Responsibility			36.00

⑭ --TOTALS--   Total Charges: 211.00

Ins. Paid: 150.00 Discnt: 25.00

Patient Payment: 0.00

	CURRENT	> 30 DAYS	> 60 DAYS	> 90 DAYS	> 120 DAYS
Patient Responsibility **⑮**	36.00	0.00	0.00	0.00	0.00

DATE	PATIENT NAME	ACCOUNT NUMBER
12/18/XX	STATEMENT SAMPLE	43056123

The amount shown in the "PLEASE PAY THIS AMOUNT" box is due and should be PAID IMMEDIATELY.
If you would like to speak with a Customer Service Representative, please contact our Customer Service Center at (415) 353-XXXX
Business hours are 9:00 a.m. to 4:00 p.m. Monday-Friday.

⑯ IMPORTANT MESSAGES REGARDING YOUR ACCOUNT

Fig. 18.2 Sample physician bill.

ENRICHMENT ACTIVITIES

You are not expected to be able to code inpatient hospital procedures at this point; however, these resources may be helpful in providing a basic understanding of ICD-10 procedure coding system:

A. Explore the contents of this website, which provides extensive information on ICD-10-PCS coding: https://www.cms.gov/Medicare/Coding/ICD10/Downloads/2016-Official-ICD-10-PCS-Coding-Guidelines.pdf.

B. Download and study the ICD-10-PCS coding guidelines from https://www.cms.gov/Medicare/Coding/ICD10/Downloads/2017-Official-ICD-10-PCS-Coding-Guidelines.pdf.

C. Download the PowerPoint presentation using this URL: http://www.cms.gov/Medicare/Coding/ICD10/Downloads/ICD-10OverviewPowerPoint.pdf.

Note: If any of the listed URLs are no longer available, use applicable search words to locate information regarding ICD-10-PCS guidelines and PowerPoint presentations.

INTERNET EXPLORATION

A. The National Committee on Vital and Health Statistics (NCVHS) has developed a set of data elements with standardized definitions that can be used to collect and produce standardized data for inpatient and outpatient hospitalization. Visit the NCVHS website for more information on the NCVHS Core Health Data Elements Report: http://www.ncvhs.hhs.gov/ncvhsr1.htm.

B. For informative articles on hospital billing, go to the CMS website at http://www.cms.gov and type "hospital billing" or "hospital claims" in the search box. Peruse this list of articles and choose one that interests you. Prepare a brief oral presentation or written report on your article of choice.

C. Log on to the American Health Information Management Association (AHIMA) website at http://www.ahima.org and click on "Schools/Jobs" or "Professional Development" to learn more about career opportunities in health information technology and health information management.

Chapter 18 has three Performance Objectives. You will follow a patient's complete hospital experience from admission to discharge and billing. To complete these objectives satisfactorily, use the health records of patient Julius R. Flowers and the blank forms presented in Figs. 18.3 through 18.8. After you have completed each Performance Objective, remove the scoring sheet from the workbook and attach your completed exercise to it for submission.

Special Notes

Broadmoor Medical Center is a participating provider for Medicare and Blue Cross and Blue Shield.

- All patients have a current release of information on file.
- All claims are assigned.
- Dr. Robert L. Jones is the operating surgeon.

Provider Block	
Broadmoor Medical Clinic	Clinic EIN #42-1898989
4353 Pine Ridge Drive	Dr. Robert L. Jones NPI 1234567890
Milton, XY 12345-0001	Dr. Marilou Lucero NPI #2907511822
Clinic NPI X100XX1000	Group #GRW0000
Telephone: 555-656-7890	Date claims 1 day after hospital discharge
Fax: 555-656-7899	

Performance Objective 18.1: Completing a Preadmission Form

Conditions: Student will complete a preadmission form (Fig. 18.3) using the information listed on the patient information sheet (Fig. 18.4).

Supplies/Equipment: Pen or computer, patient record, and preadmission information form

Time Allowed: 30 minutes

Accuracy Needed to Pass: 90%

Procedural Steps	Points Earned	Comments
Evaluator: Note time began: _____		
1. Carefully read and study the patient information sheet for Mr. Flowers. (0)		
2. Complete all required information on the preadmission form. (40)		
3. Proofread the form for accuracy, legibility, and completeness. (10)		
Optional: May deduct points for taking more time than allowed.		

Total Points = 50

Student's Score: _____

Evaluator: _____

Comments: _____

_____

_____

_____

_____

Broadmoor Medical Center
4353 Pine Ridge Drive
Milton, XY 12345-0000

Everything for life℠

PRE-ADMISSION INFORMATION FORM

Phone: 555-656-XXXX Fax: 555-656-XXXX

SURGERY ☐ Yes ☐ No   ACCIDENT ☐ Yes ☐ No   PREGNANCY ☐ Yes ☐ No   OTHER_____

DATE OF ADMISSION OR DUE DATE_____ PRIMARY CARE PHYSICIAN / PHYSICIAN NAME_____

LAST NAME_____ FIRST NAME_____ MIDDLE INITIAL_____

DATE OF BIRTH_____ MAIDEN NAME_____ PRIMARY LANGUAGE_____ SEX M / F

ADDRESS_____ CITY_____ STATE_____ ZIP_____

PHONE_____ RELIGION_____ HOUSE OF WORSHIP_____

MARITAL STATUS_____ SOCIAL SECURITY #_____ OCCUPATION_____

☐ I am currently unemployed

EMPLOYER'S NAME_____ EMPLOYER'S ADDRESS_____

CITY_____ STATE_____ ZIP_____ PHONE_____

PATIENT'S RACE ☐ Hispanic   ☐ Non Hispanic   ☐ Unknown

PATIENT'S ETHNICITY ☐ White ☐ Black ☐ Native American ☐ Asia / India / Pacific Isles ☐ Other

NEWBORN'S RACE (if applicable) ☐ Hispanic ☐ Non Hispanic ☐ Unknown

NEWBORN'S ETHNICITY (if applicable) ☐ White ☐ Black ☐ Native American ☐ Asia / India / Pacific Isles ☐ Other

EMERGENCY CONTACT / NEXT OF KIN

LAST NAME_____ FIRST NAME_____ MIDDLE INITIAL_____

ADDRESS_____ CITY_____ STATE_____ ZIP_____

HOME PHONE_____ WORK PHONE_____ RELATIONSHIP_____

PATIENT'S INSURANCE INFORMATION

☐ PPO ☐ HMO ☐ EPO ☐ POS ☐ Medicare ☐ MediCal ☐ Other ☐ I am currently uninsured

INSURANCE COMPANY NAME_____

ADDRESS_____ CITY_____ STATE_____ ZIP_____

PHONE_____ GROUP #_____ POLICY #_____

HMO MEMBER #_____ MEDICAL GROUP NAME_____

PRIMARY CARE PHYSICIAN OR PHYSICIAN NAME_____

MEDICARE #_____ MEDICAL CIN #_____

EFFECTIVE DATES_____ SUBSCRIBER'S DATE OF BIRTH_____

SPOUSE'S INFORMATION (if applicable)

LAST NAME_____ FIRST NAME_____ MIDDLE INITIAL_____ PHONE_____

DATE OF BIRTH_____ SOCIAL SECURITY #_____

EMPLOYER_____ OCCUPATION_____

EMPLOYER ADDRESS_____ CITY_____ STATE_____ ZIP_____

SPOUSE'S INSURANCE INFORMATION (if applicable)

☐ PPO ☐ HMO ☐ EPO ☐ POS ☐ Medicare ☐ MediCal ☐ Other ☐ My spouse is currently uninsured

INSURANCE COMPANY NAME_____

ADDRESS_____ CITY_____ STATE_____ ZIP_____

PHONE_____ GROUP #_____ POLICY #_____

HMO MEMBER #_____ MEDICAL GROUP NAME_____

PRIMARY CARE PHYSICIAN OR PHYSICIAN NAME_____

MEDICARE #_____ MEDICAL CIN #_____

EFFECTIVE DATES_____ SUBSCRIBER'S DATE OF BIRTH_____

UPON ARRIVAL IN ADMITTING, PLEASE HAVE YOUR VALID PHOTO ID AND INSURANCE CARD READY. PATIENT'S DEDUCTIBLE AND EST. CO-PAY ARE REQUESTED AT TIME OF ADMISSION. ALL MAJOR CREDIT CARDS ACCEPTED.

Fig. 18.3 Preadmission information form.

PATIENT INFORMATION SHEET

Today's date: __10/12/20XX__

HEAD OF HOUSEHOLD

Head of household: __JULIUS R. FLOWERS__

Occupation: __RETIRED FARMER__

Social Security # __098-87-6655__

Employer's name __N/A__

Sex: __M__   Date of birth __03/29/1933__

Employer's address __N/A__

Address: __25387 GLENBROOK ROAD__

Employer's City, St: __N/A__   Zip ____

City, St: __MILTON, XY__   Zip __12345__

Employer's phone # __N/A__

Home phone # __555-656-0110__

PATIENT INFORMATION

Patient's legal name __JULIUS R. FLOWERS__   Nickname __JUBE__   Relationship to head of household __SAME__

Date of birth __03/28/1933__   Age ____   Sex __M__   Marital Status __MARRIED__

Employer name __N/A__   Social Security # __098-87-6655__

Employer address __N/A__   Employer phone # __N/A__

City, St: __N/A__   Zip ____   Workers' Compensation Carrier (If applicable) __N/A__

Referring Physician __TEREZ__   Allergies __SULFA DRUGS__

EMERGENCY INFORMATION

Other contact not living with you: __BETHANY PORTER__   Home phone# __555-656-4433__   Work phone# __555-659-8818__

Address __8614 PARKWAY__   City __MILTON__   St __XY__   Zip __12345__

Patient relationship to other contact __DAUGHTER__   If patient is a child, parent name ____

INSURANCE INFORMATION

Primary insurance __MEDICARE__   Subscriber ____

ID # __098876655A__   Relationship to subscriber __SELF__

Secondary insurance: __BCBS SENIOR BLUE (MEDICARE SUPPL)__   Subscriber __JULIUS R. FLOWERS__

ID # __006SPF4491__   Relationship to subscriber __SELF__

OTHER FAMILY MEMBERS:

Name __BEVERLY T. FLOWERS (WIFE; RETIRED TEACHER)__   SAME ADDRESS & PHONE NO.   Date of birth: __05/20/1939__

Name ____   Date of birth: ____

Name ____   Date of birth: ____

Name ____   Date of birth: ____

I understand that it is my responsibility that any incurred charges are paid.

To the extent necessary to determine liability for payment to obtain reimbursement, process claim forms, I authorize the release of any medical information necessary to process claims.

I hereby assign all medical and/or surgical benefits, to include major medical benefits to which I am entitled, including Medicare, private insurance, and other health plans to Broadmoor Medical Center.

This assignment will remain in effect until revoked by me in writing; a photocopy of this assignment is to be considered as valid as an original. I hereby authorize said assignee to release all information necessary to secure the payment.

Signed __Julius R. Flowers__   Date __10/12/20XX__

If patient is a minor, parent or guardian signature.

Fig. 18.4 Patient information sheet.

Performance Objective 18.2: Completing a UB-04 Claim Form

Conditions: Student will complete the required sections of a UB-04 claim form (Fig. 18.5) using the information listed in the patient record for Julius Flowers (Fig. 18.6), patient information sheet (see Fig. 18.4), and hospital billing summary (see Fig. 18.8).

Supplies/Equipment: Pen or computer, patient record, and UB-04 claim form

Time Allowed: 45 minutes

Accuracy Needed to Pass: 90%

Procedural Steps	Points Earned	Comments
Evaluator: Note time began: _____		
1. Carefully read and study the documents from Mr. Flowers' record. (0)		
2. Using the information in the patient record, complete the required sections on the UB-04 form. (60)		
3. Proofread the form for accuracy, legibility, and completeness. (10)		
Optional: May deduct points for taking more time than allowed.		

Note: Student must complete these form locaters: **1, 3b, 5, 6, 8b, 9a-d, 10, 11, 12, 38, 42, 43, 44, 46, 47, 50, 58, 60, 63, 69.**

Total Points = 70

Student's Score: _____

Evaluator: _____

Comments: _____

_____

_____

_____

_____

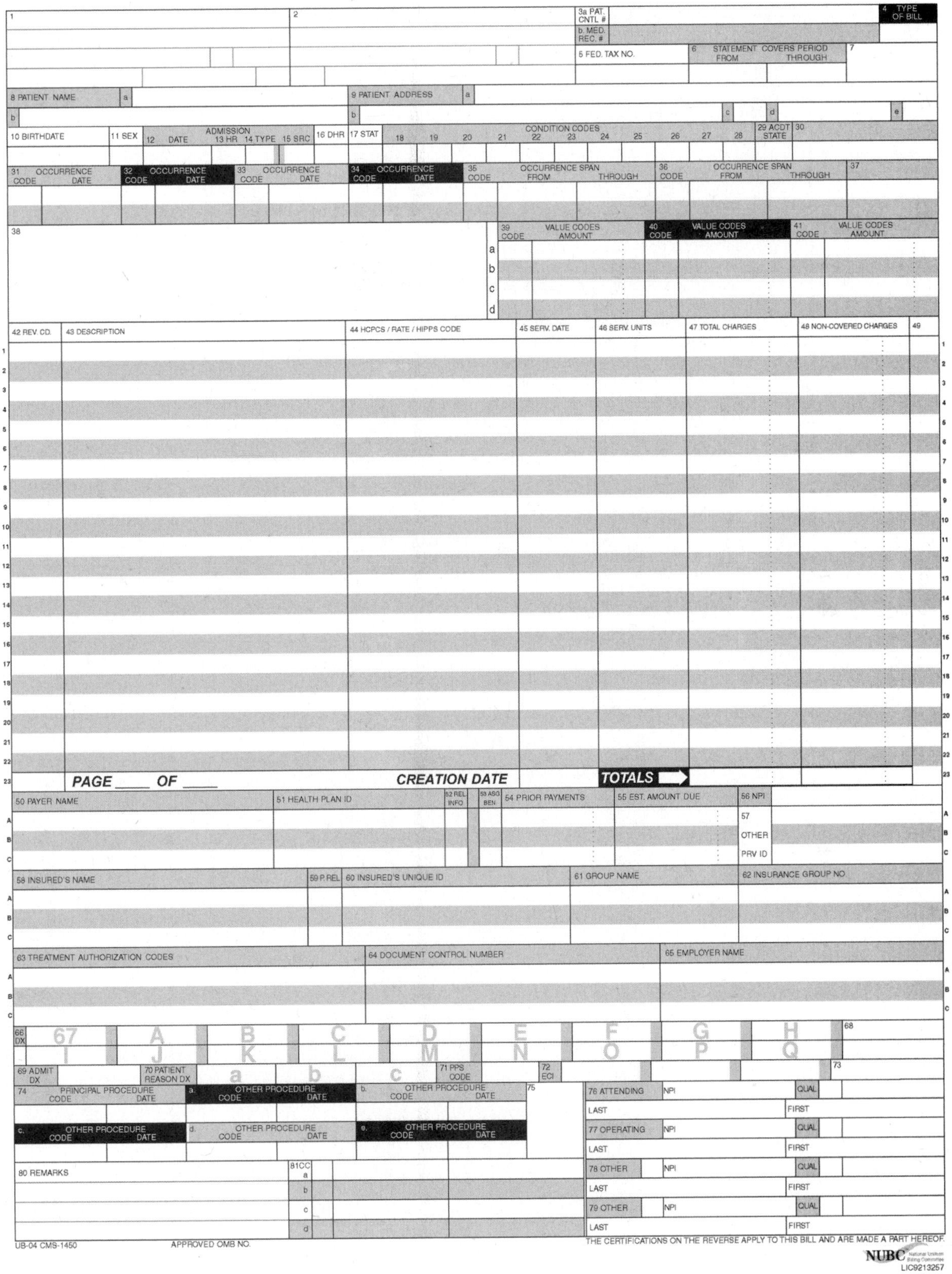
1
2
3a PAT. CNTL #
b. MED. REC. #
4 TYPE OF BILL
5 FED. TAX NO.
6 STATEMENT COVERS PERIOD FROM THROUGH
7
8 PATIENT NAME a b
9 PATIENT ADDRESS a b c d e
10 BIRTHDATE
11 SEX
ADMISSION 12 DATE 13 HR 14 TYPE 15 SRC
16 DHR
17 STAT
CONDITION CODES 18 19 20 21 22 23 24 25 26 27 28
29 ACDT STATE
30
31 OCCURRENCE CODE DATE
32 OCCURRENCE CODE DATE
33 OCCURRENCE CODE DATE
34 OCCURRENCE CODE DATE
35 CODE OCCURRENCE SPAN FROM THROUGH
36 CODE OCCURRENCE SPAN FROM THROUGH
37
38
39 VALUE CODES CODE AMOUNT
40 VALUE CODES CODE AMOUNT
41 VALUE CODES CODE AMOUNT
a b c d
42 REV. CD.
43 DESCRIPTION
44 HCPCS / RATE / HIPPS CODE
45 SERV. DATE
46 SERV. UNITS
47 TOTAL CHARGES
48 NON-COVERED CHARGES
49
1 2 3 4 5 6 7 8 9 10 11 12 13 14 15 16 17 18 19 20 21 22 23
PAGE ____ OF ____
CREATION DATE
TOTALS
50 PAYER NAME
51 HEALTH PLAN ID
52 REL INFO
53 ASG BEN
54 PRIOR PAYMENTS
55 EST. AMOUNT DUE
56 NPI
57 OTHER PRV ID
A B C
58 INSURED'S NAME
59 P. REL
60 INSURED'S UNIQUE ID
61 GROUP NAME
62 INSURANCE GROUP NO.
A B C
63 TREATMENT AUTHORIZATION CODES
64 DOCUMENT CONTROL NUMBER
65 EMPLOYER NAME
A B C
66 DX
67 A B C D E F G H
I J K L M N O P Q
68
69 ADMIT DX
70 PATIENT REASON DX a b c
71 PPS CODE
72 ECI
73
74 PRINCIPAL PROCEDURE CODE DATE
a. OTHER PROCEDURE CODE DATE
b. OTHER PROCEDURE CODE DATE
75
76 ATTENDING NPI QUAL LAST FIRST
c. OTHER PROCEDURE CODE DATE
d. OTHER PROCEDURE CODE DATE
e. OTHER PROCEDURE CODE DATE
77 OPERATING NPI QUAL LAST FIRST
80 REMARKS
81CC a b c d
78 OTHER NPI QUAL LAST FIRST
79 OTHER NPI QUAL LAST FIRST
UB-04 CMS-1450
APPROVED OMB NO.
THE CERTIFICATIONS ON THE REVERSE APPLY TO THIS BILL AND ARE MADE A PART HEREOF.
NUBC National Uniform Billing Committee
LIC9213257

Fig. 18.5 Blank UB-04 claim form.

PATIENT ER RECORD

PATIENT NAME: Julius R. Flowers   DOB: 03/28/1933
DATE: 10/12/20XX   RECORD NO: 2910388
PRIMARY CARE PHYSICIAN: R.L. Jones, MD

S: Mr. Flowers is a 74-year-old Native American, English-speaking male who was
admitted to Broadmoor Medical Center through the Emergency Department at
7:45 a.m. today after sustaining a head injury from a fall down the porch steps at
his home, hitting the right side of his head. Patient's wife reported that the patient
suffered a brief loss of consciousness—but "only a minute or so." After the fall,
he seemed confused but was able to walk with some help. The ambulance was
called, and he was transported to Broadmoor Medical Center.

O: Upon admission to the Emergency Department, Mr. Flowers exhibited weakness
and tingling to the left upper extremity, mild headache, and confusion. There was
some bruising and minor bleeding above his right ear. Denied double vision and
nausea. Reflexes were diminished on the left; balance and gait were unsteady.
Patient's ability to answer questions was somewhat compromised, as he was
somewhat incoherent. His wife answered most of the questions regarding the
details of the accident. B/P: 112/68; Pulse: 66. PERRLA. Patient is currently on
Captopril, 25 mg., bid. **He is allergic to all SULFA DRUGS.** A CT scan was
ordered.

A: Subdural hematoma

P: Surgical evacuation of subdural hematoma

(s)   Emelio R. Terez, MD
Emergency Room Physician

ICD-10 code: I62.01

Fig. 18.6 Patient record (Flowers).

Performance Objective 18.3: Complete a Billing Form

Conditions: Student will complete a hospital billing form (statement) (Fig. 18.7) using the information listed on the hospital billing summary (Fig. 18.8). Assume that Medicare paid all but the first $1184 (2013 deductible), which his Medigap policy paid. List only the total charges using the date of discharge, the payments, and the balance due, if any. Statement date should be the day after the last payment was received.

Supplies/Equipment: Pen or computer, patient record, and preadmission information form

Time Allowed: 30 minutes

Accuracy Needed to Pass: 90%

Procedural Steps	Points Earned	Comments
Evaluator: Note time began: _____		
1. Carefully read and study information and forms associated with this Performance Objective.		
2. Enter all pertinent information on the form provided in Fig. 18.7. (10)		
3. Calculate the total charges for patient's hospitalization. (5)		
4. Medicare payment date: 11/12/XX (5)		
5. Medigap payment date: 12/02/XX (5)		
6. Current balance, if any (5)		
7. Proofread the form for accuracy, legibility, and completeness.		
Optional: May deduct points for taking more time than allowed.		

Total Points = 30

Student's Score: _____

Evaluator: _____

Comments: _____

_____

_____

_____

_____

Chapter **18** Hospital Billing and the UB-04

HOSPITAL BILLING FORM (STATEMENT)

Broadmoor Medical Center

4353 Pine Ridge Drive
Milton, XY 12345-0000   Phone: 555-656-7890 Fax: 555-656-6890

THIS IS YOUR HOSPITAL BILL		
Patient Name & Address	**Account #**	**Primary/Secondary Insurance(s)**

Dates of Service	**Activity**	**Amount**	**Balance**

Statement Date: **Due Date:**   **Balance Due:**

If you have billing questions, telephone 555-656-7890 Ext: 3210

Fig. 18.7 Hospital billing form.

```
HOSPITAL BILLING SUMMARY

Patient Name: Flowers, Julius R.        Acct. # 200200546

Discharge Date: 10/16/20XX at 11:45 a.m.

Hospital Charges:

Rev CD    Description           HCPCS/Rates    Serv Units    Total Charges

121       2-Bed Room (Med/Surg)  $2010.00          4          $8040.00
250       Pharmacy                                               187.45
260       IV Therapy                                             144.90
272       Sterile Supplies                                        65.00
301       Lab/Chemistry                                         2314.12
305       Lab/Hematology                                         201.30
351       CT Scan                                  1             612.50
424       Phys. Therapy/Eval.                                    176.00
450       Emergency Room                           2             562.25
730       EKG                                                    105.00


Primary Payer:              Medicare
Provider No.                0976540
Treatment Authorization Code  36378833
Principal Diagnosis Code    ICD-10 Code: S06.371A
```

Fig. 18.8 Hospital billing summary.

APPLICATION EXERCISES

Health Insurance Professional's Notebook

Assemble information and example forms for the Health Insurance Professional's Notebook regarding claims, such as:

- Blank UB-04 form
- Current guidelines for completion of the UB-04
- Typical sample forms associated with patient hospitalization

SELF-EVALUATION

Chapter Checklist

Student Name: _____

Chapter Completion Date: _____

Evaluate your classroom performance. Complete the self-evaluation and submit it to your instructor. When your instructor returns this form to you, compare your self-evaluation with the evaluation completed by your instructor.

1.	Record	Your start time and date: _____
2.	Read	The assigned chapter in the textbook
3.	View	PowerPoint slides (if available)
4.	Complete	Exercises in the workbook as assigned
5.	Compare	Your answers to the answers posted on the bulletin board, website, or handout
6.	Correct	Your answers
7.	Complete	All tests and required activities
8.	Read	Assigned readings (if any)
9.	Complete	Chapter performance objectives (competencies), if any
10.	Evaluate	Chapter performance and submit to your instructor
11.	Record	Your ending time and date: _____
12.	Move on	Begin next chapter as assigned

Student Name: _____

Chapter Completion Date: _____

Evaluate your classroom performance. Compare this evaluation with the one provided by your instructor.

Skill	Student Self-Evaluation			Instructor Evaluation		
	Good	Average	Poor	Good	Average	Poor
Attendance/punctuality						
Personal appearance						
Applies effort						
Is self-motivated						
Is courteous						
Has positive attitude						
Completes assignments in timely manner						
Works well with others						

Student's Initials: _____

Date: _____

Points Possible: _____

Points Awarded: _____

Chapter Grade: _____

Instructor's Initials: _____

Date: _____